A Guide to Transgender Health

Recent Titles in
Sex, Love, and Psychology
Judy Kuriansky, Series Editor

A GUIDE TO TRANSGENDER HEALTH

State-of-the-Art Information for Gender-Affirming People and Their Supporters

Rachel Ann Heath, PhD,
and Katie Wynne, PhD, FRACP

Sex, Love, and Psychology
Judy Kuriansky, Series Editor

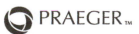 PRAEGER™

An Imprint of ABC-CLIO, LLC
Santa Barbara, California • Denver, Colorado

Library of Congress Cataloging-in-Publication Data

Names: Heath, Rachel Ann, author. | Wynne, Katie, author.
Title: A guide to transgender health : state-of-the-art information for gender-affirming people and their supporters / Rachel Ann Heath, PhD and Katie Wynne, PhD, FRACP.
Description: Santa Barbara, California : Praeger, an Imprint of ABC-CLIO, LLC, [2019] | Series: Sex, love, and psychology | Includes bibliographical references and index.
Identifiers: LCCN 2019005407 (print) | LCCN 2019005892 (ebook) | ISBN 9781440863097 (e-book) | ISBN 9781440863080 (cloth : alk. paper)
Subjects: LCSH: Transgender people—Medical care.
Classification: LCC RA564.9.T73 (ebook) | LCC RA564.9.T73 H43 2019 (print) | DDC 362.1086/7—dc23
LC record available at https://lccn.loc.gov/2019005407

ISBN: 978-1-4408-6308-0 (print)
       978-1-4408-6309-7 (ebook)

23 22 21 20 19   1 2 3 4 5

This book is also available as an eBook.

Praeger
An Imprint of ABC-CLIO, LLC

ABC-CLIO, LLC
147 Castilian Drive
Santa Barbara, California 93117
www.abc-clio.com

This book is printed on acid-free paper ∞

Manufactured in the United States of America

CONTENTS

SERIES FOREWORD

A GUIDE TO TRANSGENDER HEALTH: STATE-OF-THE-ART INFORMATION FOR GENDER-AFFIRMING PEOPLE AND THEIR SUPPORTERS

My appreciation for this book, and recommendation of it to readers, is not only based on my current professional support of gender diversity, but on my longtime experience with the trans issue reaching back over 40 years. As a young senior research scientist and psychologist who was part of the first group of experts in the field of sexuality diagnosis and treatment, I was approached by a pioneer in gender reassignment surgery. Very concerned about whether those requesting his services were really psychologically prepared for the drastic change in their lives—or instead were looking to solve life's problems or, worse, were depressed and at risk for suicide—he asked me to assess his candidates. I clearly remember one young man who cried that he was "born in the wrong body"—affirming a critical determinant of gender incongruence necessary for reassignment eligibility—but who also shared severe and long-lasting misery about his life, including tragic past physical and sexual abuses, and a distinct belief that if only he were a woman, he would be taken care of and finally happy. Clearly, other issues had to be resolved.

At the time, I was also on the committee drafting sexuality criteria to be included for the first time in the third edition of the famous *Diagnostic and Statistical Manual*, and working with senior psychiatrists considering the condition "gender dysphoria."

While research today still shows that transgender persons have "co-occurring" psychiatric conditions, and the current federal administration does not allow transgender individuals to serve in the U.S. military, many advances have been made that do respect and support the rights and choices of transgendered people.

So, how far have we come as a society facing trans issues and needs, and where are we headed? How much do we understand?

This book offers rich answers to those questions. Readers get a comprehensive and holistic picture from medical, social, and psychological perspectives. For even the most informed of professionals, there is something to learn, from enlightened terms such as "trans or gender-diverse (TGD) person," to the longing for and science of fertility for transgendered people.

This volume is an important companion to other books in the Sex, Love, and Psychology series from Praeger Publishers, including one by first author Rachel Ann Heath, *The Praeger Handbook of Transsexuality: Changing Gender to Match Mindset* (2006).

Transgender people themselves, their loved ones, and their supporters will find an extensive understanding of gender identity in these pages. So, too, all mental health professionals, clinicians, and researchers, as well as those involved in any field related to sexual identity, from professionals to politicians, will find this book valuable, insightful, and timely.

Judy Kuriansky, PhD
Series Editor, Sex, Love, and Psychology

PREFACE

As soon as a pregnancy is confirmed, thoughts lead inevitably to the question, *Will my baby be a boy or a girl?* Either the excited couple keeps this question a secret until the baby is born, or else they become so curious about whether they will have a son or daughter that they use modern medical technology to resolve the issue, the sooner the better!

This is no idle request as the first question most people ask is whether a newborn child is a boy or a girl. Once the new baby's sex is known, in Western societies 75 percent of girls are given pink clothes and 79 percent of boys are given blue clothes.[1]

Although the baby's sex is usually confirmed before or shortly after birth, occasionally the medical team is uncertain whether the baby is a boy or a girl. Uncertainty and distress then follow as medical experts wonder how to tell the parents that they are unsure about the baby's sex. Ambiguous sexual organs contribute the most to the confusion, leading to difficult medical and ethical decisions for the doctors and the child's family, sometimes with harmful consequences for the individual.

Even when a child's sex is accurately determined, a few years later an even more disturbing situation for parents might occur when their young child insists on behaving like a child of the opposite sex. Little boys insist that they be dressed like their sister and play with dolls, whereas tomboy girls detest the thought of frilly frocks and head straight for the comfort of baggy trousers and short hairstyles. These girls prefer rough-and-tumble play with boys, and trucks and trains over dolls and cooking utensils. Such behavior may demonstrate exploration of

gender or it may indicate a difference between born sex, as defined by the genitals, and gender identity as shown by the young person's behavior.

These days, people can be any gender they like, not just the two genders,
male and female, that many societies demand. And the gender they display
may have nothing to do with their genitals. They can have a gender that
is anywhere between male and female, or they can have no gender at all.
A person's gender might change from one day to the next—this is OK too. We
refer to the gender a person chooses as their *affirmed gender*. If the person's
affirmed gender and *birth-assigned sex* are the same, then that person is *cisgender*, a *cisgender man* or a *cisgender woman*. If a person's birth-assigned sex and
affirmed gender do not correspond, for example one is female and the other
male, we say that this person is *trans*, or whatever term the gender-diverse
person might use to describe themselves. But please ask them first, because
every gender-diverse person has their own preferred label.

How often, when asked to specify your sex as male or female, have you hesi-
tated before ticking the appropriate box? For people who are trans or whose
gender is *none of the above*, it always feels wrong to tick the male or female box.
For some people, this bureaucratic requirement never coincides with their
individual balance between feeling male or feeling female, even if they are not
trans or gender-questioning.

We may even wonder why telling someone about our sex is necessary, especially if they are never likely to be our sexual partners! So, imagine how difficult it must be for people of both sexes who have a deep, possibly lifelong,
commitment to being treated as, and living the role of, a gender that differs
from their birth-assigned sex. Many trans people suffer enormously from distress caused by society's response to their gender difference. Trans people can
benefit enormously from love and support from family and friends, and from
acceptance by the communities in which they live. It is our responsibility to
make sure that these brave people live happy and productive lives.

Living in a gender that is different from one's birth-assigned sex, either permanently or temporarily, has been common in most human societies throughout recorded history. From Native American two-spirit people to the *hijras* of
India, people have been enthralled by, and respectful of, gender-variant people.
Media reports of a person's transition from a gender corresponding to their
birth-assigned sex to their affirmed gender often incite public interest. Also,
autobiographies that offer fascinating insights into their trans authors' lives
provide interesting reading for many of us. Few can avoid questioning their
own gender feelings after reading about the anguish of another's search for
happiness and a better life, especially when the hostile environments of family
upheaval, employment prejudice, and other barriers need to be overcome.

This book provides an up-to-date account of current knowledge about
gender difference, when people affirm that their gender does not reflect the sex

recorded on their birth certificate, when they seek happiness by being true to themselves, and when supportive others, their family, friends, community, and dedicated professionals, provide what is needed for them to have a safe and productive life. The information we provide is based on published research, as well as the experience gained by living the life and helping gender-diverse people achieve their goals. Our account of recent research provides readers, especially those in the trans communities and their supporters, with a valuable resource to inform their own decisions, and to assist others in understanding the complex issues involved in gender affirmation. We examine important aspects of gender diversity as it relates to the needs of trans people and their supporters. Throughout, we emphasize the new roles that medical and other professionals can play so that trans people can attain happiness and an identity they can call their own without ever being diagnosed with a mental illness, as was a common prerequisite for medical treatments not so long ago.

The book begins with a brief historical account of gender diversity, its prevalence in a variety of cultures, and people's attitudes toward trans people. Next follows a summary of how biologists, psychologists, and sociologists explain gender. Then we consider how people can differ in how they feel about their gender. This is called *gender diversity*. In the following chapter we discuss the various ways that gender-diverse people can tell us about their gender. We call this process their *gender affirmation*.

The next topic involves a more detailed look at how people of different genders behave in various life situations. Are men better at reading maps than women? Are women more empathic than men? How do men's and women's brains differ? Does that difference have any bearing on how they act or feel? What about trans people's brains? Are they different from the brains of birth-assigned men and women who do not identify as trans?

The next part of the book examines the needs of children and adolescents, especially those whose affirmed gender is different from their birth-assigned sex. How can we help these young people enjoy happy and successful lives as their true selves? We discuss the process of puberty and what happens when you pause this process using blockers. What can we do to reduce the high self-harm and attempted suicide rate for these young people? What is the evidence for starting hormone therapy and what effects does this have?

In a chapter on gender affirmation by adults we learn how some people can choose a medical route to achieve happiness and comfort in their own body using hormone therapy and various surgeries. We discuss in detail how hormones work and their potential implications for long-term health, and we describe the current surgical techniques. These medical procedures, which are available for those who desire them, have required assessment and diagnosis of a medical condition known as gender dysphoria contained in the American Psychiatric Association's compendium of mental illness. More appropriate procedures are now being employed that consider every gender-affirming person's right to self-evaluation and control of their own destiny. This strategy has been reinforced by the World Health Organization considering gender affirmation as a part of sexual health—it is no longer an illness but a situation in which a person employs medical interventions to better fit their body and mind. In most situations, the person's family doctor can receive training on how to respectfully assist these people.

In the next chapter we describe how trans people can preserve their eggs, sperm, or fertilized embryo so that they can have children with their own genetic material. These procedures have been quite successful. They offer hope to those who might later regret their inability to have a family of their own. We describe what is known about the experiences of trans and gender-diverse people during pregnancy and in feeding their newborn. Before long, a wider range of options will be available to meet fertility needs.

Some, but not all, trans people might wish to undergo various kinds of surgeries to make their daily lives a lot easier and to offer them a sense of body validation in their affirmed gender. These surgeries range from genital reconstruction to breast enhancement or reduction, removal of internal reproductive organs for masculinization, as well as facial and voice-box surgery for feminization. We discuss a variety of other lifestyle aids that assist trans people's daily lives. These procedures for affirmed women include voice and deportment training, as well as scalp hair replacement and body hair removal using laser and electrolysis.

It is so important that trans people of all ages and all genders are well supported by family, friends, and everyone else around them. Evidence suggests that young trans people who have loving support from family and friends show no more distress than any of their cisgender friends. We also consider the discrimination, rejection, bullying, and violence to which trans people are often subjected in their daily lives. These awful events can cause great distress that impacts on how safe trans people feel. We include a section on trans aging, a topic of increasing importance as many older affirmed men and women are reaching retirement age and beyond. It is not clear whether these people will have problems navigating the fraught processes of aged care, the risk of dementia, chronic disability, and end-of-life preparation.

The book concludes with a summary of the current guidelines for a successful transition as well as some crystal-ball gazing as we consider what the future holds for gender-diverse people. Will they achieve their just human rights under all circumstances? Will governments worldwide recognize gender diversity as a natural part of the human condition and allow gender-diverse people the same rights enjoyed by every citizen in their country? We will restate our mission that centers the care of trans people in the family primary care medical network, which plays such an important role in maintaining a healthy and productive society. We mention Internet and social media resources so that readers can explore new developments and comment on the book's contents. We will also use these resources to correct the occasional error that might remain in the final version of the book. We are only human!

TERMINOLOGY

Trans people can be offended when they read controlling recommendations for their own lives written by nontrans authors. As Kate Bornstein of "gender warrior" fame has written,

> The literature to date on the transgender experience does not help us to establish a truly transgender world view in concert with other transgender people, because virtually all the books and theories about gender and transsexuality to date have been written by non-transsexuals who, no matter how well-intentioned, are each trying to figure out how to make us fit into *their* world view.[2]

As one of us has a transgender background and the other extensive experience helping gender-diverse people of all ages, we can write credibly on these issues. We have both immersed ourselves in the trans world seeking to understand the challenges such people face from one day to the next, as well as doing all we can to make that passage as smooth as possible within our own community in Newcastle, Australia, and by extension everywhere else.

We have adhered to Hale's rules[3] according to which trans people are experts on their own condition. Authors should avoid expressing views that do not represent the experiences of trans people but rather recognize that trans people are especially well qualified to comment on issues affecting their lives. Appropriate terminology should be used, although these definitions may change with time. Authors should be familiar with debate within the trans communities and address current issues of concern. Authors should consider the needs of all gender-diverse people no matter their affirmed gender and their sexual preferences. Ideally, writers should immerse themselves generously in the fabulous world of trans people before airing their views publicly. Luckily for you, dear reader, we are such authors!

Many gender-diverse people are sensitive to the labels used to describe them. Some detest being called *transsexual*, especially when they have no intention of undergoing medical treatments to change their bodies to conform to a binary gender such as male or female. For such people, the term *transgender*, for example, may be used by those gender-diverse people who enjoy enacting a part-time trans lifestyle. Such is the consternation caused by inappropriate terminology that we will undoubtedly be criticized for the terminology used in this book. We apologize in advance should our choices cause offense. For the title of this book we have preferred the term *transgender health* with a subtitle that recognizes the work's usefulness for members of the broader gender-diverse community and their supporters. The more general term *trans* covers all people who might consider themselves transgender or transsexual or some other label that the person prefers.

When discussing sexual orientation as opposed to gender identity, the terms *homosexual* and *heterosexual* are awkward, especially when the former is used with, or instead of, *gay* and *lesbian*. To be more accurate in our choice of descriptions we use *gynephilic* and *androphilic* to refer to a sexual preference for women or men, respectively. Gynephilic[4] derives from the Greek for *love of a woman* and androphilic derives from the Greek for *love of a man*. So, a *gynephilic man* is a man who likes women, that is, a heterosexual man, whereas an *androphilic man* is one who likes men, that is, a gay man. For completeness, a lesbian is a *gynephilic woman*, that is, a woman who likes other women. A *gynephilic transsexed woman* refers to a woman of transsexual background whose sexual preference is for women. Unless *homosexual* and *heterosexual* are the more readily understood terms in certain contexts, this more precise terminology will be used throughout the book. As the terms homosexual, gay, and lesbian are often associated with bigotry and exclusion in many societies, the emphasis on sexual affiliation is both appropriate and socially just.

Details of the statistical analyses have been ignored throughout the book. The terms *statistically significant* and *not statistically significant* can be assumed whenever a finding is expressed in either the affirmative or negative, respectively. The minimum odds that a difference is wrongly claimed to be true are 1 in 20, in accordance with scientific convention. Rather than report the average ages of research participants, the terminology *25-year-old*, say, implies that the average age is 25 for all participants in that group.

Research methodology is an important consideration when the literature employs small populations that cannot be sampled randomly. Just because a finding has been published in a peer-reviewed journal does not mean that it will be accepted unqualified. Rather, each outcome is evaluated using the scientific and ethical criteria demanded by contemporary medical, social, and psychological research. In many places in the text we refer to properly conducted literature reviews that employ statistical methods known as meta-analysis. This allows the results of similar research projects to be combined in order to better assess the scientific validity of the phenomena being considered.

When research findings conflict with the impressions of trans people, the practical value of these findings is correspondingly downgraded. The trans community has suffered too long at the hands of uninformed "experts" for this book to serve as a platitudinous reiteration of distorted truths. For this reason, we have ignored the many papers in the literature that have now been confirmed as representing bogus and discriminating science, a process of dogma acquisition that is not in the spirit of a disinterested enquiry based on facts and ethical justice.

ACKNOWLEDGMENTS

Rachel Heath is indebted to the School of Psychology at the University of Newcastle, Australia, for her appointment as an honorary staff member, and for her colleagues' encouragement and assistance in completing the research for this book.

Katie Wynne is grateful to the Endocrinology and Diabetes Department at John Hunter Hospital, Newcastle, Australia, for their support in her professional development as a transgender health specialist and their assistance in the development of local services. She thanks her family, Peter, Hannah, Zac, and Jess, for their inspiration and patience. Many thanks to Jane Coffey (MA, Royal College of Art), design director of Future Shelter, for donating her time and expertise to create our "gender diversity" book cover.

We appreciate the dedicated assistance from our editor at ABC-CLIO, Debbie Carvalko, who offered encouragement and prompt advice on editorial aspects of the project.

It was impossible to research a book of this kind without referring to the extensive Internet resources on gender diversity. Spending many hours communicating with gender-diverse people and others, both in person and on the Internet, has informed much of the book's contents. It is impossible to write a credible account of these complex issues without considering the collective experience and wisdom of these courageous community members.

ABBREVIATIONS

ADHD	Attention deficit hyperactivity disorder
AIDS	Acquired immunodeficiency syndrome
AND	Androsterone
BSRI	Bem Sex Role Inventory
BSTc	Central region of the bed nucleus of the stria terminalis
CCEI	Crown-Crisp Experiential Index
DHT	Dihydrotestosterone
DSM	*Diagnostic and Statistical Manual*
EEG	Electroencephalogram
EST	Estrogen-like substance
FSH	Follicle-stimulating hormone
GIDAAT	Gender identity disorder of adolescence and adulthood—nontranssexual type
GnRH	Gonadotrophin-releasing hormone
HIV	Human immunodeficiency virus
ICD	International Classification of Diseases
IQ	Intelligence quotient
LGBTIQ	Lesbian gay bi trans intersex queer
LH	Luteinizing hormone
MMPI	Minnesota Multiphasic Personality Inventory
MRI	Magnetic resonance imaging
P300	Event-related potential related to decision-making

PET	Positron emission tomography
SCL	Symptom Check List
SDN-POA	Sexually dimorphic nuclei in the preoptic area
SOM	Somatostatin expressing
SRY	Sex-determining region Y protein gene
TAT	Thematic Apperception Test
TGD	Transgender and gender-diverse
U.K.	United Kingdom
U.S.	United States
VIP	Vasoactive intestinal polypeptide
WHO	World Health Organization
WPATH	World Professional Association for Transgender Health

Chapter 1

INTRODUCTION

Being trans means being assigned male and living one's life as a female or as some other gender, or else being assigned female and living one's life as a male or as some other gender. Some people do not identify with a gender at all. Some trans people undergo medical treatments to align their body with their gender identity to become more comfortable in their life and relationships. But not all gender-diverse people want to make a medical change.

Unconventional gender expression often attracts the attention of significant others in the person's family and community. It can challenge some of the foundations of many modern societies, such as marriage, the workplace, and peer relationships. To minimize the burden imposed upon alternatively gendered people, their supporters need to devise an easier path so that their loved ones can enjoy happy and fulfilling lives.

When writing about sensitive matters such as trans people's aspirations, their sexuality, and gender diversity, the temptation to right the wrongs of the past is always present. However, it is equally important to offer readers a summary of the facts. This is necessary because gender-diverse people and their supporters should not be deluded by half-truths. It is important for all professionals and researchers who work with gender-diverse people to be provided with accurate information. Otherwise, these supporters might be deterred from doing their very best to help their possibly disenchanted clients. This book treads a fine line between upholding the human rights of a downtrodden minority while ensuring that what is known about the trans experience and gender diversity is presented accurately.

Before embarking on a detailed survey of gender, sex, and the trans experience, we provide a brief history. Then follows an account of people's largely positive attitudes toward trans people based on surveys conducted in Sweden and more widely over the Internet. This material is tempered somewhat by disturbing incidents of prejudice against gender-diverse people. The chapter concludes with information on the number of gender-diverse people in population studies, a contentious and difficult matter.

Between 1900 and 2017, there were 5,772 peer-reviewed articles published on transgender health, with a dramatic increase in the number of papers being published in the last decade. Most of these recent papers have investigated the prevalence of human immunodeficiency virus infection, mental health, and discrimination. The oldest article, published in the German journal *Zeitschrift für die gesamte Neuologie und Psychiatrie* in 1913, was about neurological and psychiatric aspects of *transvestism*, or crossdressing. Much of this research (43%) has been performed in the United States, with stigma, transphobia, assault, and violence being the most often researched topics, especially with respect to the resulting elevated levels of depression and anxiety observed in trans people. Another study published in 2019 indicated that the most important research areas were therapeutics and surgeries, gender identity and expression, mental health, biology and physiology, discrimination and marginalization, physical health, sexual health, HIV and sexually transmitted infections, health and mental health services, social support, relationships and families, and resilience, well-being, and quality of life.[1]

1.1 A BRIEF HISTORY OF GENDER DIVERSITY

Gender diversity has been a common human trait since ancient times. In old Mesopotamia, the god Innana could change a person's gender from male to female and vice versa. However, this particular change in gender may have been temporary because in some of these ancient societies gender roles appear to have been strictly enforced.[2]

According to Green,[3] the Greek goddess Venus Castina reacted sympathetically to feminine souls locked up in male bodies. One of the earliest examples of living as the opposite gender is the Assyrian king Sardanapalus, who dressed in women's clothing and spun thread with his wives. In Ovid's *Metamorphoses* the male Tiresias was transformed into the woman Teresa when two copulating snakes were struck with a stave. When Teresa strikes the snakes again, she is transformed back into a male, so that gender identity in this case was fluid. This is an early example of someone being able to change from one gender to another.[4] A more permanent change of sex and perhaps gender occurred among the Galli in Rome a few centuries before the current era. These worshippers of the goddess Cybele castrated themselves and lived the rest of their lives without penis and testicles.[5]

The book of Deuteronomy in the Bible contains a passage that is often interpreted as meaning that a man cannot wear women's clothing and vice versa. However, when the exact meanings of the original Hebrew words are considered, a more accurate translation would be something like this:

> A woman shall not be associated with the instrument of a superior man, and a superior man shall not wear the garment of a woman, for whoever does these things is a cultic abomination to Yahweh your God.[6]

This suggests that the biblical restriction on crossdressing only applies to the most masculine of men, those who are destined to fight in battle under the guidance of Yahweh, their God.

Gender diversity during the Middle Ages is illustrated by the sixth-century story written by Gregory of Tours. A man, Poitevin, dressed in nun's clothing who lived secretly in a nunnery was forgiven for his indiscretion provided he agreed to be castrated. Since childhood he had worn female clothes as he suffered from "an incurable disorder of the groin," possibly an indication of genital ambiguity resulting from a difference in sexual development.

In the 13th century, Pelagia originally lived as a woman dressed in a monk's outfit so that her previous life as a prostitute would not be discovered. She then lived as a man, Pelegius, whose female sex was only discovered after she died. Around the same time, another woman assumed a male role to escape an unhappy marriage. Although women can often get away with dressing as men, even today the idea that men can dress as women is frequently taboo. This is partly due to a perception that the status loss from living as a woman might also apply to all other men.[7] This is especially the case in societies that devalue women and by implication their impersonators.

It is interesting that in a medieval Hebrew text, *Evan Bohan (Touchstone)*, Kalonymus bemoans the fact that he was born a boy with all the responsibilities that entails. He would have preferred to have been a girl. As he says, "happy is she who know [*sic*] how to work with combed flax and weave it into fine white linen." He proceeds to imagine life as a woman, pleading with his maker why it wasn't so.[8]

One of the earliest examples of a surgical procedure to correct a genital anomaly was performed on a seven-year-old child in 1779. The child was thought to be a girl but had enlarged labia majora and clitoris. The surgery was conducted to release the large clitoris and produce what appeared to be a small penis and scrotum.[9]

Chevalier d'Eon (1728–1810), a French diplomat who spent the second half of his life living full-time as a woman, was a mistress of King Louis XV of France. D'Eon was so attractive that he rivaled Madame Pompadour for the king's attention. In a newspaper article reporting his death in 1810, Chevalier d'Eon was considered famous "on account of his questionable gender." Although some 36 years earlier a large amount of money was paid to obtain a surgical certificate to say that d'Eon was female, when he was on his deathbed a French surgeon had confirmed that he was indeed male.[10]

Eonism, a term first mentioned by the famous sexologist Havelock Ellis, has been used ever since as a synonym for cross-gendered behavior in nonhomosexual males.[11] Around the same time as d'Eon, the first colonial governor of New York, Lord Cornbury, came from England fully attired as a woman and remained so during his time in office.

A loss of social status for men who crossdress as women, when compared with their female counterparts, is not new. Richard von Krafft-Ebing, a 19th-century German psychiatrist, considered men who crossdress to be *failed men,* whereas women who crossdress were accomplished, intelligent, and independent women [*sic*]. In his hefty book, *Psychopathica Sexualis*, von Krafft-Ebing reports on the gender-diverse behavior of first peoples, such as *mujerados,*[12] members of the Pueblo people of New Mexico, where high status was given to effeminate men. These men served in roles usually designed for women, such as looking after children, performing household chores, and so on.

In the 1860s, Ulrichs regarded the homosexual, a term proposed by Kertbeny in 1869, as a person with a brain that was of one sex and a body that was another. So, homosexuality could be considered a type of gender inversion or *third sex* unrelated to the male and female sexes.[13] Important for our current thinking about trans people and gender diversity, Ulrichs's ideas could only explain his observations of gender-diverse people if sexual and gender feelings resided not in the genitals but in the brain. Sex and gender can be easily confused when, for example, a *sissy*, who represents undesirable male qualities such as weakness, dependency, and helplessness, is considered a threat to maleness. The confusion of masculine femininity with male homosexuality still exists today.

Magnus Hirschfeld (1868–1935), the famous German pioneer in sex and gender research, considered sex and gender to both lie on a continuous scale as does length, weight, and time. Significantly for his era, Hirschfeld believed that physiology, especially the hormones, plays a key role in causing these variations in sex and gender. Hirschfeld coined the term *transvestism* in 1910 to refer to what we prefer to call crossdressing. Later in 1923, he used the term *transsexualism* as a diagnostic label in psychiatry for the first time, more than a quarter of a century before Cauldwell used the same term in 1949. These days we prefer not to use such a term to describe those gender-diverse people who wish to undergo medical treatments due to its implication that the person may be mentally ill.

In 1918, Hirschfeld reported that the first genital reconstruction surgery had already occurred in Berlin as early as 1912. This pioneering surgery resulted in an incomplete female-to-male genital conversion, to be followed in 1920 by crude genital surgery performed on a male-to-female client.[14] So, Hirschfeld identified the clinical category of transsexualism that was later developed and popularized by Benjamin. Cauldwell stated rather pessimistically that "to attempt to medically treat transvestism [as opposed to transsexualism] would be as foolish as to try to treat some star to make it behave differently in its relation to the solar system."[15] Clearly Cauldwell had confused the terms *transvestism* and *transsexualism* and must surely have been referring to the latter. The importance of medical and surgical procedures for trans people since these early days has proven Cauldwell wrong.

Hirschfeld maintained that crossdressing is an innate affliction that becomes more intense with age. Any sudden stress that a person suffers may lead to its full expression as a more permanent form of gender-diverse behavior. Hirschfeld distinguished nine types of transvestite: the extreme, the partial, a transvestite in name alone, a constant transvestite, a periodic transvestite, a narcissistic transvestite, a metatropic transvestite (defined as being attracted to mannish females in the case of males), and the last two categories, bisexual and homosexual transvestites.[16] This detailed categorization of gender-diverse people was elaborated much later by Benjamin and, more recently, by others.

The sudden appearance of full-blown gender diversity in middle age and beyond is a common phenomenon that is seldom recognized. In this respect and in many others, Hirschfeld was way ahead of his time. For example, Inez, Benjamin's ninth client, first made contact when she was 52 years old. She subsequently underwent a three-stage genital surgical procedure involving castration, removal of the penis, and then vaginoplasty, the construction of a vagina using, most commonly, the inverted skin of the penis. This is basically the same technique used in quite a few present-day genital surgery procedures for trans women.

Lili Elbe, born as a male named Einer Magnus Andreas Wegener in Denmark in 1882, was one of the first recorded genital surgery cases. Unfortunately, she died in Dresden, Germany, in 1931, a year after an attempt was made to surgically remove rejected ovaries that were placed in her abdomen during the original surgery. Lili's feminization probably resulted from Klinefelter syndrome, a condition in which testosterone levels are quite low and estrogen levels are relatively high. If this is true, then Lili would have had a 47, XXY sex chromosome karyotype containing an extra X chromosome. So, one of the first trans people publicized widely in the media probably had a difference in sexual development.[17] Lili's life story is contained in her diaries, edited by Niels Hoyer. It was dramatized with some license and community criticism in the 2015 movie *The Danish Girl*.[18]

Abraham performed the United States' first genital reconstruction surgery for trans women in 1931.[19] However, such surgical solutions only became widely known after media publicity of Christine Jorgensen's successful surgery in Denmark in 1952. Christine was formerly a GI in the American army before becoming the "blonde bombshell" seen in newspaper photos.

In the 1960s, it was realized that hormonal treatment without risky surgery might provide relief for some trans people. Psychotherapy, although beneficial for some trans people, did not provide a complete resolution of their problems. Despite this realization, during the 1960s and 1970s, many trans people suffered at the hands of psychiatrists who tried to "cure" them using electric shock therapy and other invasive, cruel treatments.

1.2 DR. HARRY BENJAMIN'S LEGACY

In her historical review of transsexuality in the United States, Randi Ettner[20] highlighted Harry Benjamin's outstanding accomplishments in the field of transgender health. Benjamin started his lengthy career as an endocrinologist and gerontologist. Benjamin's colleague, Professor Steinach from Vienna, introduced him to *gerontotherapy* techniques for hormone replacement in older people and offered him experience in surgical techniques required for sex-organ transfer between animals.

In 1948, Kinsey, perhaps the United States' most famous sexologist, introduced Benjamin to a youth named Van who had requested genital reconstruction surgery. Due to the lack of surgical expertise in the United States, Van eventually had surgery in Europe in the mid-1950s, thanks to Benjamin's sympathetic concern. Christine Jorgensen, who was treated by Benjamin before heading to Denmark for her surgery, and who enjoyed considerable fame upon her return to the United States, began a lifelong correspondence and friendship with Benjamin.

Benjamin first used transsexualism as a diagnostic category for patients who requested medical interventions in a talk he gave at a December 1953 symposium conducted by the Association for the Advancement of Psychotherapy.[21] Benjamin's Sex Orientation Scale, one of the first quantitative measures of sexual behavior, was used to discriminate the so-called *true transsexuals* from others. The true transsexuals, who score V and VI on a 6-point scale using Benjamin's test, are also more likely to score at the homosexual end of the Kinsey Scale. This suggests they should be classified as nonheterosexual and attracted to men, a contentious situation given recent trans politics decrying any necessary association between sexual orientation and gender diversity. Benjamin believed that this group would need to have genital surgery to live happy and fulfilling lives.

The distinction between *true* or *primary transsexuals* who usually transition at a relatively young age, and *secondary transsexuals* who live an apparently unremarkable masculine life prior to transition in midlife or beyond, persists as a diagnostic concern for some practitioners today. However, the scientific evidence supporting this proposition is dubious, a fact made clear by those who claim the distinction is an example of transphobia, an abnormal fear of anything or anybody associated with gender diversity. A more detailed account of sexuality is contained in Chapter 4.

A review of Benjamin's first 10 transsexual cases, whom he cared for between 1938 and 1953, reported that he had helped more than 1,500 gender-affirming clients during his long career. Many of these early clients came to Benjamin self-diagnosed based on early cross-gendered behavior, secret crossdressing, purges, isolation, and lots of guilt. The first 10 clients included one crossdresser, as well as six category V and VI trans people. Three category IV trans people who may not necessarily request genital surgery included a German citizen who inspired some of Hirschfeld's early writings on transvestism. Benjamin introduced the term *transgender* to refer to crossdressing behavior before eventually using *transsexual* and *transvestite* to describe various aspects of his clients' behavior. Evidently, problems with appropriate terminology existed even in Benjamin's time, as of course they still do today.[22]

A review of the correspondence between Benjamin and 21 adolescents aged 16 to 19 who requested Benjamin's help from 1963 to 1976 mostly mentioned issues such as same-sex attraction, family rejection, experiencing gender variance, and being in the wrong body. A few of these young people mentioned that they had experienced forced rehabilitation treatment that also included admission to a locked ward in a psychiatric hospital. Benjamin most often sent readings in reply to the letters he had received and even offered to discuss the situation with these young people's parents. In his replies, Benjamin mentioned issues that are important for young trans people today, such as the need to be affirmed as their gender of choice, problems with parents, delays in obtaining treatment, and the issue of parental consent. However, in the 1960s and 1970s there was little information available about trans issues other than Benjamin's book and Christine Jorgensen's autobiography. At issue was the need to disown homosexuality as it was considered a criminal offence in the 1960s and 1970s. So, it was natural for some young people to reframe their story of same-sex desire by saying that they would indulge in a new heterosexual relationship following transition. These young people already knew about the availability of hormone therapy and genital surgeries, which were requested in most of the correspondence Benjamin received.[23]

Meanwhile, the Americans were working hard to allow trans people to live successful and happy lives. The Gay and Lesbian Historical Society of Northern California[24] reviewed transgender activism in the Tenderloin district of San Francisco between 1966 and 1975. The Tenderloin, located within San

Francisco's red-light district, had been a refuge for trans people who otherwise had no proper support.

The radical transgender movement in the United States started after a riot at Compton's Cafeteria in the Tenderloin district in August 1966. Many of the bars and clubs in this part of San Francisco were frequented by *queens*, trans people who lived full-time as women and who were sexually active with men. Some of the queens underwent hormonal and surgical procedures to pass more successfully as women. Although trans women, many of whom were sex workers, used to come to Compton's Cafeteria as a welcome refuge from a difficult life elsewhere, they were still discriminated against, a situation that came to a head when the cafeteria owners called the police to remove them early one morning. Rather than accept further abuse, these trans women, supported by gays and lesbians, fought to protest their situation. A documentary film was made in 2015 to celebrate this early instance of trans activism in the United States.[25]

The Methodist Church was the first religious organization to care for homosexual and trans people in the Tenderloin district, successfully reducing police brutality and serving as a safe meeting place for these needy people. Some of these women engaged in sex work to survive economically as they had no other employment opportunities. Sadly, a similar situation exists today due to the prohibitive cost of genital surgeries and associated feminization procedures, especially for otherwise destitute trans people.

Benjamin, who based his practice on the innovative ideas developed by Hirschfeld in Germany, advised his first trans client in the Tenderloin during a summer visit in the late 1940s. Benjamin's clinic, which operated during the 1950s and 1960s, attracted many trans people who sought information and access to hormones and surgery. This allowed genital surgeries to be conducted in the United States even when there was no physical deformity, a necessary ethical requirement at that time before any type of surgery could be performed. It is worth noting, however, that genital surgeries were also conducted at that time, controversially, to correct what used to be called a physical *intersex* condition, better described nowadays as a difference in sexual development. It was unfortunately common to operate on baby boys with indeterminate genitals and have them neutered and reassigned as girls.

The Erickson Educational Foundation, funded in 1964 by Reed Erickson, promoted the education and treatment of trans people in the San Francisco and Los Angeles regions of California. Prior to 1966, genital surgeries, breast enhancement, and hormone therapy for trans people were not generally available in the United States, although the urologist Belt performed genital surgery in Los Angeles in the 1950s and 1960s. Also, three genital reconstruction procedures were performed on trans women in San Francisco between 1954 and 1964.

The first gender counseling service in the Tenderloin was set up in 1971 by Laura Cummings. Her technique discriminated drag queens and crossdressers from trans women since the latter would benefit from female hormones, whereas the others could not tolerate the disruption to their sexual activity from erection problems resulting from hormone treatment. As is commonly experienced, only those women who wish to transition can celebrate the loss of their libido following hormone therapy. These days, those people on the feminine spectrum who identify as nonbinary have a more difficult challenge when it comes to medical interventions if they wish to maintain libido and erectile function. In the 1970s, hardly anyone thought of gender as anything other than binary.

In 1972, the Salmacis Society began organized meetings of lesbian cisgender and trans women for exclusive femme-femme discussions. This enlightened period for trans people did not reappear until the 1990s when a new generation became actively involved in reevaluating their social situation, leading to a period of staunch trans activism that continues today.[26]

1.3 THE PATHOLOGIZATION OF GENDER DIVERSITY

Cohen-Kettenis and Gooren[27] have reviewed modern aspects of the presumed medical condition of transsexualism, including its origin, diagnosis, and treatment. Transsexualism first appeared as a psychiatric diagnosis in the third edition of the American Psychiatric Association's *Diagnostic and Statistical Manual of Mental Disorders*, DSM-III, in 1980. *Transsexualism* was subsequently replaced in the fourth edition, DSM-IV, by the term *gender identity disorder*. In the 1970s, Fisk[28] had proposed a similar term, *gender dysphoria syndrome,* to represent the distress experienced by those whose gender identity does not correspond to their birth sex.

In 2013, the gender identity disorder diagnosis was replaced in DSM-5 by the somewhat less pathologizing diagnosis *gender dysphoria.* In a recent update of the more inclusive *International Classification of Diseases*, version 11, published by the World Health Organization in 2018, a new diagnosis, *gender incongruence,* appeared, not in any mental illness section, but in one involved with sexual health. Many community members and others have been awaiting this improvement for a long time.[29]

Beginning in the late 1960s and early 1970s, gender identity disorder clinics were opened in the United States, Australia, the United Kingdom, Canada, the Netherlands, and elsewhere. Most of these clinics, often associated with university medical schools, employed similar diagnostic and treatment protocols for clients who were observed to express dysphoria, that is, discomfort, with their gender feelings. John Money opened the first gender clinic in the United States in 1965 at the Johns Hopkins University medical school in

Baltimore. Following a controversial and unscientific adverse report on its operation, the clinic closed in 1975.[30]

In 1987, a publicly funded Monash Gender Dysphoria Clinic began operation in Melbourne, Australia. Its staff consisted of two psychiatrists, a gynecologist, a plastic surgeon, an endocrinologist, a psychologist, a speech therapist, and a social worker. Referrals to the clinic came from general practitioners, specialists, and other health professionals. Also, some clients self-referred. All new clients were screened by a psychiatrist for accompanying psychiatric conditions such as delusions, psychosis, and mood disorders, and a life history was taken. After evaluation by an endocrinologist, and possibly a clinical psychologist, the assessment team met to determine a candidate's suitability for entry into the program. Successful clients partook in a real-life experience that required them to live full-time in their preferred gender role for at least 18 months. During this time, hormone therapy commenced, as well as ancillary requirements such as speech therapy and facial hair removal for trans women. Further counseling was offered, including possible consultations with families. This clinic continues to successfully evolve; a survey of 127 patients in a revamped clinic conducted during a one-month period in 2014/2015 showed a satisfaction rate of about 88 percent.[31]

In the United Kingdom, trans people can use both public and private avenues to assist their gender affirmation. Even today, the operation of the U.K. public system is both interesting and inconsistent in the delays experienced for initial treatment and surgery, and the various facilities that exist in some parts of this densely populated country. Some gender-affirming clients can avail themselves of alternative private means to achieve their goals, usually with far less scrutiny than in the public hospital systems.

In the early 2000s, questionnaires were sent to directors of U.K. health authorities seeking information on services for trans people, obtaining an 82 percent response rate. Twenty percent of authorities reported a local transgender service, although not all had surgical facilities. Sixty percent of the remainder had no services for trans people but instead referred cases to other health boards for assessment and treatment, most commonly the pioneering clinic at Charing Cross Hospital in London. Three local health boards reported no facilities for treating trans people due to a reported lack of demand. The number of gender centers has increased over the last decade, but there are not nearly enough to cater to such a large population.[32]

The earlier absence of a comprehensive system of care in the United Kingdom meant that some clients were obtaining hormone therapy without sufficient medical resources for surgery, an unsatisfactory situation. Some trans people had to travel long distances for treatment, and delays were long. It was claimed that some of these people began hormone therapy with insufficient counseling and without a psychiatrist and/or psychologist confirming that they were sick. Only six gender clinics in the United Kingdom offered comprehensive services, there being no standardized protocols for assisting trans people. These days, the clinics employ the World Professional Association for Transgender Health (WPATH) Standards of Care to guide their treatment protocols, which are uniform throughout the United Kingdom.

In their desperation, some U.K. trans people sought a private and more expensive route to obtain hormone therapy and various surgeries. This attractive alternative includes surgery in overseas locations, such as the United States, Canada, and, commonly, Thailand. If proper care for trans people was so difficult to obtain in an advanced medical system such as that in the United Kingdom, how much more difficult must it be in poorer, less organized countries? It is unfortunate that there have been reports that some people in the U.K. National Health Service have made it difficult for private doctors to offer an alternative, possibly more efficient, form of medical assistance for trans people. Hopefully, things will improve for the large number of trans people in the United Kingdom who seek medical assistance to facilitate their transition.

The availability of proper medical treatment for trans people differs between countries depending on their cultural, social, and legal environments. For example, during the first 10 years of operation of the German Transsexuals' Act, which operates similarly to the Gender Recognition Act in the United Kingdom and requires a psychiatric diagnosis for people to be recognized as transsexual, trans women diagnosed with gender identity disorder were slightly older, at age 34, than trans men with a similar diagnosis whose average age was 30. The average delay between a legal name change in a German law court and change of sex status following genital surgery was two years, about the same as in most Western countries.[33]

Cultural, political, and religious considerations determine the availability of surgical options for trans people. For example, the first genital surgery case in China, a 20-year-old birth-assigned male, did not occur until the 1980s. She had been reared as a girl and had avoided traditional masculine pursuits such as rough-and-tumble play.[34] Although genital surgery has been available in other Asian countries such as Thailand for some time, the first such surgery in Japan occurred as late as 1998.

1.4 TRANSGENDER POLITICS

Being transgender might be usefully defined as "changing the social perception of one's everyday gender through the manipulation of non-genital signs."[35] This criterion distinguishes being transgender from the possibly dated idea of transsexuality, which almost always implies that the person has undergone or intends to undergo genital surgery.

As trans people have received such a rough deal from people in power, those brave enough to out themselves have campaigned unceasingly for improved rights, especially since the 1990s. Trans activists, such as Leslie Feinberg and Riki Wilchins, proclaim that trans people should take responsibility for their own histories and political initiatives, including ownership of a unique shared identity. Whereas transgender politics seeks to challenge and destabilize the binary gender system, gender identifiers still exist in such terminology as *trans men* and *trans women*. Perhaps the terms *trans masculine* and *trans feminine* reflect some variation around the absolute binary man and woman. However, it is difficult to situate those who have no gender feelings within this terminology.[36]

Over the last decade, more people have identified as nonbinary, especially when offered an opportunity to do so in surveys and on social media. DSM-5 has made special provision for the medical diagnosis and treatment of those identifying as nonbinary, although at present there has been insufficient research to evaluate the most appropriate procedures for people who do not identify with one of the binary gender categories, male or female, but rather feel that their gender is perhaps some combination of both. Such people challenge biological, sociological, and legal experts to devise a more appropriate gender classification for everyday use.[37] At present, there is no clear passage for nonbinary people should they seek medical interventions, although several countries, including Australia, Canada, Germany, India, Nepal, and New Zealand, allow nonbinary designations on birth certificates and passports.

As we have seen, gender diversity in its various forms has a colorful past, harking back to our earliest recorded history. The modern realization of a medical transition path for trans people occurred when relatively safe genital surgical procedures became available in a small number of locations in the 1950s. Since then, there have been considerable advances in assistance to trans people, as well as in the recognition of trans people as normal, productive members of society. The situation continues to improve with an increase in social tolerance accompanied by advances in surgical and other medical procedures. Even so, news about a sex change gets immediate media attention, especially in cases of regret. It is easy for the public to believe that regret following medical intervention is a routine event.[38] However, this is not the case. Skilled treatment leads to a marked improvement in the trans person's quality of life and their ability to make beneficial contributions to society. A good indicator of a society's maturity is how well it treats a stigmatized group such as the trans community. The next section discusses the cultural basis of gender-diverse behavior by comparing the approaches of traditional and Western societies.

1.5 SOCIAL AND CULTURAL ASPECTS OF GENDER DIVERSITY

Gender-diverse behavior was recorded in early human records. Laquer[39] suggested that some premodern European tribes consisted of one sex and two genders, the basic sex being male. These people considered the vagina, a defining characteristic of the female, to be an inverted internal penis. This idea contrasts with the modern concept of a person's sex based on external, rather than internal, genitals.

Considered in its broader cultural context, gender is "a complex, temporally extended system in which issues such as renown, age, and rank are all at work."[40] Gender is something people do—a way they behave—rather than a quality they possess. Every society has people who display gender differently from their society's norm. For example, the Burmese Dayaks consider universal humanity to be feminine, a gender role assumed by shamans and other religious people who are considered women with a penis. In Kenya's Turkana society, a child is initially neuter or androgynous until the appropriate sex is determined at puberty during initiation rites. According to traditional belief, Turkana women undergo removal of inappropriate male parts in the interests of sexual purity.

Since gender expression is a performance or imitation, transgendered behavior can occasionally represent an "imitation of an imitation."[41] So, drag shows and temporary crossdressing survive, provided the performance adheres to acceptable male or female behavior. Medical treatment of trans people sometimes adheres to this same gender divide, especially when successful passing in one's preferred gender role is deemed important. Whereas ambiguous gender behavior is scorned in Western societies, for example, this is not the case in other societies within which third-gender people play important cultural roles.

The *third-gender* concept was originally introduced by Martin and Voorhies, who suggested that in some cultures gender is not partitioned into two categories. In general, the third gender represents any gender embodiment that does not lie within the binary gender scheme of man and woman, rather than implying that there are only three different genders. Although third-gender people are generally revered, they often suffer similar levels of prejudice as that endured by trans people everywhere else.[42] This is certainly the case for the *sistergirls*, trans indigenous Australians. Whereas sistergirls are revered within traditional Aboriginal society and perform important female duties within their families, they suffer many forms of discrimination in the wider community that can adversely affect their mental health.[43] Sistergirls suffer transphobia within traditional Australian indigenous communities, and even more abuse and discrimination when they move to the larger cities such as Sydney where the population is predominantly white. The response of the indigenous community to social deviance may be to issue payback, a form of verbal and physical assault including rape, not only toward the sistergirl herself but also toward her immediate family.[44]

Chevalier d'Eon, the famous French crossdresser, experienced an increase in religious experiences following a change in gender presentation. Such spiritual conversions occur in traditional societies such as the two-spirit people in North America, who mediated between physical and spiritual aspects of their people's lives. Other spiritually esteemed trans people include the *acault* (trans women) in Myanmar, and the *maa khii* (trans men) in northern Thailand.[45] In Thailand, masculine women and feminine men are called *tom* and *kathoey*, respectively. Such people are often sexually attracted to people of their same birth-assigned sex. Perhaps Thai culture does not appear to distinguish between homosexuals and trans people.[46]

The *sworn virgins* are trans women who assume a male role in rural Albania and Kosovo. These women become honorary males; they do not marry but assume the role of household head. They exhibit a masculine speech style as well as masculine activities and body language. They also change their name to reflect their new masculine social role. Few if any of these women participate in lesbian activities, suggesting a dissociation between gender identity and sexual orientation in their community.[47]

Gender diversity in Japan is widespread. Both male female-role and female male-role actors partake in stage shows, suggesting that the Japanese entertainment industry is tolerant of homosexual and trans behavior with sexual activities being common. Trans women who work in the Japanese sex and entertainment industry are called *new-half* people. Although they communicate using female speech patterns, some new-half people adopt an intermediate sexual identity that is not entirely female. In Japan there is a sanctioned departure from the binary gender norm that is mainly limited to entertainment and discrete communication.[48]

Most *Aravanis*, a trans *hijra* community in Tamil Nadu, India, accept the Hindu belief that the female gender is the starting point, and transformation into a male gender is only needed to provide fatherly roles in their society. Aravanis are invited to bless newborn babies because their third-gender status offers its own special spiritual significance.

Aravanis are men who dress as women and work in nontraditional occupations such as cooks and dancers. Although they occasionally provide sexual services to men, they dress differently from men, avoid sexual relationships with women, and do not indulge in sexual relationships within their own community. The Aravanis assume a female sexual identity and refer to each other using female terms. As they are often shunned by male family members, they offer both material and emotional support to each other. Many Aravanis take hormones and have genital surgery to more adequately fulfil their female role.

They occasionally assume a monogamous liaison with a man they call their husband.[49]

The gender beliefs of Aravanis were investigated by asking them to judge the appropriateness of gender transgressions in one of two stories, one involving a boy who behaves like a girl, the other involving a girl who behaves like a boy. Aravanis tolerate all types of gender transgression. They believe that a girl is more likely to become a boy in the next life than a boy will become a girl because of the boy's good karma. However, in their current life, they believe that a girl could not become a boy whereas a boy could easily become a girl. Gender presentation is important because if a boy dresses and behaves like a girl, then he would be expected to become a girl. But even if a girl dressed and acted like a boy, a gender transformation from female to male was considered impossible. So, for the Aravanis, a male gender identity is more fluid than a female one. In most Western societies the opposite applies, there being greater tolerance of girls dressing and behaving like boys than vice versa. Whereas men who adopt a different gender role may lose status in many Western countries, it is a male prerogative in some parts of India. So cultural factors are important determinants of gender expression and tolerance.

Many trans people respond to society's stigma by maintaining the traditional male–female gender divide, with a binary gender attribution being suitable for those who value passing. Perhaps feminist authors should be tolerant of individual differences and eliminate the pathological labeling of trans women as has been done by some radical feminists who restrict *womanhood* to birth-assigned women, thereby explicitly excluding trans women. The situation has not changed over the last few decades as more radical feminists strive to preclude trans women from taking part in all aspects of the feminine way of life, an extreme attitude that despite a vicious social media campaign has been doomed to failure. Such an attitude has caused considerable distress among fair-minded gender-diverse people and other members of the wider community.

1.6 HOW DO PEOPLE VIEW GENDER DIVERSITY?

Gender-diverse behavior has been considered variously as abnormal, anomalous, and scandalous in many Western societies. This negative attitude toward trans people's lifestyles reflects long-term sanctions based on religious, cultural, and legal constraints. However, such negative attitudes have softened, especially in the entertainment industry where drag queens, men who impersonate women, and drag kings, women who impersonate men, have provided comic relief for the masses. Perhaps the best-known exponent of this art is Dame Edna Everage, the mature-age female persona developed by the Australian actor Barry Humphries. Despite its popularity, such lampooning of cross-gendered behavior incites incredibility in those trans people who must live permanently in their affirmed gender without the convenience of being able to slip back into a gender role based on their birth-assigned sex when the going gets tough. This situation was not helped by the aging Humphries's explicit denunciation of trans people in comments he has made in the right-wing U.K. media.[50]

The attractiveness and seductiveness presented by some trans women can occasionally threaten male values. Movies with a transgendered theme such as *Some Like It Hot* and *The Silence of the Lambs* invoke both amusement and horrified repulsion in viewers, leading to an ambivalence in people's attitudes toward trans people. Television, and more recently social media, have brought trans people into the public gaze. These shows range from the outlandish representation of trans people on the *Jerry Springer Show* to the more refined interviews that occasionally occurred on the *Oprah Winfrey Show*.

Recently, documentaries with a trans theme have appeared on television as well as in a few notable feature-length movies involving trans characters. The popular films *Priscilla Queen of the Desert* and *Mrs. Doubtfire* and the rather disturbing *Boys Don't Cry* are noteworthy, despite the first two being about crossdressed characters rather than trans people who have transitioned. Felicity Huffman's winning of a Golden Globe award in 2006 for her starring role of Bree, a trans woman, in *Transamerica* was a notable achievement, even though these days it is considered important that trans characters be portrayed by trans actors. People were either amused or outraged by the TV show *There's Something About Miriam* in which a group of unsuspecting young men become infatuated with an attractive woman who, unbeknown to them, was trans. The participants' subsequent outrage indicated the disservice such a show does to thoughtful people, especially members of the trans community.

These days there are lots of videos on YouTube with a trans theme, notably those about Jazz Jennings, a young American trans woman who has become a media star in her own right. Of special significance are the videos and stories about Sarah McBride, who in 2016 was the first trans woman to address the national conference of the U.S. Democratic Party. She has written a notable book, *Tomorrow Will Be Different*.

The public can now read autobiographies written by trans people.[51] More than any other medium, the written word, accompanied frequently by life-history photographs, has described the agonies and joys experienced by those trans people who have been brave enough to share their experiences with others. Of special significance is the way partners, family, and work colleagues have accommodated themselves to the changes transition imposes upon their loved ones. Inevitably, such stories provide a glimpse of humanity that is scarcely experienced by most people in a lifetime.[52]

The Internet has provided more information on trans people and issues of interest to trans people and their supporters than was previously available. Nowadays, people can explore their gender feelings by reading informative web pages on the Internet. There are also lots of instructional videos on medical aspects of transition as well as many personal stories. Open and closed groups on Facebook provide access to experiences and advice from fellow trans people and their knowledgeable supporters. They can also communicate directly with trans people in public and in private using chat rooms, by email, and more frequently via the numerous social media platforms including Facebook and Twitter.

1.7 ATTITUDES TOWARD TRANS PEOPLE

As in many other matters of social interest, Sweden is an ideal place to conduct a survey of attitudes toward trans people. Since 1972, genital surgeries have been covered by that country's national health scheme, postoperative people being able to live as their affirmed gender and to enjoy the same rights as other citizens, including marriage and adopting and raising children. In 1998, a questionnaire designed to explore people's views on transsexualism was sent to almost 1,000 Swedish people aged between 18 and 70, obtaining a good response rate of 67 percent.[53] For the purposes of this survey, the now-obsolete medical condition of transsexualism was defined as follows:

> *Transsexualism* occurs in both men and women and is characterized by a gender identity of the opposite sex. A transsexual person is often said to be trapped in the body of the wrong sex and have a strong desire to live and be accepted as a member of the opposite sex and to *change sex*. A sex change implies a new name, treatment with the hormones of the opposite sex, and surgery of the genitals to make his or her body as congruent as possible with the preferred sex. *Transsexualism* is not the same as *transvestism*, which refers to men who occasionally dress in women's clothes. A *transvestite* does not wish to change sex.[54]

The survey produced several interesting findings. More women than men returned the questionnaire. Interestingly, 65 percent of respondents, the Biological group, believed that transsexualism has a biological cause, whereas for the remainder, the Social group, a socially determined cause was considered more likely.

In terms of medical and social implications, only 22 percent considered transsexualism to be a treatable disease; 64 percent supported a trans person's desire for a name change; 52 percent approved a change in identity; and 53 percent approved of access to hormone treatment. Fifty-six percent supported trans people's desire for genital surgeries. Sixty-three percent of respondents believed that the individual should pay for their own medical treatment;

56 percent approved of marriage following genital surgery; and 52 percent opposed the idea that single trans people should be allowed to adopt and raise children, whereas 43 percent approved the trans person's right to raise children provided they were married. Sixty-one percent of respondents considered that a trans person, no matter their affirmed gender, could work with children. Seventy-one percent would be pleased to work with a trans person and 60 percent would be prepared to have such a person as their friend. However, 84 percent of respondents would not want a trans person as their partner. People agreed that the media provides adequate, but not excessive, attention to trans people. Only 8 percent of respondents knew a trans person, and 38 percent of people believed that the incidence of transsexualism had increased in Sweden over the last 20 years. Interestingly, 53 percent of people considered that trans people were born that way, reinforcing slight majority support for a biological basis for the condition.

Searching for a biological basis for transsexualism, rather than assuming that the lifestyle is socially determined, may be worthwhile as fewer of the people who consider transsexualism to be biologically determined believe it is a disease. More women than men thought that transsexualism was not a disease. Similarly, more young people than older people thought transsexualism was not a disease. These results suggest community support for the removal of medical gatekeeping from the medical assistance provided to trans people.

Biological group respondents of all ages, including more women and younger people, supported a change in name and identity for a trans person. They also thought that trans people should be treated with hormones followed by genital surgery, if they so desire. Biological respondents preferred that trans people use their own financial resources to pay for their medical treatments, as also did the younger respondents. More Biological respondents thought trans people should be able to marry in their affirmed gender, as also did more women and younger respondents. Nevertheless, Biological respondents were not so keen for single trans people to adopt and raise children by themselves. However, this situation changes dramatically if the couple are married, the Biological respondents supporting the idea that trans people should be allowed to look after children, an attitude they shared with female respondents in general. Biological respondents favored postoperative trans people being allowed to work with children, a liberal view they shared with women. More Biological respondents, as well as most women, would be prepared to work with a trans person and have such a person as their friend.

The Swedish survey demonstrated that country's liberal attitudes toward gender-diverse people's desire for a normal life. Overall, women and those who believed that transsexualism has a biological basis were the most supportive of trans people. Such findings, if replicated in other Western societies, would

provide considerable encouragement to those trans people who wish to proceed to genital surgeries and other necessary medical treatments.

Heath and colleagues conducted a 2005 Internet survey that was similar in
content to the Swedish study.[55] Eighty-four percent of the 413 mostly female
people who answered the survey came from Australia and the United States,
and more than the expected number were nonheterosexual (39%). The North
Americans were younger, mostly female, and more religious whereas the Australians were older and less religious. Most people (61%) considered transsexualism to have a biological cause, especially older, partnered, transgendered,
and nonreligious respondents. Religious people who were regular churchgoers
preferred a social origin for transsexualism, and partnered, heterosexual, and
nontransgendered people exhibited negative attitudes toward trans people.
Nevertheless, most people thought that transsexualism was not a disease, but
that trans people and those with a difference in sexual development, which
was defined as *intersex* in the survey, should have access to medical treatments
such as hormones and genital surgeries.

Most people thought that trans people should have the right to marry,
change their name, and adopt children on equal terms with others in the community. While almost everyone would welcome a trans person as a coworker
or friend, most people would not like to have a trans person as their partner.
When it came to publicly funded genital surgeries, most people were more
lenient toward people who differ in sexual development compared with trans
people. When answers to a test of personal attributes were considered, supportive people tended to be more empathic and less domineering than those
with more negative views toward gender diversity.

One biological correlate for transsexualism has been identified based on a
discrepancy between brain sexual differentiation and born sex. In an old study,
the central region of the bed nucleus of the stria terminalis (BSTc) in the
hypothalamus appeared female in appearance for deceased trans women, using
as evidence postmortem brain micrographs. This difference cannot result from
estrogen exposure as men treated with estrogen for medical conditions other
than transsexualism had a male BSTc size. Other studies have demonstrated
both genetic and finger-length ratio differences between trans people and others, although these differences are small and controversial. Such discoveries
bolster the hopes of those trans people who believe that their condition might
have a firm biological basis, especially when tolerance is enhanced when people believe that transsexualism has a biological basis, as was the case in both
surveys. A more up-to-date account of evidence for the biological basis of the
trans experience is contained in Chapter 2.

Much of the research into sex differences maintains the superiority society
attaches to heterosexuality. Rogers[56] criticized the unconfirmed, biased view-
points of both evolutionary psychologists and sociobiologists who have made

unsubstantiated claims about the ancestral differences between men and women. Such claims demean women and lower their social prestige. Such an injustice can be doubly damaging to trans people, who should not have to suffer the consequences of a society that preferences heteronormativity, the privilege granted those who do not identify as members of the LGBTIQ communities. More pointedly, Cordelia Fine has proposed that there is scant evidence for gender differences in the brain, with many of the differences we observe between men and women being socially conditioned.[57]

The most devastating outcome for trans people is transphobia, defined as "skepticism about the existence of the transsexed or a dislike or hatred of, and occasionally hostility toward, them." Transphobia is not limited to the general public but is exhibited by members of the psychological and medical professions, sometimes even by those who assist trans people. Raj outlined various forms of clinical transphobia, the irrational attitudes of clinicians directed toward their trans clients. These include unethical treatment strategies applied to those who do not experience any psychological disability, such as:

a. pathologizing clients by suggesting that their gender-affirmation is a symptom of serious psychiatric illness;

b. insisting upon client compliance toward therapy based on outdated ideas about the causes of gender diversity;

c. employing unethical and unproven diagnostic methods such as physiological responses to erotic stimuli;

d. using unproven techniques such as psychoanalysis to effect a cure, the unethical *conversion therapy* approach;

e. using behavior modification techniques with young people who exhibit gender-atypical behavior to deter them from what the clinician believes will be an undesirable lifestyle;

f. discriminating against gynephilic trans women, that is, those who are sexually attracted to women, but not applying this restriction to androphilic trans men, that is, those who are sexually attracted to men;

g. excluding from [social transition], that is, living full-time in their preferred gender, those people who are unemployed or not studying full-time, and who cannot pass in their affirmed gender role;

h. showing prejudice toward those trans people, mainly women, who engage in sex work;

i. only providing hormone therapy for those who intend pursuing genital surgery when some trans people [do not] undergo such surgery for personal, health, or financial reasons; and

j. frustrating trans people by imposing excessive gatekeeping.

A shift in focus toward all forms of gender diversity being considered normal behavior rather than toward it being a pathological condition is required. The therapist's role should change from clinical provider to client facilitator.

Improvement in support for trans people requires a more diverse client population, more therapists with trans backgrounds, improved access to surgery and other medical procedures by government and insurance companies, and better training of professionals who assist trans clients.[58]

Fearing an incorrect and unexpected misdiagnosis, trans clients are often antagonistic toward their medical advisers, at the same time challenging the need for expensive clinical assessment. Some advisers serve as *gatekeepers* by setting up eligibility criteria and clinical thresholds, while the client demands hormones and surgery. Such opposition can be moderated by offering greater decision-making responsibility to the client. Cooperative strategies emphasize client-directed, collaborative, self-determined medical management based on a demedicalized, socially acceptable approach.

Whatever the treatment strategy, it should be person-centered and solution-focused using the most appropriate procedure for each client. Not enough professionals have certified training in trans counseling to serve as informed and innovative counselors. Often, trans clients know more about their needs than do their therapists.

People who believe that gender diversity has a biological basis are more understanding and sympathetic to the needs of trans people. On the other hand, when professionals treating trans people are as antagonistic to their needs as are some members of the public, trans people can be justifiably aggrieved at this infraction of their human rights. Education is needed to achieve a change in people's attitudes toward gender-diverse people at the professional adviser level and throughout the community.

1.8 HOW MANY TRANS PEOPLE ARE THERE?

Controversy exists regarding how many trans people there are, due to the earlier measures indicating its relative rarity, and the tendency for some trans people to transition in stealth without medical supervision. A largely hidden population of people who have not attended gender clinics or trans events further complicates the task of assessing prevalence. Most of the early prevalence estimates were obtained from gender clinic clients who had been pathologized with a medical condition of transsexualism, gender identity disorder, or more recently, gender dysphoria. So it is nearly impossible to determine the wider incidence of gender diversity.

A retrospective study of 1,285 trans people who attended a Dutch gender clinic between 1975 and 1992 included 949 men and 336 women.[59] The annual number of applicants increased over time with numbers stabilizing in the late 1980s, the ratio of trans women to men of about 3:1 remaining relatively constant over this 17-year period. Seventy-seven percent of the men and 80 percent of the women progressed to hormonal and/or surgical treatment.

Sixty-seven percent of trans women and 78 percent of trans men were young, having presented for treatment in their late teens or early twenties. A smaller proportion of older trans women, who transitioned in middle age and beyond, underwent genital surgeries than was the case for the younger trans women. Of those who progressed to genital surgery, only five trans women regretted their decision. This small number, representing 0.7 percent of the applicants, was composed of older trans women. Overall, the prevalence in the Netherlands of transsexualism as a medical condition was estimated to be 1 in 11,900 for birth-assigned men and 1 in 39,400 for birth-assigned women, values substantially greater than the 1 in 30,000 for birth-assigned males and 1 in 100,000 for birth-assigned females published in DSM-IV, the *Diagnostic and Statistical Manual* used by psychiatrists and clinical psychologists worldwide until 2013.

Prevalence rates can vary depending on how people are measured and what society they live in, and these rates may change over time. In 2000 in the Czech Republic, the incidence of transsexualism for both males and females was 1 in 10,000, the average age for genital reconstruction surgery (GRS) being 29.[60] In West Germany between 1981 and 1990 there were only 1,422 cases of diagnosed transsexualism. Most of these trans people were in the 25 to 34 age range, the next most common age range being the following decade between the ages of 35 and 44. Here, the estimated prevalence of transsexualism was 1 in 36,000 for trans women and 1 in 131,000 for trans men, a sex ratio favoring trans women of about 3:1.

Other observations, recently confirmed, suggest a much higher prevalence of transsexualism as a medical diagnosis. Issues related to gender are occasionally masked by other conditions such as anxiety, depression, bipolar disorder, conduct disorder, substance abuse, dissociative identity disorders, borderline personality disorder, other sexual disorders, and differences in sexual development. This means that people presenting with these other conditions will not be counted in medical estimates of prevalence. Some crossdressers, female impersonators, and homosexual people may also exhibit gender variance but not be included. As the intensity of a trans person's gender feelings can fluctuate over time, some people may not present for intervention and so will be excluded from prevalence studies. Finally, gender variance among birth-assigned females was relatively invisible in Western societies so that many trans masculine people would not have been counted.[61]

A recent study of trends in the use of trans diagnostic codes in the U.S. National Inpatient Sample Data Set has shown an almost fourfold increase in prevalence over the decade 2004 to 2014 from 4 in 100,000 to 14 in 100,000. The median age was 38 and 54 percent were birth-assigned male. Forty-one percent had been hospitalized for mental health issues, 10 percent had genital surgery, and 1 percent had chest or breast surgery.[62] These numbers may seem to be the wrong way around as breast surgery is much more common than genital surgery for trans men. However, these statistics only refer to hospitalization in public medical centers in the United States, so they would not include many cosmetic procedures.

Because an unknown number of trans people are not counted in prevalence studies, the true prevalence must be much higher than any of these published figures suggest. Lynn Conway[63] has argued that transgender prevalence is up to 100 times greater than the figures quoted in the literature. Such a gap in visibility is reasonable as many people never undergo gender-affirming surgeries and so never appear in the medical records of psychiatrists and surgeons. Many people never seek medical help because they can obtain black-market hormones, or else have family and job commitments that deter them from approaching a gender specialist.

Although precise estimates are difficult to obtain and tend to vary from one country to another, as we have seen, the current best published estimate of the prevalence of the medical condition of transsexualism is about 1 in 10,000 for birth-assigned men and 1 in 30,000 for birth-assigned women, based on data collected from specialist clinics mainly in the Netherlands. These figures are about three times larger than those quoted in the latest edition of the American Psychiatric Association's *Diagnostic and Statistical Manual* (DSM), version 5. The prevalence of self-identified trans and gender-diverse people is far higher than those diagnosed in the medical system.

The Massachusetts Behavioral Risk Factor Surveillance System surveyed 28,176 adults aged 18 to 64 between 2007 and 2009 and found that 0.5 percent identified as transgender. This finding suggests that it is almost inevitable that health workers will meet quite a few trans people in their work.[64] This significantly higher result was confirmed by a recent study of a general population. When high school children were randomly sampled, the incidence of transgender people was found to have increased substantially to about 1.2 percent.[65]

Clearly, a more carefully conducted epidemiological study is required, not only to inform trans people how very special they are, but to allow health and support agencies to estimate current and future demands for their services. If Conway is correct and the prevalence of gender diversity expressed in all its forms as gender variance among birth-assigned men alone is 1 in 250, we have a major public health issue on our hands.

SUMMARY

Following a brief review of the historical origins of gender diversity, the rapid advances in recognition, assessment, and help provided for the associated medical conditions were summarized. This review highlighted the important contributions made by medical pioneers such as Harry Benjamin, and trans pioneers such as Lili Elbe and Christine Jorgensen. These people encouraged medical professionals to expand their skills into a challenging and potentially stigmatized field while simultaneously paving the way for the many trans people who would follow in their footsteps. A few examples of pioneering gender clinics were provided.

Although many trans people comply with socially prescribed gender roles and pass if they can, others live their lives either in an androgynous way, or in a more radical form akin to the third-gender role that is tolerated in many non-Western societies. A Swedish survey, reinforced by a similar study conducted in Australia, confirmed that people's attitudes toward trans people and their desire for proper treatment indicated a high level of tolerance, especially among those who believed that, rather than being merely some social whim, there is a biological basis for the condition. This positive approach is dampened somewhat by those professionals who exhibit similar prejudice toward trans people as do some members of the public. Prevalence studies indicated that, despite the large variability between estimates, the latest figures suggest that requests for medical treatment may be many times more prevalent than is recognized in the most recent version of the DSM. Sampling difficulties and the tendency for many trans people to live in stealth ensure that such estimates are highly unreliable in the absence of properly conducted epidemiological studies. However, common sense suggests that the prevalence of gender diversity is rather high, greater than for many recognized medical conditions that attract generous research funding and medical facilities from governments and other agencies.

Chapter 2

WHAT IS GENDER?

In this chapter we consider the biological, psychological, and developmental bases of gender as an important human characteristic.

2.1 SEX AND GENDER

Sex refers to biological aspects whereas *gender* is affected by social and cultural influences and may not necessarily be biologically determined. Trans people have the body and genitals of one sex, and the gender identity of another. Any reconciliation of the two, if desired, can only be achieved by changing one's body rather than one's mind since brain-sex is more deeply rooted than are the bodily manifestations of sex.[1] Even when we suspect that a person's trans status might be related to their brain-sex, as we will see when we discuss the biological evidence, the official diagnostic category for the medical condition of *gender dysphoria*, according to the American Psychiatric Association's *Diagnostic and Statistical Manual*, version 5 (2013), is a psychological condition with no reference to brain structure or function.[2]

Sex has been defined as "the biologically-based categories of male and female," whereas gender involves "the psychological features frequently associated with these biological states, assigned either by the observer or by the individual subject."[3] In the following discussion we use the term *gender* instead of *sex* as many gender differences cannot be biologically verified. *Sex* is used when referring to biological entities such as the brain and other aspects of human body function, including hormones.

Interpreting gender differences is complicated, especially if masculinity and femininity do not lie on opposite ends of a single dimension but need to be represented by more than one dimension. Most gender differences in psychological characteristics and behavior are small with a large overlap between the scores obtained by men and women. For example, although some people consider boys to excel at mathematics when compared with girls, even this small gender difference is probably culturally determined and can be affected by the social environment in which the study is undertaken.

The existence of stereotypes suggests that male behavior represents authority, status, competence, and social influence, whereas female behavior is characterized by low status, lack of confidence, and limited influence. Nevertheless, stereotypical female behavior is often nurturing and adaptive, whereas male behavior is occasionally associated with negative consequences such as violence. Although gender stereotypes might have a firm basis in our psychological and biological makeup, they mask the similarities in behavior between men and women, leading to social injustice and prejudice for those who violate society's gender norms. A comprehensive review of the evidence could only find substantial gender differences in childhood play and adult aggressive tendencies, such is the extent of the overlap between the behaviors of males and females.[4]

Any attempt to capture all the aspects of sex and gender would have to include biological sex, legal sex, affirmed gender, sexual orientation, social behavior, outward presentation, and preferred sexual activity.[5] This of course suggests that sex and gender are quite complicated, as can be seen by examining their biological basis in the next section, and their many other aspects in later chapters.

2.2 THE BIOLOGICAL BASIS OF GENDER IDENTITY FORMATION

Of the gender differences occurring in humans, perhaps the most essential are those occurring in the brain, resulting possibly from the prenatal exposure to hormones and genetic effects. These average differences between males and females are likely causes of human variability in gender identity. We now consider the biological basis of gender identity, revealing some interesting differences in brain structures between men and women, as well as between trans people and others of their birth-assigned sex.

2.2.1 Prenatal Development of Sex Differences

Sex differences originate in the differentiation process that determines whether the human embryo will become male or female. During the first six weeks of fetal development, male and female embryos are indistinguishable. The major sex determination event is the transformation of a rudimentary structure, the gonad, at around seven weeks' gestation, into either a testis or an ovary, a process initi-ated by the SRY gene located on the Y chromosome, the one usually associated with being male. In the male fetus, the testes will gradually start to release the hormones Mullerian-inhibiting substance from Sertoli cells and testosterone from Leydig cells.[6] Testosterone increases in concentration within testicular tis-sue, fetal blood, and amniotic fluid, attaining a peak concentration around week 16.[7] The development of external male genitals requires the further transforma-tion of testosterone to dihydrotestosterone (DHT) by the enzyme 5-α-reductase.

During this process, two pairs of genital ducts develop within the urogenital ridge. Testosterone promotes development of one system, the Wolffian ducts, to form the epididymis, vas deferens, seminal vesicles, and ejaculatory duct. The production of Mullerian-inhibiting substance in males causes the other system, the Mullerian ducts, to regress. In females, the absence of Mullerian-inhibiting substance allows these ducts to eventually form the fallopian tubes, the uterus, and the upper portion of the vagina.

At two critical periods during early development, males are exposed to greater levels of testosterone than are females. The first critical period occurs during the middle of gestation, and the second period occurs during the first six months after birth when another testosterone surge occurs, sometimes called *mini-puberty*.

Could these processes lead to gender diversity as well as sex differences? Could this be due to changes in the brain? A sexually dimorphic brain region is one that shows clear differences between men and women. Sexually dimorphic neural structures are not necessarily determined by sex differences in gonadal hormone levels but could be determined by genetic differences.[8] Although genetics may affect brain-sexual differences, it has not been easy to establish a genetic basis for the trans experience when compared with differences in sexual determination, for which genetics plays a major role. Using genetic material from 30 trans women and 31 trans men, no association was found between the outdated diagnosis of transsexualism and any chromosomal variations.[9]

However, genetic effects may be rather subtle. When the genetic structures of 29 trans women were compared with those of 229 birth-assigned women, there were differences in the genetic sequences that govern the function of the sex hormones estrogen and testosterone, as well as in genetic sequences for aroma-tase, the chemical that converts testosterone to estrogen.[10] A recent review of twin data and generic markers of the trans experience did not find consistent results, leading to some doubt about whether being trans is coded in our genes.[11]

2.2.2 Sex Differences in Brain Function

There are interesting differences in the brains of men and women that may be responsible for some gender differences in behavior. Newer imaging techniques such as magnetic resonance imaging (MRI) have revealed interesting sex differences in the living brain. It was thought that these differences must be set before birth, but it is now known that some of these areas, for example the size of the posterodorsal nucleus of the medial amygdala, an emotional center that is larger in males than females, are also modifiable after birth. Experiments using rats have shown the adult brain continues to change in response to hormonal influences.[12] For example, testosterone acts on the spinal nucleus of the bulbocavernosus, which enervates the penis in order to change the size and connectivity of neurons that control penis function. In females, estrogen causes the ventromedial nucleus of the hypothalamus to produce new synapses. As well as hormonal stimuli, environmental influences such as stress cause changes in the hippocampus, a midbrain structure that is also involved in memory and learning. Therefore, life experiences affect behavior by interacting with the effects of hormones.

Sex differences exist in brain regions outside of the amygdala and hippocampus regions such as the corpus callosum, the nerve tissue connecting the two brain hemispheres. The corpus callosum is more richly connected in females than in males, suggesting that the brain hemispheres might have fewer lateralized functions in women than in men.[13] Although the female brain weighs about 100 grams less than that of males, the metabolic activity per unit volume is about the same. The corpus callosum has a larger area in males than in females, but this anatomical difference, which is rather small, does not result in measurable sex differences in behavior.[14]

The hypothalamus, a small lower brain region that controls functions such as hunger, thirst, reproduction, and sleep, as well as regulating hormone release by stimulating the pituitary gland, is also sensitive to sex differences. Specific hypothalamic nuclei[15] are sexually dimorphic; the preoptic area (SDN-POA) in men is more than twice as large as it is in women, this sex difference fluctuating with age. There is a correspondingly larger number of androgen and estrogen receptors in this site for men than for women. The central section of the bed nucleus of the stria terminalis (BSTc) is a small region of the hypothalamus defined by its dense vasoactive intestinal polypeptide (VIP) innervation, probably originating in the amygdala. The BSTc is also characterized by its somatostatin nerve fiber network and associated neurons that exhibit clear sex differences. The BSTc is 40 percent larger in men than in women and has almost twice as many somatostatin neurons in men.[16] Somatostatin is a peptide chemical involved in nerve message transmission. For example, deficits in somatostatin accompany both epilepsy and Alzheimer's disease.[17]

Data obtained from ten 47-year-old men and fourteen 41-year-old women indicated that males have a higher somatostatin density in both the temporal and frontal cortical regions of the brain than do females, suggesting that somatostatin receptor density in the cerebral cortex may be related to sex.[18]

Sex differences in the SDN-POA first become evident around four years of age when the number of cells decreases for girls but stays relatively constant for boys. There is a rapid decrease in cell numbers for men over age 50 and a corresponding decrease in cell numbers for women over age 70. In men, the reduction in SDA-POA cell count occurring between 50 and 60 years leads to a small sex difference. Thereafter, a decrease in cell count occurs for women over 70 but not for men, resulting in older men having a larger SDA-POA cell count than older women.

The VIP-containing subnucleus of the human suprachiasmic nucleus, a region of the hypothalamus that controls hormone cycles, is twice as large in young men as in women of comparable age. This sex difference reverses beyond 40 years of age when the subnucleus size for women becomes larger than that for men. Therefore, age can be a crucial factor affecting the direction of brain-sex differences.

Vasopressin is responsible for body fluid retention and may cause an increase in blood pressure. Young males exhibit greater vasopressin nerve activity in the supraoptic nucleus than do women. This sex difference disappears after age 50, suggesting that a region with no sex differences in its structure can nevertheless reveal a sex difference in how it functions.

Interesting sex differences have been observed in intact living brains using MRI, which can display brain structure in living organisms. Although the brain is 10 percent smaller in women than in men, relative to overall brain size, compared with men, women have a greater cortical gray matter volume as well as larger volumes in brain regions associated with language such as Broca's area and the superior temporal cortex. Relative to men, women have larger hippocampus volumes, larger caudate and thalamic nuclei, as well as a larger anterior cingulated gyrus, dorsolateral prefrontal cortex, right inferior parietal lobe, and a greater volume of white matter in the corpus callosum. Men, on the other hand, have larger brain volumes in the limbic and paralimbic regions, the hypothalamus, and in the paracingulate gyrus.[19] So many brain regions are sensitive to a person's birth-assigned sex.

The limbic system, the part of the brain responsible for our emotions, consists of the anterior cingulate, the amygdala, the hippocampus, and the insular cortex. When selectively stimulated, the limbic system's activity can be measured using positron emission tomography (PET). Men have a greater insula response on the left side of the brain than do women, whereas women have a greater amygdala response on the left side of the brain than do men.[20] These sex differences might be related to women's generally greater emotional responsiveness than men.

Using similar MRI technology, the caudate, part of the brain's reward structure, and possibly the globus pallidus and hippocampus are larger in female than in male brains, whereas the amygdala is smaller in female brains. This finding is possibly due to there being mostly androgen receptors in the amygdala and mostly estrogen receptors in the hippocampus. The smaller amygdala in women might explain their greater proneness to emotional disorders, whereas the larger caudate nucleus in women might protect them from typically male diseases such as attention deficit hyperactivity disorder (ADHD) and Tourette's syndrome.[21] However, behavioral correlates of sex differences in brain regions are difficult to demonstrate for certain.

Differences in brain function may be responsible for sex differences in the prevalence of physical and mental disorders. For example, predominantly female disorders include anorexia nervosa, bulimia, senile dementia, multiple sclerosis, anxiety disorder, post-traumatic stress disorders, and unipolar depression. Predominantly male disorders include Kallmann syndrome that involves a delayed puberty, sleep apnea, autism, ADHD, dyslexia, schizophrenia, stuttering, substance abuse, and learning disability.

When men and women are matched on age, handedness, education, and IQ, MRI data reveal larger sex differences in regions having a greater number of sex hormone receptors. Women have larger brain volumes than men in the frontal and medial paralimbic regions, in the precentral gyrus and the fronto-orbital cortex, as well as in the superior frontal and lingual gyri.

The studies of trans women that have included only those women sexually attracted to women and who were imaged prior to commencement of estrogen therapy do not show consistent evidence of feminization in these brain regions. Many areas of their brain resemble those of cisgender men. However, some regions are different from cisgender men and women such as reduced thalamus and putamen volumes and larger gray matter volumes in a few areas in the frontal region of the brain that are involved in body perception. These studies, which are summarized in Section 2.4, do not provide evidence for brain activity in areas associated with any distress that might be linked to gender identity. These findings raise doubts about the biological validity of a diagnosis such as gender dysphoria.

2.3 GENDER DIVERSITY AND BRAIN DIFFERENCES

Prior to undergoing hormone therapy, trans women's brain gray matter volume, white matter volume, cerebrospinal fluid volume, and intracranial volume all resemble those of their birth-assigned sex, which in this case is male, rather than their affirmed gender identity. In each case, the volumes are lower for birth-assigned females than for trans women. By contrast, using brain fractional anisotropy, a measure of the extent to which nerve fibers in the brain are aligned in one direction with an anisotropy value equal to 1.0 or spread out, in which case the anisotropy value equals 0.0, showed that trans women had anisotropy values between that of birth-assigned women and birth-assigned men. This intermediate result for trans women applied to six distinct parts of the brain, the left and right superior longitudinal fasciculus, the right forceps minor, the right inferior fronto-occipital fasciculus, the right corticospinal tract, and the right cingulum, suggesting a consistent intersex brain fractional anisotropic structure for trans women. It is interesting to note that all but one of these differences occur in the right hemisphere of the brain.[22]

Compared with birth-assigned females, trans men who had not started testosterone therapy show higher fractional anisotropy values in the anterior and posterior parts of the right superior longitudinal fasciculus and the forceps minor. Fractional anisotropy values in the corticospinal tract were lower for trans men than for birth-assigned males but higher than values recorded for birth-assigned females.[23]

The bed nucleus of the stria terminalis (BSTc) exhibits a female form in trans women, whereas a more male-like BSTc was observed in one trans man. These differences did not depend on whether the people had already been on hormone treatment. During its development in animals, the BSTc is sensitive to the effects of testosterone. One explanation could be that a reduction in prenatal androgens is responsible for this difference, and perhaps this could be a factor in gender-diverse behavior in birth-assigned men. Using postmortem brain samples from six trans women collected over an 11-year period, the volume of the BSTc was found to be similar in size and shape for birth-assigned women and trans women. BSTc size was not affected by sex hormones in adulthood nor was it related to sexual orientation. A small BSTc volume was found in the trans women that was 52 percent of that observed for gynephilic males and 46 percent of the value for birth-assigned males.[24]

When considered together with animal data, these results suggest that gender diversity may result from interactions between brain development and sex hormone concentrations. However, such a claim is impossible to evaluate empirically as causal influences cannot be inferred when there is no experimental manipulation. Furthermore, it remains challenging to prove a direct link between brain anatomy, function, and human behavior.

Sex differences in BSTc size might result from differences in its nerve connections with the amygdala, which forms part of the limbic, or emotional, system of the brain. The number of somatostatin-expressing (SOM) neurons in the BSTc was determined using postmortem brain samples from 42 men and women with varied sexual orientation, differences in sexual development, and gender identities. The number of SOM neurons for men was 71 percent larger than for women. The number of SOM neurons was similar for trans women and birth-assigned women, the data for one trans man being located within the birth-assigned male range. The number of neurons for trans women was 40 percent less than that found for birth-assigned men. There was no difference in the number of BSTc neurons for young compared with middle-aged trans women, suggesting that BSTc size depends on gender identity rather than age at transition. Except for a relatively recent tendency for them to transition earlier, young trans women usually start their transition from male to female in their late teens or early twenties, whereas other trans women would start their transition when they were middle-aged or beyond.

The number of SOM neurons in the BSTc was not affected by hormone levels, suggesting that hormone therapy may not affect neuron numbers, especially in trans women. The findings from an elderly man with a strong untreated cross-gender identification whose BSTc neuron count lay in the female range indicated that hormone therapy has no effect on the BSTc neuron count. A 31-year-old man with a feminizing adrenal tumor still had a BSTc neuron count that was within the male range. Estrogen treatment, orchidectomy that involves testicle removal, antiandrogen treatment that minimizes the effect of testosterone, and hormonal changes in adulthood do not influence BSTc neuron numbers. Perhaps BSTc neuron numbers are determined by testosterone exposure during brain development, leading to sex dimorphic brain regions that determine one's gender identity. This inference is complicated by the observation that a greater concentration of α-estrogen receptors occurs in the BSTc for males than for females.[25]

Anatomical properties of the BSTc have been examined using postmortem evidence from 25 males and 25 females whose ages ranged from about 27 weeks after conception to 49 years. Data from these 50 brain samples showed that BSTc volume increased with age for both males and females, so that at its maximum the adult BSTc volume was 39 percent larger for males than females. BSTc volume was only larger for males from about puberty onward, suggesting that differences in sex hormone concentrations around puberty might be responsible for final BSTc size. This sex difference might depend on activity produced by the SRY gene located on the sex-determining region of the Y chromosome. This gene is expressed in the hypothalamus of adult males, but not in females. The later development of nerve connections from the amygdala might also produce sex differences in BSTc size in adults. These data indicated that the greater relative volume for males only occurs in late adolescence. Interestingly, this is a time when prior to the availability of puberty-blocking medications, many young trans people first seek help for their gender diversity. However, many trans people report feelings of gender difference much earlier than this when they are children, suggesting that other brain structures might be responsible for gender diversity. Although a developmental change in gender identity might be responsible for later changes in BSTc structure, further brain-sex differentiation and possibly hormonal effects persist well into adulthood.

These findings raise interesting questions about the proper role of BSTc, especially among those trans people who experience gender incongruence before puberty. Doubt exists regarding the significance of BSTc as a causal influence on gender identity, given the clear sex reversal effect that occurs on its anatomy around 16 years.[26]

Evidence from brain studies has shown that men have more androgen receptors in the brain than women, the highest receptor concentration occurring in the mamillary body complex, a region of the hypothalamus involved in sexual behavior and cognition. Androgens regulate aromatase activity, which is responsible for converting testosterone into estrogen, in several brain regions. So androgens indirectly affect estrogen concentrations in the brain. The clearest sex difference in androgen receptor concentrations occurs in the medial nucleus of the mamillary body, a brain region involved in sexual arousal. Here the density of such receptors is much greater in males than in females. The relatively weak androgen receptor density compared with estrogen receptor density, especially in the BST region of the hypothalamus, suggests that the process that converts a form of testosterone into estrogen more likely controls sexual behavior rather than gender identity. Therefore, any difference in BST size for trans people is probably not the result of androgen activity in this part of the brain, as has been claimed in the above-mentioned BSTc studies.

Nonreproductive organs in any physical sense, including the brain and especially the hypothalamus, are sensitive to the effects of sex hormones. The greater prevalence of estrogen receptors in blood vessel walls may explain why women are protected against cardiovascular disease when compared with men. On the other hand, women have a greater concentration of estrogen receptors in the ventromedial hypothalamic nucleus of the lower brain region than do men. Perhaps trans women also have a lower density of α-estrogen receptors in the ventral perimamillary part of the histaminergic tuberomammillary nucleus of the hypothalamus, a small brain region associated with arousal, sleep, and energy balance, than do birth-assigned men, another interesting brain difference.[27]

Difference in brain anatomy may not reflect differences in brain function, which can be better assessed using cognitive testing. Neuro-olfactory processing was measured when 12 preoperational trans women and an equal number of cisgender men and women were asked to smell two different steroids, a progesterone-like androsterone (AND) that is present in male secretion such as sweat, saliva, and semen, and the estrogen-like substance (EST) that is present in the urine of pregnant women. The trans women exhibited anterior hypothalamus responses to AND but not to EST. They differed from cisgender males in this respect. However, interpretation of the results of these studies is difficult due to problems associated with statistical evidence for detecting real differences in positron emission tomography (PET) image comparisons. It is also unclear whether the findings reflect differences in gender identity or sexual orientation.[28]

Brain responses to stimulation differ between trans women and others. The P300 event-related expectancy response detects brain signals obtained from electroencephalogram (EEG) recordings when a stimulus is presented. The signal is detected about three-tenths of a second after the stimulus onset when auditory stimuli are presented during a memory test. The P300 response is usually associated with expectancy and decision-making processes. Trans women who were tested after having undergone genital surgery were shown to have a reduced P300 amplitude in the left frontal and temporal-parietal regions of the brain and a P300 delay in the central frontal brain region when compared with the average scores of birth-assigned men and women.[29]

When trans and cisgender men and women were asked to discriminate between nonsense syllables such as *ged-ped* and *dod-dop* presented to either the left or right ear in an auditory discrimination task, cisgender males discriminated better between syllables presented to the right ear than those presented to the left ear. Cisgender females' recognition of the nonsense syllables was similar for both ears. Trans women resembled cisgender women rather than cisgender men, as they did not show the right-ear advantage typical of men.[30]

Table 2.1 shows brain regions, especially in the hypothalamus, that exhibit clear sex differences. Many of these differences may result from prenatal hormone influences. However, the available evidence is circumstantial because the consequences of some biological processes that are sex-related can only be revealed in adults. Such evidence provided by the similarity between brain structures for birth-assigned women and trans women in the BSTc region of the hypothalamus is interesting. Whether this result is moderated by age is difficult to evaluate as only postmortem samples have been analyzed. In the following sections we examine psychological influences on gender identity development. Eventually, we may be able to link psychological effects and behavior with their associated brain structures.

2.4 BRAIN IMAGING DISCOVERIES RELATED TO GENDER IDENTITY AND BODY DYSMORPHIA

Brain imaging using PET and MRI has shown that there are differences in some parts of the brain between trans people and cisgender people. Cisgender females have thicker cortex than cisgender males in the frontal and parietal regions of the brain whereas cisgender males have a larger right putamen, a lower central part of the brain that is responsible for movement regulation. For example, for those who have not started hormone therapy, trans women tend to have thicker cortex in the parietal and occipital lobes than cisgender men, a pattern that is more like the brains of cisgender women. Trans men have a cortical thickness similar to that of cisgender females and a larger cortical thickness than cisgender males in the parietal and temporal regions of the

Table 2.1 Documented Sex and Gender Identity Differences in Brain Structures

Brain Region	Sex Difference	Gender Identity Difference
Posterodorsal nucleus of medial amygdala	M > F	
Corpus callosum connectivity	F > M	
Corpus callosum volume	M > F	
Sexually dimorphic nucleus	M > F	
BSTc	M > F, age > 15	TF = F, TM = M ?
VIP subnucleus	M > F	
BNST-dspm	M > F	
Suprachiasmic nucleus	M > F	
Left insula of limbic system	M > F	
Left amygdala	F > M	
Androgen receptor immune response	M > F	
Cortical gray matter volume (location-dependent)	F > M	F < TF
Cortical white matter volume (location-dependent)	F > M	F < TF
Ventricle volume		F > TF
Broca's area and superior temporal cortex	F > M	
Hippocampus volume	F > M	
Caudate and thalamic nuclei	F > M	
Anterior cingulated gyrus	F > M	TF < F, TM < M
Posterior cingulate		TF < F, TM < M
Precuneus and cuneus		TF < F, TM < M
Dorsolateral prefrontal cortex	F > M	
Right inferior parietal lobe	F > M	
Limbic and paralimbic volume	M > F	
Hypothalamus	M > F	
Paracingulate gyrus	M > F	
Fronto-orbital cortex	F > M	
Somatostatin density (temporal and frontal)	M > F	
Brain fractional anisotropy (right hemisphere)		F < TF < M F < TM < M
Better recognition of words presented to right ear	M > F	M > TF = F

M = male, F = female, TF = trans female, TM = trans male.

Source: This table is an expanded and updated version of Table 2.1 in Heath, R.A. (2006). *The Praeger Handbook of Transsexuality*. Westport, CT: Praeger.

brain. Trans men also had a larger right putamen than cisgender females but did not differ in this part of the brain from cisgender males. Trans women did not differ in cortical thickness from cisgender females, but they had larger cortical thickness than cisgender males in the orbitofrontal, insular, and medial occipital regions of the brain. So, prior to hormone therapy, trans males showed evidence of subcortical gray matter masculinization, whereas there was feminization of brain cortical thickness in trans women. These differences between trans people and those of their same birth-assigned sex were only evident in the right hemisphere of the brain.[31]

After testosterone treatment, trans men showed increases in cortical thickness on both sides of the brain around the postcentral gyrus, an upper part of the brain responsible for interpreting touch sensations. There were increases in cortical thickness in several areas of the left hemisphere, as well as in the middle frontal and the occipital region of the right hemisphere, the part of the brain associated with vision. There was a positive relationship between changes in testosterone level and changes in cortical thickness in the mid-region and posterior regions of the brain. Trans women, on the other hand, showed a decrease in cortical thickness following estrogen and antiandrogen treatment. This decrease in cortical thickness for trans women was accompanied by an increase in the volume of the ventricles, the internal spaces in the lower regions of the brain.[32]

It may be that trans people's physical traits, such as those that relate to their birth-assigned sex and their affirmed gender, are represented differently in those parts of the brain that are responsible for a person's self-image. This part of the brain allows people to know that the body about which they are aware through their senses, the *body detection network*, corresponds to their own self-image, the *body referential* or *body ownership network*. Any discrepancy between their own body image as indicated by the body detection network and that represented by the body referential network in trans people might produce feelings of body image incongruence. Any distress produced by this body incongruence may lead to a trans person's desire to reconcile body self-image and body perception by requesting medical interventions such as hormone therapy and surgeries.

The parts of the brain responsible for self-image representation, the anterior cingulate, the middle prefrontal cortex, the posterior cingulate, precuneus, and the cuneus, tend to be smaller in trans people than in cisgender people as was confirmed in a recent study that compared brain structures in trans men with those observed for cisgender men and women. The authors proposed that trans people might experience a conflict between their perceived and desired body images accompanied perhaps by an associated emotional response that can only be resolved by transgender affirmation. Of special significance, there were no differences between the trans men and cisgender people in those parts of the brain associated with distress or depression. This makes one wonder whether gender dysphoria as a diagnosis has any relevance to brain function in trans people.[33] Clearly, any distress related to anxiety and mood is more likely a reflection of society's adverse response to the trans person's deviations from accepted gender norms rather than to any inherent psychopathology related to the trans person's own gender affirmation.

Intracranial volume is larger for men than women, but women have a thicker cortex than men in the frontal, parietal, and occipital lobes of the brain. In older people there is no sex difference in the volume of the amygdala and hippocampus, both of which decrease with age. In several regions of the right hemisphere, the cortical thickness of untreated trans women does not differ from that of birth-assigned women. However, it is larger than the cortical thickness of birth-assigned males. In some aspects of the brain's white matter, untreated trans women lie somewhere between birth-assigned men and women. Brain regions involved in cognitive and emotional behavior appear to be masculinized in trans men, whose brain fiber density is greater than that of birth-assigned females but less than that for birth-assigned males. These differences are mostly confined to the right hemisphere. Trans men and trans women also differ in the connections between different brain regions, these differences being also more evident in the right hemisphere than the left hemisphere. There is a hint from these results that transsexuality, as represented by those trans people who undergo medical transition, represents a kind of "brain intersex" condition due to a diversity of brain function in trans people when compared with people who identify with their birth-assigned sex.

The prominence of the right hemisphere changes in brain-imaging results suggests that differences between cisgender and trans people of both sexes might reflect the role of body perception and its emotional consequences. Early on, trans people would have had perceptions and emotions associated with their body self-perception as male or female that are mediated by the inferior parietal and premotor cortices. Any differences in how these parts of the brain function may reflect a disruption of the link between a person's perceived physical body and their psychological self. The discovery of a disconnect between the perceived body and the desired self, and the associated emotional response to this mismatch will force us to reevaluate the basis of the trans experience in terms of a brain-based condition, primarily located in the cortex, rather than exclusively being related to gender identity and any associated distress.

There was reduced cortical thickness in some brain regions for trans women and an increase in cortical thickness in other cortical regions for trans men. It could be that long-term estrogen therapy in trans women can induce a type of brain atrophy that is evident in those over 65 years old and is a side effect of the replacement of testosterone by estrogen.[34]

For an individual, we cannot be sure that a person's brain is distinctly male or female as it is more likely to contain a combination of male and female sex characteristics that are distributed throughout the brain. Sex hormones affect the organization of brain gray matter, the cell structure of the brain that does not contain the neural communication channels that appear white due to their insulating myelin covering. In particular, testosterone causes changes in gray matter in the amygdala and in the hippocampus, brain regions with specific locations, whereas estrogen has its major effect on gray matter that is distributed throughout the brain. There are similarities between trans women and cisgender women in gray matter volumes within the insular cortex of both hemispheres, a part of the brain believed to be involved in emotion and body homeostasis.[35]

It is possible that for trans people the birth-assigned gender traits are differently integrated into the person's representation of self in the brain, as was suggested above for trans women. Some of the structures responsible for this conflict may be sexually dimorphic so that trans men and trans women may differ in how their self-concept is represented in the brain. These are the parts of the brain that activate differently depending on whether a person is viewing their own body or a simulated version of it. Damage to these areas of the brain often result in out-of-body experiences, such as a feeling of floating outside one's body. To properly perceive your body as your own requires activation of a part of the brain known as the pregenual anterior cingulate cortex, an arc of brain tissue around the lower central region of the brain. Links with the emotional centers of the brain, such as the amygdala, may be responsible for the felt disconnect with body features, leading to many trans people's need to medically transition.[36]

2.5 PSYCHOLOGICAL ASPECTS OF GENDER IDENTITY FORMATION

As indicated already in this chapter, the difference between sex and gender is difficult to define, especially when we consider the functions of various brain regions. Mostly, *sex* is limited to biological differences between males and females, such as the sex chromosomes, gonads, genitals, hormonal balance, and differences in brain structures. *Gender*, on the other hand, commonly refers to our feeling masculine or feminine or some other feeling unrelated to these binary gender categories, depending on our own identity and society's expectations of our behavior.

Chromosomal sex usually involves XY chromosomes for the male sex and XX chromosomes for the female sex. However, the situation is not that simple. Variations of the more common sex chromosome combinations result in a difference in sexual development. For example, some XX individuals have a male genotype, or behavioral expression, and similarly a few XY people have a female genotype, due to unusual arrangements of sex-determining genes.

As we have seen, gonadal sex involves organs producing germ cells, ovaries producing eggs, and testicles producing sperm. Hormonal sex represents the different combinations of hormones that characterize the two sexes. Generally, men have mostly testosterone and women estrogen. However, for good reproductive and homeostatic reasons, both sexes have a little of the other sex's hormone. For example, testosterone in females is important for libido. Although brain-sex, defined as sex differences that occur in the brain, is important for all aspects of human behavior, it is little recognized as a major contributor to our sexual behavior and gender identity.

Gender, the psychological and social correlate of our sexual existence, includes the concepts of gender identity and gender role. *Gender identity* refers to a person's feeling of being either a man or a woman, or some combination of both, or perhaps no gender feeling at all. *Gender role* refers to characteristic gendered behavior sanctioned by society, such as the antiquated idea that women should be responsible for child-rearing and other domestic duties while men should work to support their family.

Gender identity can be defined as "the structured set of gendered personal identities that results when the individual takes the social construction of gender and the biological 'facts' of sex and incorporates them into an overall self-concept."[37] Gender identity also refers to a person's awareness of, and feelings about, their own gender category, whether that be man, woman, some combination of the two, or neither.

Forming a gender identity is different from being male or female based on a person's birth-assigned sex. Like the development of our self-identity, gender identification takes time. It is influenced by our physiological and sexual endowments as well as by what we learn from parents and significant others. Gender identity may correspond with birth-assigned sex. Assigned females are expected to develop a feminine gender identity whereas males will develop a masculine gender identity. However, diversity is common in nature and for some people there is a discrepancy between assigned sex and the development of their gender identity, leading to a need for reconciliation.

During the gender identity phase of development, all children learn to label themselves according to their own self-affirmed, often binary, gender. Next, the child learns about gender stability, that is, once you are a boy or a girl, you will grow up to be a man or a woman, respectively. In the gender constancy stage, the child realizes that gender does not change too much and cannot be affected by cultural and personal whims, such as temporary changes in hairstyles and clothing.[38]

A child's first acceptance of a consistent gender descriptor, such as *I am a boy no matter how I present myself*, requires the attainment of concrete operational thought, a cognitive process that usually occurs when the child is between four and six years old. Children are said to have attained concrete operational thought when they understand that a quantity of fluid remains the same irrespective of the dimensions of containers into which it is poured. So, a simultaneous process of cognitive and gender identity development occurs. After children have discovered their own gender identity and realize that this identity does not change over time, they reach a stage of *gender stability*. Finally, the child recognizes that gender identity is unaffected by changes in circumstances such as wearing gender-inappropriate clothing, leading to the experience of *gender consistency*.[39] Attainment of gender consistency depends on mental age, or general intelligence, rather than chronological age, confirming a nexus between gender identity development and cognitive development. In other words, constancy reflects a type of thinking that is mature enough to know that things do not change when the context is shifted, as is the case when a child's gender feelings do not change from one moment to the next even when their circumstances might.

A child acquires a gender identity by actively engaging with environmental cues arising from interaction with their parents and other people around them. Children can also create their own gender-consistent environment by selecting appropriate same-sex playmates and sharing experiences during play activities. In this way, the child becomes aware of the gender stereotypes that often guide their future behavior.

Acquiring a consistent gender identity requires the eventual attainment of gender constancy via developmental stages starting in infancy. By six months, babies can discriminate male voices from female voices, indicating their rudimentary categorization ability as well as their better hearing than vision. The baby can distinguish male and female faces by nine months when they are more sensitive to visual cues. Interestingly, gender categorization occurs before the learning of language. Finally, by the time they are one year old, toddlers can associate male or female faces with corresponding male or female voices, thus expanding further their concept of gender.

A two-year-old child usually displays gender-consistent toy preferences as well as an ability to recognize their own gender from photographs, an ability that first appears when the child is about eighteen months old.[40] Accurate verbal labeling of males and females occurs when the child is between two and two and a half years old. When they are two, children prefer socializing with other children of their own gender. Spontaneous gender-based toy choice, girls playing with dolls and boys playing with cars, for example, also occurs around this time. Sixty-seven percent of 27-month-old children can correctly identify their own sex. Fifty-six percent successfully completed a gender-labeling task with girls outperforming boys, and 23 percent labeled toys correctly in terms of gender stereotype, such as dolls for girls and trucks for boys. However, only 13 percent of these children could correctly categorize gender-identified activities, such as boys playing rough-and-tumble sports and girls wearing pretty dresses. When children could choose their preferred toys, girls spent more time playing with dolls than did boys.[41] Furthermore, three-year-old children can sort photographs into their appropriate gender categories without assistance.

Developing a stable gender identity depends on acquiring an understanding of one's own gender identity. By the time they are three, most children begin understanding society's gender stereotypes such as using words like *big*, *fast*, and *strong* to describe boys and *small*, *scared*, and *slow* to describe girls. A child's initially rigid conception of gender becomes more flexible as they get older.[42]

The expression of gender-specific behavior depends on socioeconomic status, upper-class children exhibiting behavior that is more flexible. Working-class children, on the other hand, are more likely to behave traditionally in terms of expressiveness for girls and goal achievement for boys.

When children can correctly tell whether someone is a boy or a girl, they spend much more time playing in same-sex groups. This preference for same-sex play increases with age and becomes firmly established during the first few years at school. Such in-group affiliation reinforces both their own gender identity and the expected behavior of children in same-sex groups.

Girls can become more cooperative in the presence of others once they can label another child's gender properly. Although groups of boys tend to play in larger groups and have more physical contact than do groups of girls, girls are generally less domineering than boys and more readily form within-group friendships. Boys tend to dominate their own-group conversations, whereas girls form good relations with their peers by communicating equitably. Whereas boys maintain a circle of friends, girls tend to have a single best friend to whom they show considerable support and devotion.[43]

The Pre-School Activities Inventory assesses gender role development, gender-role preference, and acquiescence in preschool children. The average gender-role score for boys is higher than that for girls. The difference between boys' and girls' scores almost doubles between the ages of two and a half and five years, indicating a progressive increase in gender-role discrimination ability during this period.[44]

Gender-role attitudes have been measured for children between four and six years old, a period of gender development that progresses from a generally well-established own-gender identity to acquiring gender constancy. When a girl's gender-role attitudes are assessed using structured doll-play and storytelling, they select a doll that is the same gender as the subject of a story. Male gender-typing is evident in boys by the time they are four, this ability improving with age. However, four-year-old girls take longer to achieve the same degree of male gender-role knowledge as boys. Between four and six years, children attend more to members of their own birth-assigned sex, but this preference declines with age.[45] Six-year-old children play with children of their own birth-assigned sex more often than they do with children of the opposite sex.

Attaining a stable gender identity relies on forming gender schemas defined as "dynamic knowledge representations that show age-related development as a function of interactions between the individual and his or her environment as well as changes in response to situational variations."[46] A *gender schema* refers to one's own gender identity, the role expected of someone of that gender, and how gender determines appropriate behavior, both individually and in response to social influences. When children rely primarily on same-sex interactions, their gender schemas are less flexible than when children are also free to explore cross-sex relationships.

The key factor in gender schema development is physical appearance. Young children readily categorize tall, short-haired people as males and short, long-haired people as females, irrespective of other discriminating characteristics. Once gender identification has occurred, children consider a newly learned fact about one of their girlfriends as pertaining to all girls, a typical stereotypical response. For example, once a child discovers that a girl has *estro*, a fictitious reference to estrogen, in her blood, she will think that all girls have this quality, possibly including herself. Children also pay greater attention to, and have better memories for, gender-appropriate tasks than gender-inappropriate ones.

The formation of gender schemas has been studied in 11-year-old children as well as in adults. The most gender-typical scenarios reported by children are their interests in childcare that is typically female, mechanical tasks that are typically male, and cooking that is typically female, boys showing more gender-stereotypical behavior than girls. For adults, a scenario involving male and female executives can elicit gender stereotypes. The proportion of imagined female leaders is higher for those who saw a videotape showing women in management than it is for participants who did not view the video.[47] Stereotypes can be modified, indicating that environmental influences affect both gender roles and the formation of gender schemas. Parents' and their children's gender schemas are similar, the parent-child similarity being greater for mothers than for fathers. Gender stereotypes are less prevalent in single-parent families and in those families in which both parents work,[48]

Kristina Olson, who is conducting a national Trans Youth Project from the University of Washington in the United States, has shown that quite young gender-affirming children can recognize themselves in their affirmed gender when asked to categorize photographs of people as *me* and *them*. When asked about their futures, these children are even more affirmative about their gender constancy. These young people have little doubt that their affirmed gender will ever revert to their birth-assigned sex, such is the solidity of their gender identity. It is so important that these young transgender children be allowed to make a social transition in a supportive home environment.[49]

SUMMARY

Several brain regions, particularly the hypothalamus, provide evidence for reliable sex differences in brain structures that appear to be related to gender identity. The discovery of a small region of the hypothalamus that may be related to gender diversity was quite an achievement, even though more research is needed to assess any causal relationship. More recent research has considered MRI imaging data from many brain regions, including such variables as cortical thickness and the extent of gray matter. There have been tentative findings suggesting differences between trans and cisgender people, especially in brain activity occurring in the right hemisphere.

There is emerging brain imaging evidence suggesting that those trans people who seek medical interventions may do so not because of any distress with their own affirmed gender identity but because of a mismatch between those parts of the brain that encode their self-image and other brain regions that provide perceptual information about their body. If this proposition is confirmed by further brain imaging data, a better understanding of why some trans people need to transition using hormones and surgery will occur, one that is not necessarily based on gender distress or an incongruity between birth-assigned sex and affirmed gender.

After explaining the differences between what we mean by sex and gender, we examined developmental aspects of acquiring a stable gender identity. Gender recognition occurs in infants as young as six months, well before the acquisition of language and before the process of forming a gender identity that starts when the child is about two years old. Gender identity development progresses in parallel with cognitive development through several stages of increasing abstraction until gender constancy is reached when the child is about six years old. At this stage, the child's gender identity is unaffected by peripheral changes such as clothing and choice of toys. Further development of gender identity occurs when the child understands gender schema that incorporate not only the child's own identity but also their understanding of gender-role behavior in response to environmental demands. This information is especially important for our understanding of gender-affirming processes that occur in young people who transition socially at elementary school or a little later.

Chapter 3

GENDER DIVERSITY

This chapter discusses the differences between people with various gender identities, including gender differences in cognition and personality as well as in social and emotional behavior. Once we have understood these gender differences, we discuss gender diversity in some detail.

But first, some definitions: *Transgender* describes "the community of all self-identified cross gender people whether intersex, transsexual men and women, crossdressers, drag kings and drag queens, transgenderists, androgynous, bi-gendered, third gendered or as yet unnamed gender gifted people."[1] Such gender diversity has been classified in terms of four types: migrating, oscillating, negating, and transcending.[2] *Migrating* involves moving from one extremity of the male–female gender divide to the other on a permanent basis. *Oscillating* involves moving back and forth between male and female polarities as illustrated by the part-time crossdresser and anyone with a fluid gender identity. *Negating* indicates processes that eliminate binary gender categories, a stance adopted by *gender warriors* and those who are nonbinary or who have no gender. Finally, *transcending* presupposes going beyond binary gender categories toward a new experience involving an indeterminate number of gender possibilities. One way to visualize this process is to locate gender at any point within a sphere rather than at either end of a line representing female at one end and male at the other. This book's cover represents gender diversity as interlocking multicolored circles. Surely gender contains a rich tapestry of possibilities and every one of these is to be valued.

In the early stages of their transition, some trans people fashion a new sense of self by socializing with members of support groups and others in the trans community. This helps a trans person's adjustment by allowing them to tell their own unique story and listen to others' stories. For example, in one such group a trans person claimed to have a "girl-brain in a boy-body." Others reported feeling different for as long as they could remember. A common narrative in birth-assigned boys is crossdressing in a female role, or thinking about crossdressing, when they were a child. This process symbolizes the *true self* before it can be influenced by authority figures such as parents and teachers. Perhaps a trans woman recalls an ineptness at sports from an early age, whereas trans men were generally admired for their athletic prowess as well as tomboyish behavior such as climbing trees.[3] In the sections that follow we discuss differences in the thoughts, personalities, and behavior of trans people.

3.1 PERCEPTUAL AND COGNITIVE DIFFERENCES

Rather than observing their respective genitals, the Old Testament's King Solomon determined the sex of two twins using gender-discriminating behavioral measures, such as how they would catch an apple and how they would throw the apple back. Catching and throwing differs between men and women as any comparison of male and female softball players will reveal.[4] This example illustrates how reliable the behavioral expression of gender can be. As we have pointed out in Chapter 2, the only substantial differences in gendered behavior were found in childhood play and aggressiveness, these being examples of differences in gender role rather than in gender identity. However, there are other interesting smaller differences in perception and cognition that add to our understanding of gender diversity.

Gender differences in cognition may not depend on fixed attributes that are present at birth, but may depend on hormone influences that occur throughout the lifespan. It has been commonly reported that men are better than women on mathematical reasoning tasks, in solving mental rotation tasks, in the perception of the horizontal, and in targeting accuracy, whereas women perform better on verbal memory tasks and tasks requiring finger dexterity, as well as having larger color vocabularies. Women also generally obtain higher scores than men on tests of object location memory. In this task, people are shown randomly located objects and are required to recall which objects have been moved.[5]

Gender differences in cognitive performance depend on hormonal influences. For example, the level of testosterone required for men's best performance in spatial tasks, such as determining whether two objects are the same when they are rotated, is a value in the low male range. Women's performance on spatial and verbal fluency tasks depends on the phase of their menstrual cycle. During the postovulation stage, when estrogen levels are lower, women's performance tends to improve on spatial tasks but is worse than usual when they are asked to perform verbal fluency tasks, such as reciting all the words that rhyme with *gender*. Men perform better on spatial tasks in the spring when their testosterone level is low and worse early in the morning when their testosterone levels are high.

On the other hand, only small gender differences occur for verbal ability, mathematical ability, visual-spatial ability, and aggression when these abilities are measured by standard psychological tests. Although gender differences in mathematical ability appear from adolescence onward, only 1 percent of test score differences in mathematics can be attributed to gender. Men and boys with high mathematical ability perform better than women and girls on difficult algebra problems, but both groups perform similarly on easier mathematical problems.[6] A gender stereotype might be operating here because some women might be led to believe that they cannot be as good as men at mathematics, resulting in a lower test score.

Only about 5 percent of the individual differences in spatial ability are gender dependent. Better performance by men is limited to tasks such as mental rotation and horizontal–vertical discrimination. Gender differences in cognitive abilities have decreased over time, suggesting that environment and learning play important roles in moderating these differences. Women score higher than men in work motivation, but men score higher in both job mastery and competitiveness.[7]

Before starting hormone therapy young trans men perform better than cisgender females in mental rotation and visualization tasks, but more generally there is no difference between trans people and others, suggesting that cognitive ability is unrelated to gender identity.[8] A study of trans men before and three months after they started testosterone therapy showed an increase in their spatial ability, as indicated by performance on the rotated figures test. This was accompanied by a decrease in verbal scores, as measured by word and sentence production tests.[9] Trans women's performance decreased on spatial ability tasks after hormone initiation, whereas that of trans men improved over a one-year period. So, hormone therapy has a limited effect on performance in spatial and verbal tasks with some small differences between trans men and trans women occurring.[10]

Girls use a greater variety of colors than boys when drawing. Girls prefer warmer colors such as pink and red. Boys concentrate their attention on object movement and location, whereas girls concentrate on form and color. Female vision is biased toward using the parvocellular visual system that is specialized for identifying objects (*what is it?*), whereas male vision makes greater use of the magnocellular visual system that is specialized for locating objects (*where is it?*). Women are also generally better at recognizing faces than are men.[11]

Human attractiveness is thought to be associated with a biologically determined preference for healthy and fertile mates. People rate appearance by grading samples of arbitrarily selected faces as the most attractive. Women rate men with slightly feminized faces as more caring, cooperative, and honest. They also consider such men as potentially better parents. On the other hand, women prefer more masculinized faces during the fertile period of their menstrual cycle. Large eyes and small noses are more attractive in women, as also are larger lips and more fatty deposits in the upper cheek area. Generally, men judge a smaller lower facial region in women as more attractive.[12]

People determine a person's gender using face shape, mouth size, cheek position, and eye size. Judgments of male faces rely on eye spacing, nose size, and eyebrow shape, whereas judgment of female faces use nose size and a combination of eye spacing and eyebrow shape. When distinguishing between male and female faces, all features except the nose are useful, with greater emphasis being given to the eyes and chin. However, the situation is not that simple as removing the eye region makes it difficult to detect female faces, whereas removing the nose makes it hard to recognize male faces. So different facial features are used to determine gender in males and females.

Male faces are wider and longer than female faces. Important correlates of gender are eyebrow thickness, nose width, mouth width, eye-to-eyebrow distance, forehead height, and the distance between the inner corners of the eyebrows. Measures of 24 facial features can be reduced to five basic facial dimensions that distinguish between male and female faces. These dimensions are the distance between the outermost corners of the eyes (E3); the distance between the two cheekbones (W4); the width of the nose (N2); the distance between the eyes and eyebrows (B2), which is larger in women; and the distance between the eyes and mouth (L1). When these five dimensions are substituted into the following Facial Masculinity Index equation, male faces are correctly classified 87 percent of the time, and female faces 92 percent of the time.

$$\text{Facial Masculinity Index} = -0.9E3 + 0.2W4 + 0.5N2 - 0.4B2 + 0.2L1$$

A positive Facial Masculinity Index indicates a masculine face, whereas a negative value indicates a feminine face. Femininity is indicated by a larger distance between external eye corners and between the eyes and eyebrows, as well as by a small nose and a narrow, rounded face. Masculinity is characterized by a large nostril-to-nostril width, wide cheekbones, a long face, a small distance between the eyes, and a short distance between eyes and eyebrows. Most gender-discriminating distances in the human face involve horizontal and vertical directions rather than diagonals.[13]

The Facial Masculinity Index might be used to determine whether trans women who wish to be recognized as female should consider facial feminization surgery.[14] Too masculine a face might be problematical for those trans women who wish to pass in their affirmed gender. The effect of facial feminization surgery should be to transform the Facial Masculinity Index from a positive value to one in the female range. More information about facial feminization surgery for trans women is contained in Chapter 9.

Gender differences in speech processing may depend on differences in brain hemisphere asymmetry. For example, the left side of the brain is responsible for gender differences in speech recognition ability. Since brain lateralization, the tendency for one hemisphere of the brain to process information differently from the other, is greater in men than in women, the extent to which one brain hemisphere processes speech more effectively than the other would be greater for men than for women.[15]

Prenatal exposure to high levels of testosterone causes a slowing in the development of the left hemisphere of the brain and augmented development of the right hemisphere. This results in a greater prevalence of left-handedness in males, as well as conditions such as stuttering and dyslexia.[16] So, there is a close relationship between hormonal influences on brain development and cognitive performance in later life.

Gender differences in how people use language have biological as well as developmental and social causes. There is a sufficient difference in their average voice pitch range for men and women to be distinguished on that basis alone, even though the voice pitch ranges for men and women overlap to some extent. Gender differences in intonation pattern are a far more important cue for gender identification than are most other linguistic forms. Such speech differences complement other cross-culturally universal gender identifiers such as hairstyle and dress, body posture, facial expression, and gesture patterns, especially those involving hand and finger movements. Voice training for trans women is described in greater detail in Chapter 9.

Some commonly used linguistic conventions differentiate male and female speech. Women tend to use words that men rarely use, for example, ancillary adjectives such as *divine*, *cute*, and *sweet*, as well as tag questions at the end of statements, such as "We're staying, *aren't we?*" Women tend to be polite in their choice of words, and invoke more uncertainty in their speech by using phrases such as *I guess*, *I hope*, and so forth. Women are more likely than men to use intensifiers, such as *so*, *very*, and *really*, as well as the correct grammar when they speak. Women's speech is characterized by a rising intonation at the end of phrases. Some of these linguistic features suggest that women are more interested in maintaining good social relationships than are men. It is also noteworthy that men tend to interrupt women's speech more often than women interrupt men in mixed-sex groups.[17]

An important distinguishing feature of text written by female authors, when compared with that of male authors, is their more frequent use of pronouns.

Female authors tend to involve their reader more in their writing, whereas male authors use the text primarily for presenting facts. The pronouns *I*, *she*, and *you* are used more often by women than men, whereas men tend to use words such as *a*, *the*, and *that* more frequently. Fiction is normally written in a feminine style, whereas nonfiction is more likely to be expressed with a masculine writing style, irrespective of the author's gender.[18]

In electronic communication, just as in speech, women are more likely than men to use emotional references, to use intensive adverbs such as *really* in "the game was *really* good," to make compliments, and to use minimal responses such as *mmmm*. Women are also more likely to ask questions and employ polite language. In same-sex email messages, women express more emotions, personal information, hedges such as *it was sort of OK*, and adverbs that indicate intense feelings than do men. Recently, there has been a tendency for women to use social media more than men when they wish to maintain an online friendship network. The use of computers has become more gender-neutral as more women undertake computer training and have their own computers and handheld devices.[19]

Most female and almost all male Internet users can be identified by how they phrase email messages.[20] Such fundamental differences in how men and women use language in conversation make it difficult for trans people to adopt the speech patterns of their affirmed gender later in life if they wish to do so, even after they have mastered changes in average pitch and frequency modulation.

3.2 EMOTION AND PERSONALITY DIFFERENCES

Gender accounts for about 5 percent of the individual differences in provoked aggression. About 1 percent of the individual differences in conformity can be accounted for by gender, women being more easily influenced than men. Although women are generally better than men in their use of nonverbal cues, such as changes in their facial expression, this gender difference is small.

Hormone levels generate differences between men and women in their emotional responses to environmental events. Estrogen depletion in women often produces depression and anxiety that can be alleviated by hormone replacement therapy. Following menopause, there is a greater prevalence of serious anxiety and depressive disorders in women. Such gender differences in emotional response may result from sex differences in the brain's neurotransmitter systems that control the flow of nerve messages.[21]

Instrumental behavior, as indicated by competitiveness and aggression, is usually associated with masculinity, whereas expressive behavior, such as gentleness and nurturance, is more often associated with femininity. A positively androgynous person, that is, someone who scores highly on both femininity and masculinity, tends to display independence, compassion, ambition, and tolerance. On the other hand, a negatively androgynous person, that is, someone who has low scores on both masculinity and femininity, tends to be less independent and more self-involved in whatever activity they are doing. Positively androgynous people exhibit better mental health and adjustment than those with either positive masculinity or positive femininity.[22]

Gender differences can be measured using personality test scores, with women generally scoring higher on neuroticism and agreeableness than men, and lower than men on self-esteem. In other tests of personality, women score higher than men on warmth, gregariousness, and positive emotions but lower on assertiveness and excitement-seeking. Gender differences in personality are greater in healthy and prosperous cultures in which women enjoy a greater level of education and a variety of career opportunities. However, these personality differences are not especially large. More substantial differences occur within populations of men and women rather than between them due to the large overlap of scores whenever we compare individual men and women on any of these personal attributes.[23] Trans people have been found to show some differences in vocational interests from those typically chosen by people of their birth-assigned sex, such as wanting to become a nurse or an engineer. There appears to be some genetic link that influences these differences in career interests.[24]

The three most characteristic aspects of femininity reported by young people are being critical of one's own appearance, being concerned with outward appearance, and emotionality, whereas the two most characteristic aspects of masculinity are being career-oriented and independent. Masculinity is less diversified, less unstable, and less subject to change than is femininity. *Sex seen as power/empowering* is a masculine rather than feminine trait, whereas *reading for pleasure* is a typically feminine pursuit. Being family-oriented is especially feminine, whereas being career-oriented is a masculine trait. Perhaps gender unites men but divides women due to the larger diversity of feminine personality attributes. These characteristics are changing over time. In a study spanning a five-year period, women were less dependent on a partner for maintaining social status than was the case in previous generations.[25]

Crying is a uniquely human characteristic that has its origins early in life when it is a baby's only way to signal distress. Gender differences in emotionality are revealed when women cry more easily and for longer periods than do men. A lot of crying occurs when people are alone, and when they lack social and emotional support. There are two types of crying: an emotional outpouring that is intense, long-lasting, and persistent, and a more short-lasting type that is easily controlled, as sometimes occurs when we are watching a sad movie. Crying results from a complex interaction between biological, social, and cognitive processes. From the biological viewpoint, crying is associated with both parasympathetic and sympathetic arousal. The sympathetic nervous system prepares us for action, whereas the parasympathetic nervous system prepares us for feeding and rest. How readily a person cries seems to be more biologically based, whereas crying frequency is mainly determined by environmental needs.[26]

3.3 DEVELOPMENTAL ASPECTS OF GENDER DIVERSITY

In this section, we consider the development of gender-expansive and gender-incongruent behavior in boys and girls. Gender-expansive behavior occurs when the child's gender expression and behavior do not correspond to that most frequently observed in children of their same birth-assigned sex. There is an exploration of expressive behavior that is more typical of a person who identifies with a different birth-assigned sex. In other words, boys may experiment with behavior that is more typical of girls and vice versa. However, none of these behaviors need indicate that the child will adopt a more permanent identification with a gender that is different from their birth-assigned sex. If this is the case, the child may be exhibiting behavior that might be classified as gender-expansive. In what follows we do not necessarily claim that cross-gendered behavior differences are likely to be permanent. Each individual child and in many cases their parents will know when that is the case.

For example, the most common cross-gendered behavior exhibited by girls, such as dressing in boys' clothes, playing boys' games, and playing with boys' toys, increases in frequency from when the girl is between two to three years of age to when they are four or five. Thereafter, cross-gendered behavior declines, only to increase again when the child is six or seven. The decline in cross-gendered behavior when the child is about five years old may result from peer pressure when the child starts school.[27]

Gender-conforming behavior requires children to develop and understand social norms for acceptable behavior as exhibited by parents and significant others. Related aspects of gender constancy include gender-stereotypical norms imposed by the wider society for appearance and conduct, as well as stereotype flexibility so that any violation of social expectations does not affect the person's core gender identity. For example, even though boys play football, it is acceptable for girls to play football too. This behavior by girls does not mean that they have suddenly changed gender role unless there is a consistent preference for behaving more typically like boys. So normal fluctuations in behavior do not imply that gender constancy has been violated, yet some of these children's behavior may be gender-expansive, as previously defined. Once gender constancy has been attained, we can assume that a child's affirmed gender might also remain the same, particularly once they have reached early adolescence.

Gender incongruence occurs when the child does not identify with their birth-assigned sex. In the past, parents of children with this normal variation in gender identity have not usually sought specialist assistance until the child is about seven years old. However, these days help is being sought for even younger children. Birth-assigned boys with gender incongruence may internalize their feelings more and exhibit less social competence than other boys. However, it is difficult for parents to distinguish between gender incongruence and gender expansiveness, a child's desire to explore gender roles and experiences that are not consistent with their birth-assigned sex, until the young person can communicate their own developed sense of gender identity.

Masculine behavior in girls is more common than feminine behavior in boys, simply because many societies believe it is more acceptable. Categories used to classify early cross-gendered behavior include rough-and-tumble play; toy and activity preference; imagined roles; crossdressing; preference for male or female friends; social reputation as a sissy, tomboy, or loner; as well as the child's gender identity. Parents have reported that feminine seven-year-old boys can be distinguished from their nonfeminine peers by being more likely to wear girl's clothing, to wish to be a girl, to play with dolls, and to be interested in women's clothing. These children are less likely to partake in rough-and-tumble play and to want to grow up to be like their father. However, except for the feminine boys being more attractive, there are no socially important family influences, such as father absence, that differ between gender-incongruent and other boys.[28]

Psychological problems attributed to gender incongruence, especially in children and adolescents, may result from stigmatization due to differences in their developmental progression through the stages of gender identity formation. Confusion sometimes occurs when the assumption is made that gender-expansive boys exhibit the early manifestations of a possibly androphilic sexual orientation. Although such an outcome can occur, it cannot explain the high level of distress experienced by gender-incongruent children, especially when they endure discrimination and bullying at home and at school.

Family issues are important as a child's cross-gendered behavior, for example an aversion to gender-typical activities such as rough-and-tumble play in boys, is often associated with emotional distance from the same-sex parent. This lack of interest in typically masculine activities might produce a self-concept characterized by inadequate masculinity, a feeling reinforced by peers and significant others. Some parents have stated their commitment to maintaining the well-being of their gender-diverse children and their need to advocate for other children and their supporters. Experiences provided by parents who see at firsthand the abuse and bullying suffered by their children are worthwhile reporting for the benefit of all those good people who care about the welfare of all trans people, irrespective of their age.[29]

SUMMARY

Gender diversity occurs in many aspects of human life. These include cognitive processes, such as spatial and verbal memory, vision, learning, and facial recognition. There are also differences between men and women in personality, language, and emotionality. Some of these differences, for example, in memory, learning, and perhaps personality, reflect differences in brain function. Other differences, such as in language and social behavior, require adherence to gender norms imposed by cultural and social influences, as well as the emotions in the case of crying. When a young person's gender identity development and expression is different from their birth-assigned sex, the young person's parents and caregivers may seek professional help to assist the young person's gender affirmation. Knowledge of such gender differences help trans people as they negotiate their transition. Especially for those who wish to pass, living in their new gender role and changing their behavior so that it is consistent with their affirmed gender is a difficult task for many trans people. Supporting a gender-diverse person as they explore, develop, communicate, and express their gender identity is vital to their future well-being.

Chapter 4

GENDER AFFIRMATION

This chapter considers the gender-affirmation process as revealed by the experiences of trans people in transition from their birth-assigned sex to their affirmed gender. First, we discuss some of the challenges and advantages associated with transition using examples from the increasing number of research reports available. Then we discuss both gender identity and sexual orientation. Relationships between sexual orientation and gender identity, as well as individual differences in sexual orientation and sexual health for gender-diverse people are mentioned. However, most of the material in the following discussion relates to the gender-affirmation process in gender-diverse people, a situation that we hope will be much clearer after we have discussed these distinctions. Rather than emphasize biological aspects of gender identity, we concentrate on important aspects of the gender-affirmation process from the trans person's perspective. Much of the health and medical aspects of transition are covered in Chapters 6, 7, and 8.

4.1 THE TRANSITION PROCESS

When a gender-diverse person is finally ready to present themselves to the world in their affirmed gender, some interesting challenges can occur. First, the person must decide whether the transition is worth the personal social risks, such as being discriminated against by family and friends, feeling obliged to conform to what is expected of members of their affirmed gender, and simply maintaining a lifestyle that is similar to what they already have in terms of established friendships, employment, and social standing. Sometimes people have a moment of enlightenment, as illustrated by the following comment from one study participant:

> The lightbulb went [*sic*] off and I went "wait a minute. This isn't really about clothes; it's about who I am." And lots of pieces just fell into place for me. I had realized I was miserable with life in general and I couldn't quite pinpoint why, but I knew I didn't feel right about who I was.[1]

Next, the gender-diverse person needs to consider what it is going to be like being a part-time or full-time member of their affirmed gender. If they choose a part-time lifestyle, how will they manage the changeover, say, from working as their birth-affirmed gender during the week to enjoying life as their true selves at other times? How will they feel when they are obliged to explain their situation to family, friends, and significant others? Will they be able to meet other people and form relationships, or will they need to be somewhat closeted to avoid the possible stigma, its associated bullying, or worse?

Young people will need to decide how they are going to present themselves to the world in their affirmed gender, as a male, a female, or as a nonbinary person. Some young people prefer a more fluid or androgynous presentation that more accurately represents their fluctuating gender feelings from one day to the next. Others refuse to commit to any gender identity at all and live their lives without consciously accommodating themselves to society's gender norms.

If their puberty has been forestalled by medical intervention, many young trans people can easily enjoy life without anyone knowing about their birth-assigned background.[2] However, they can experience difficulties when they wish to be accepted by family, friends, and at school. According to a survey conducted in Australia, trans people felt accepted when they were welcome in public places, were a valued member of society, and when they were allowed to present in public as their affirmed gender, having no restrictions placed upon them and not being avoided by others. People who accept a young trans person are pleased to work with them, can accept them as their neighbor, and are happy to be their friend. To be most helpful to trans people, mental health professionals should learn more about the trans experience and be fully qualified to practice transgender medicine. These professionals should never diagnose a client with a mental illness just because they are trans, unless it is a serious comorbid condition that is unrelated to their gender expression. They should also accept their client's affirmation as trans and always use the correct pronoun when addressing the trans person.[3]

Accompanying this Australian survey were participants' comments, examples being:

> The school counsellor was very judgmental, critical and prejudiced. He told my son that he wasn't trans but just afraid of puberty. When I went to speak with the

counsellor he made it out like I was to blame for my son's questioning. (Mother of 16-year-old trans son)

At first we thought the school counsellor was an asset, but we then learnt that they had suggested to the Principal that our child was just trying to get attention, and that what was needed was behavior management, not affirmation of gender. (Mother of 16-year-old trans daughter)[4]

But on a more positive note:

Initially the stand-out positive was just to be heard without feeling judged, specifi-cally by the school counsellor. Then our focus was on information and guidance, and the school counsellor was able to provide that to us in terms of reading materials and referrals to specialists. (Mother of 12-year-old trans daughter)[5]

A study of opinions from 29 counselors suggested that the basic needs of gender-diverse young people are that they be accepted and supported, that they be heard, respected and loved, and have professional support. They should also be allowed to express their gender, to feel safe and protected, to be allowed to live a normal life, to have peer and school support, to have access to gender-neutral facilities, and to have access to appropriate hormone therapy. The young people's parents require better information about their child's situation, as well as support from family, friends, and school and health professionals to protect their child's health and safety.[6]

Teachers and school counselors may seek answers to questions about young trans people such as: How common is gender diversity? Aren't these kids too young to know what their genders are? Are they just seeking attention and is this real? Do kids take hormones? Is it a phase and will they grow out of it? How can you tell that these kids are not going to be gay? What causes this? Can I ask whether a trans person has completed their transition and has had surgery? Is this really a mental disorder? Should I push the child one way or another if they are not sure? If there's a dress code, can a trans female student wear a bra? What about using the school and public bathrooms? Will my job be threatened if I support trans students? What about the other children? How can I get other people to use different names or pronouns if they are not legal?[7] Although the answers to these questions will depend on the context and social situation for each trans person, some possible answers are discussed in this chapter and in the rest of the book.

4.2 GENDER IDENTITY, SEXUAL IDENTITY, AND SEXUAL ORIENTATION

The distinction between gender identity and sexual orientation is important because these terms are often confused, possibly leading to some misunder-standing. Most people assume that men prefer women as their sexual partner, and women prefer men. However, some men prefer men, and some women prefer women as their sexual partner. Although some men present as women, this transgendered preference provides no information about their sexual preferences, a similar situation applying to women who present as men. Neither does this account consider those who identify as nonbinary, either as individuals or as partners. A person's sexual orientation is usually defined with respect to their birth-assigned sex.[8] If a trans woman prefers men as her sexual partners, some clinicians have considered her to be homosexual. If she prefers women, as is often the case when a married partner transitions, then she is often considered to be heterosexual rather than homosexual.

Because of this confusion between the use of the term *homosexual* to describe the sexual preferences of trans people for whom birth-assigned sex and affirmed gender are different, we use *gynephilic* to indicate a preference for woman and *androphilic* to indicate a preference for men. So, a homosexual trans woman is now called an androphilic trans woman, and a trans woman who is not homosexual is a gynephilic trans woman. Similarly, a homosexual trans man is a gynephilic trans man, and a trans man who is not homosexual is an androphilic trans man.

There is no well-known term to describe the sexual orientation of those who identify as nonbinary or more generally as *genderqueer*, a term that describes those who do not identify as purely binary in either their gender identification or sexual orientation. We can simply use genderqueer to refer to all the behavioral characteristics of this diverse group of people.

Some homosexual people have personality types akin to those of their opposite birth-assigned sex. There are interesting relationships between sexual orientation and gender identity, even though in principle the two characteristics are logically unrelated and probably rely on activity in different brain regions or circuits. Such relationships are relevant for our understanding of gender diversity, especially when we consider the sexual preferences of trans people.

Various interpretations of the differences between gender identity and sexual identity have been proposed. Gender and sexuality have been defined as follows:

> [G]ender [encompasses] both an institutionalized interpretation of what it means to live as a woman or a man (including rules of belonging) and individual interpretations of what it means to live as a woman or a man. Sexuality [is] the way we represent and enact bodily pleasures and desires, a term that engages concepts of the body (both real and symbolic) and concepts of gender, if only to negate them, and which is not reducible to [gender identity]. Sex [is] the mostly anatomical features by which social designations of female, male, and intersexed bodies are made.[9]

Many people believe that androphilic cisgender men are necessarily effeminate and, conversely, that feminine cisgender men must be sexually attracted to men. Although trans women consider themselves to be feminine, they are not always androphilic. Moreover, androphilic cisgender men do not usually have a feminine gender identity, suggesting that sexual orientation and gender identity are relatively unrelated lifestyle characteristics. In a study comparing the psychological adjustment of trans women and androphilic cisgender men, the trans women had a stronger feminine gender identity as was indicated by their earlier preference for girls' games, crossdressing, and imagining themselves as female.[10]

To evaluate a proposal that trans men have more in common with gynephilic cisgender men than with gynephilic cisgender women, interviews were conducted with six gynephilic cisgender women and 12 trans men. All the trans men had identified as gynephilic prior to their transition and none had undergone phalloplasty, the surgical construction of a penis, due to its prohibitive cost and uncertain success rate. Most of the gynephilic cisgender women had been tomboys during childhood, playing boy's games and wishing to avoid appearing in public as a girl. Although they experienced parental pressure to conform to a feminine role, they did not like wearing a dress. Even though they might look like a boy, they did not wish to be mistaken for a boy in social situations, some preferring to appear androgynously as neither a boy nor a girl.[11]

Trans men were similar in many ways to those gynephilic cisgender women who identified as tomboys when they were younger. As young people, trans men were interested in boys' games and clothes but, unlike gynephilic cisgender women, they identified as boys and wished that they had not been born a girl. The trans men were distressed by their female bodies and rejected the values and ideals of womanhood. Young trans men prefer to hide their chest and feel inappropriately attired when forced to wear a dress. In some cases, the boundary between a butch gynephilic cisgender woman and a trans man is both permeable and fluid. Despite this possibility, gynephilic cisgender women identify as women whereas trans men affirm their gender as male.[12]

There may be differences in sexual behavior between gynephilic cisgender women and trans men. It had previously been suggested that trans men avoid masturbation, preferring to obtain sexual satisfaction from a partner while feeling masculine during such activity. Although most trans men are friendly toward cisgender men, the opposite is sometimes true for gynephilic cisgender women. Sixty-seven percent of trans men report fantasizing that they are men whereas none of the gynephilic cisgender women do so. Also, a larger number of trans men have experienced a same-sex encounter before the age of 18 than is the case for most gynephilic cisgender women.[13]

Prior to their transition, up to half of trans men were androphilic, and about 10 percent had been previously married to men. A study of 45 well-educated trans men aged 37 who were undergoing hormone therapy showed that 34 had undergone chest reconstruction in a surgical procedure known as bilateral mastectomy. Twenty-one of the trans men had undergone hysterectomy but only four had completed phalloplasty. Two trans men chose metoidioplasty, a surgical procedure that takes advantage of the enlarged clitoris resulting from long-term testosterone therapy to produce a small penis. All except one of the participants were sexually attracted to women prior to transition. During intimacy, they considered themselves playing the role of a gynephilic cisgender man. The trans men decided not to become sexually involved with women owing to their perceived physical inadequacies prior to genital surgery. Either they already had a partner prior to transitioning or they had decided to start a relationship with a woman after starting their transition. Having a partner who can validate a trans man's masculinity is very important for their own self-esteem.

Some of the trans men's earlier relationships with cisgender men were considered beneficial in teaching them how to behave like men during transition. In most cases, such liaisons were initiated during the era when same-sex relationships were not socially approved, at which time a socially acceptable relationship would circumvent social stigma, and to maintain family expectations. Under such circumstances, the trans men's attitude toward cisgender men was based more on friendship than anything else, with only one of the trans men in this study finding cisgender men at all attractive. For some trans men, a sexual relationship did eventually develop with androphilic cisgender men, but this took an average of seven years to develop. It was considered particularly affirming for the trans men when their previous female partner supported them at least emotionally during the transition process.[14]

A study of sexual preferences in groups of crossdressers and trans women showed that whereas over 80 percent of male crossdressers were attracted to cisgender women, and about half of the trans women were attracted to cisgender men, a quarter of the trans women were attracted to women and the others had no sexual preference. Perhaps trans women sometimes change their sexual preferences during their transition. Most crossdressers identified either as a man with a feminine side, or simply as a person who enjoys wearing women's clothing. The trans women reported feeling like "a woman trapped in a male body," or else they just felt like a woman without reference to their physical embodiment. About a quarter of the crossdressers were taking feminizing hormones, whereas over 80 percent of the trans women were either undergoing hormone therapy or had already completed genital surgery.[15]

Differences between trans women and cisgender women in terms of their sexuality indicate that trans women are more attracted to feminine males, have greater recall of a feminine gender identity, experience less emotional jealousy, and prefer younger partners.[16] However, there are a variety of relationships entered into by trans women, including a not uncommon gynephilic relationship with another trans woman.

To summarize our discussion so far, it is somewhat difficult to discriminate between sex and gender even when we stipulate that sex is biological and gender is sociocultural. Perhaps this problem arises from the complex intertwining of gender identity and sexual orientation that pervades both the literature and popular convention. The association of homosexuality with cross-gendered behavior has been observed in many cultures, with those exhibiting such traits frequently being given a high status. Health issues are important for homosexual as well as for gender-diverse people. Some of these people find access to medical care limited and prejudice rife even though, in this more enlightened era, we might expect professionals to be sensitive to people's differences in gender identity and sexual orientation. The scourge of HIV/AIDS highlights the need for special treatment of such people within the health care system.

4.3 HEALTH ISSUES FOR TRANS PEOPLE

Trans people have been frequently exposed to health risks, especially those who work in the sex industry, either as their only source of income or to obtain social acceptance and support. Sometimes sex work is the trans person's only way to earn any money when discrimination limits their employment opportunities. Indeed, the incidence of HIV-positive respondents in one survey of trans sex workers was as high as 22 percent, highlighting their risky lifestyle.[17]

Trans women are at a greater risk of drug abuse and prostitution than are trans men. Almost twenty years ago, of 292 trans women interviewed in San Francisco in the United States, 32 percent were sex workers, 62 percent reported being depressed, 33 percent had attempted suicide, 20 percent had serious mental health problems, and 35 percent were HIV-positive. In terms of social disadvantage, 60 percent of the trans women had experienced harassment or violence and 37 percent had experienced economic discrimination.[18] In another study conducted in San Francisco in 1998, 34 percent of trans women and 18 percent of trans men reported intravenous drug use at some time in their lives.[19]

The incidence of HIV in trans sex workers was as high as 74 percent in Italy and 68 percent in the United States. Despite wishing to maintain their ability to pass as women to ensure their safety and to maintain their self-esteem, the experiences of HIV-positive trans women in health care delivery include alienation and a perception that their quality of care is less than that given to other people. Some of these trans people worried whether their HIV status would disqualify them from obtaining electrolysis and other forms of feminization, including genital surgery.[20] Trans men who tend to have unprotected sex more often than trans women are also at risk of HIV infection.[21]

The number of gender-diverse people who had suicidal thoughts is as high as 33 percent, with even higher percentages being reported in more recent surveys. Often ignored is the mental health of trans people's partners, many of whom suffer significant emotional distress similar to that experienced by people diagnosed with post-traumatic stress disorder.[22] Of concern, occasionally gender-diverse students are not well treated in educational institutions including during their studies at medical schools.[23]

Body dissatisfaction in trans men is associated with depression, anxiety, and anger. However, there is evidence that these health issues can be reduced substantially after the commencement of testosterone therapy and chest reconstruction surgery, a procedure known as bilateral mastectomy. Compared with before they had started testosterone therapy, once they had been on testosterone for a while, trans men reported feeling happier, less depressed and anxious, and more assertive and confident. As one trans man said, "I feel much more well-balanced and happier—more self-confident that [sic] I used to. I haven't had any negative mood changes."[24]

In a recent study, 233 27-year-old trans men were tested using the Minnesota Multiphasic Personality Inventory (MMPI-2), which was administered one month after starting testosterone therapy and then three months later. Differences in MMPI-2 scores at these time points showed a significant decrease in hypochondria, an unfounded concern about one's health; depression, a lack of hope about one's life situation; hysteria, an abnormal response to stressful situations; and paranoia, feelings of persecution and excessive sensitivity. These results indicated a substantial improvement in the trans men's mental health following hormone therapy. As expected, there was also an increase in their MMPI-2 masculinity score. These findings emphasize the importance of starting hormone therapy early to relieve any mental distress that might accompany a person's gender affirmation. Matched groups of cisgender males and females showed no changes in MMPI-2 scores over this four-month period. This finding showed that the effectiveness of testosterone therapy was not simply due to the passage of time. Because depression may increase suicide risk, it is important that testosterone therapy begin as soon as possible after the trans man presents for treatment with their family doctor. Any attempt to treat depression and/or anxiety using traditional psychotherapy methods will not solve the central issue for trans people. As far as we know, no similarly detailed studies have been conducted using trans women.

> When we deny or stifle parts of ourselves, we pay a heavy price: we feel a deep, amorphous sense of restriction; we are constantly on guard; we are often troubled and puzzled by internal but seemingly alien impulses that demand expression. When we are able to reclaim these disavowed parts, we experience a wholeness and a sense of liberation.[25]

In a study from the 1990s, the effects of three months of cross-sex hormone therapy was investigated in groups of trans women and trans men. Testosterone therapy for trans men was associated with an increase in anger, aggressiveness, sexual motivation, and visual-spatial ability and a decrease in verbal fluency. Estrogen therapy for trans women produced a more inward-looking sense of anger, less aggression, a reduction in sexual arousal, and an improved fluency with words. Both groups showed no change in mood over this short time period.[26]

A study of 399 trans women that examined their experiences at five different life stages showed that the older they were, the more likely they would have been outed as their affirmed gender identity to parents, siblings, friends, coworkers, and to their sexual partner, often without their expressed consent. Of course, the trans women may have garnered support from some of these people, although stigma and discrimination might have occurred for many of them. Relationships with other people were not so strong for older trans women as they were for younger trans women. Nevertheless, the older trans women were blessed with experiencing less conflict with everyone except their sexual partners, this type of conflict being most intense with close family, friends, and coworkers during late middle age. Affirming one's gender to others can be protective against the risk of major depression, especially during middle age and beyond.[27]

4.4 THE GENETIC BASIS FOR GENDER INCONGRUENCE

Discovering a biological cause for gender incongruence would be useful for understanding the origins of diversity as well as for reducing the social stigma inflicted upon the trans community. The Australian National Health and Medical Research Council Twin Register was used to study genetic and environmental influences on sexual orientation, as indicated by responses to Kinsey test items that measured sexual fantasy and attraction. Childhood gender nonconformity and childhood gender identity scores successfully predicted the degree of nonheterosexuality, suggesting that childhood gender nonconformity is a possible precursor of homosexuality. Male twins recalled their co-twin who did not identify later as heterosexual as being more gender incongruent as a child than they were. Both childhood gender nonconformity and childhood gender identity were more similar between twin pairs for male identical twins than for male fraternal twins, whereas for childhood gender nonconformity a similar finding was only found in women.[28]

A genetic analysis indicated that childhood gender nonconformity is an inherited trait for adult cisgender men and women. For cisgender women, sexual orientation, childhood gender nonconformity, and especially childhood gender identity are good predictors of a person's current gender identity. For cisgender men, on the other hand, sexual orientation and childhood gender nonconformity, but not childhood gender identity, reflect their current gender identity. Environmental variables may also be important in the development of gender identity, especially for cisgender men.[29]

A study of 7-year-old and 10-year-old twins used scores obtained for two items of the Child Behavior Checklist that measure gender-nonconforming behavior. These items seek the parent's responses when asked whether their child *behaves like the opposite sex* or *wishes to be of the opposite sex*. The prevalence of gender-atypical scores was 3 percent for boys and 5 percent for girls, percentages that are larger than current best estimates of the prevalence of gender-diverse behavior in young children. For girls, the prevalence decreased from 5.7 percent at 7 years to 3.6 percent at 10 years, and for boys the decrease with age was from 3.7 percent at 7 years to 2.7 percent at 10 years. However, compared with children who are not gender-diverse, these percentages are quite large. A higher similarity in scores on these items for identical than fraternal twins suggested substantial inheritance of gender expression of around 70 percent.[30]

The higher prevalence of gender diversity in close relatives of trans people when compared with the general population also suggests that gender incongruence may be inherited. In contrast, there is no evidence for the inheritance of crossdressing behavior. It has been suggested that some combination of genes involved in activity at androgen, aromatase, and perhaps estrogen receptors might be responsible for these genetic links.[31]

4.5 HANDEDNESS AND DEVELOPMENTAL INSTABILITY AS CORRELATES OF GENDER IDENTITY

Handedness is an interesting psychological correlate of gender identity. As handedness does not usually change with age and is unaffected by environmental and social influences, it may be associated with gender identity, once that identity has stabilized by early adolescence. Handedness is determined around week 15 in the womb. Higher than usual testosterone levels might affect development of the right hemisphere of the brain, leading to the increased chance of non-right-handedness that occurs, for example, in women with congenital adrenal hyperplasia, a condition that causes excess exposure to testosterone in the womb.

The incidence of right-handed thumb-sucking in the human fetus corresponds almost exactly with the 92 percent incidence of right-handedness in adult populations. Historically, right-handedness was considered the ideal whereas left-handedness was thought to be undesirable and awkward. Indeed, the Latin word for left, *sinistra*, is the origin of the English word *sinister*. In a few people, left-handedness is associated with a higher risk of neurodevelopmental problems including dyslexia, mental retardation, autism, schizophrenia, cerebral palsy, and epilepsy. These problems occur more frequently in men than in women as men are more likely to be left-handed.[32]

In women, non-right-handedness is associated with higher scores on masculinity, suggesting a tendency toward dominance and independence. Left-handed people of both sexes tend to show more dominance and less nurturance than right-handers. Non-right-handedness in men is associated with female-oriented occupational interests and self-rated femininity. By contrast, non-right-handedness in women is associated with male-oriented occupational interests. Trans women are more often left-handed than birth-assigned men. One study showed that 38 percent of trans women and 12 percent of cisgender men were left-handed.[33]

Other hand features also show gender differences, probably resulting from prenatal causes. Dermatoglyphics, which measures the number of finger ridges on each hand, can be obtained using ink-pad recordings. A leftward asymmetry in the number of fingertip ridges is determined during week 13 in the womb and is fully developed between weeks 16 and 19 of a pregnancy. Women exhibit this asymmetry more often than men, whereas men have a higher total ridge count on both hands. Ridge development is also affected by environmental influences such as the amount of alcohol and anticonvulsant drugs consumed during pregnancy.

Fingerprint asymmetry was measured in 270 trans women and 54 trans men, and in a comparison group containing 123 cisgender men and 99 cisgender women. Of the trans women, 31 percent were gynephilic, 22 percent were androphilic, 38 percent were bisexual, and 9 percent were asexual. Almost all the trans men were gynephilic. Fingerprints were taken from the thumb and little finger of each hand as these fingers are more likely to contain at least some ridges. There was no difference in ridge count for the cisgender male and female comparison groups, nor was there any difference in ridge count for the left and right hands. However, trans women had the higher average ridge count.[34]

Adextrality is the extent to which fingerprint ridges tend to be more prominent on the left hand than on the right hand. For those with a rightward fingerprint ridge shift, comparison group participants had a greater frequency of adextrality than did the androphilic trans men and the gynephilic trans women. By contrast, for those with a leftward fingerprint ridge shift, androphilic trans men and gynephilic trans women showed greater adextrality than did heterosexual cisgender men and woman. It appeared that dermatoglyphic characteristics depend more on a person's sexual orientation rather than their gender identity.[35]

4.6 DIGIT-RATIO AS AN INDICATOR OF GENDER IDENTITY

Digit-ratio is obtained by dividing the length of the index, or second, finger by the length of the ring, or fourth, finger. With the palm held upward, finger-length is usually measured as the distance from the basal crease, where the finger joins the palm, to the tip of the finger. Digit-ratio is a stable sexually dimorphic characteristic resulting perhaps from the effect of prenatal testosterone exposure around week 14 in the womb. The greater the exposure to testosterone, the longer will be the ring finger and the lower the digit-ratio. An individual's digit-ratio is determined by the Homeobox genes that regulate sexual differentiation and skeletal development during embryonic development. Interrater agreement when a person's digit-ratio is measured by two or more people is high.[36] As digit-ratio is a marker for prenatal testosterone, digit-ratios less than 1.0 are typical of men, whereas values greater than 1.0 are more characteristic of women. However, the overlap in digit-ratio for men and women is large, concealing to some extent any gender differences that might be present.

When digit-ratio was measured for right and left hands, the digit-ratio was less for men than women with no differences in digit-ratio being observed between the hands. The average ratios were similar, being 0.97 for men and 0.99 for women. When the data were combined for men and women, the left-hand digit-ratio was larger for those scoring high on neuroticism, a typically feminine trait, and smaller for those having high scores on psychoticism, a typically masculine trait related to aggression. However, the relationships between digit-ratio and personal characteristics were rather slight.[37]

The digit-ratios of trans men and women have been compared with those of cisgender men and women. For right-handed participants, the right-hand digit-ratio for trans women is no different from that of cisgender women, whereas the left-hand digit-ratio is similar for cisgender men and trans women. Since digit-ratio may be influenced by prenatal hormone activity, perhaps this is further evidence for a biological basis for gender incongruence. However, the greater prevalence of left-handedness among trans women together with the discovery of no differences in digit-ratio between left-handed trans women and others is a puzzling finding.[38]

SUMMARY

Evidence from both chromosomal studies and genetic analyses of twin data supports the inheritance of both homosexuality and childhood gender nonconformity. Further evidence of a biological basis for gender diversity is provided by differences between trans people and their cisgender counterparts in physical traits such as handedness, trans people being more frequently left-handed and having a leftward dermal ridge asymmetry. Evidence of a biological basis for gender incongruence is provided by similar digit-ratio values for trans women and birth-assigned women, but these differences are slight and overshadowed by the large variability in digit-ratio for people from the same gender category.

Chapter 5

PSYCHOLOGICAL ASSESSMENT OF GENDER INCONGRUENCE

In this chapter, we examine the psychological makeup of trans people, compare them with other people, and consider the psychological assessment of a newly defined medical condition, *gender incongruence*. This condition is contained in the 11th edition of the World Health Organization's International Classification of Diseases, proposed in 2018 in a section dealing with sexual health. Unlike the current medical condition, *gender dysphoria*, defined in the fifth edition of the *Diagnostic and Statistical Manual of Mental Disorders* published by the American Psychiatric Association in 2013, gender incongruence is not a mental illness but a normal variation of human behavior. However, almost all the research and clinical applications to date are for gender dysphoria and its precursors, gender identity disorder and transsexualism. To provide a suitable background we begin with a review of research on the lifestyles of gender-diverse people, including those who do not choose to transition socially or medically.

5.1 THE LIFESTYLE OF GENDER-DIVERSE PEOPLE

This section summarizes research conducted on the lifestyles of trans people. Although they are sometimes the recipients of discrimination and worse, there are numerous examples of courage and resilience that ensure that these people are to be admired.

For those who choose to transition socially into a binary gender role, the Bem Sex Role Inventory (BSRI) has been used to assess how well trans people adopt behavior that is typical of the opposite sex. This is done by examining scores on two abstract measures derived from people's self-ratings and defined as *Masculinity* and *Femininity*. People scoring high on *Masculinity* and low on *Femininity* are defined as *Masculine* and those scoring high on *Femininity* and low on *Masculinity* are defined as *Feminine*. Those scoring high on both dimensions are *Androgynous*, whereas those scoring low on both dimensions are considered *Undifferentiated*. Most of the older trans women participating in a study that used the Bem Sex Role Inventory were university educated and married, with an average age of 36, compared with the other participants whose average age was 21. As expected, cisgender men scored higher on *Masculinity* than *Femininity*, the reverse being true for cisgender women. On the other hand, trans men scored similarly to cisgender men. It was interesting that trans women, especially younger ones, scored even higher on *Femininity* than did cisgender women. Trans women and trans men were often thought more androgynous than cisgender members of both sexes.[1]

The PULSE survey conducted in Ontario, Canada, in 2015 sought lifestyle information from 433 trans people. There were approximately equal numbers of trans men and trans women, their ages ranging from 16 to 77. About 30 percent of those who responded to the survey were living as their birth-assigned gender, 23 percent were living as their affirmed gender with no medical interventions, and 42 percent were on hormone therapy. Fifteen percent of trans women and only 0.4 percent of trans men had undergone genital surgery. The survey showed that trans women were less likely than trans men to be living in their affirmed gender due to the adverse effects of transphobia, especially for those unable to access medical procedures. However, many of the latter might have been occasional crossdressers and those who identified as nonbinary.[2]

According to summary data contained in Table 4 of a recent study[3] that surveyed 2,095 transgender and gender-nonconforming young people in the United States, the overwhelming majority of those responding, 68 percent, were birth-assigned girls. It is hard to understand how people can identify as gender-diverse when for 40 percent of boys and 35 percent of girls their self-reported gender identity conforms to their birth-assigned sex. If we consider only those who are unsure whether they identify as masculine or feminine, 29 percent of birth-assigned boys and 41 percent of birth-assigned girls are in some sense nonbinary. Only 31 percent of birth-assigned boys and 24 percent of birth-assigned girls identified as a gender opposite to their birth-assigned sex. It is possible that previously the number of people identifying as nonbinary may have been underestimated.

5.2 FORMING A TRANS IDENTITY

As discussed in Chapter 2, between the ages of two and seven most children progress through the stages of forming a coherent gender identity consistent with their birth-assigned sex. However, for a few children, either gender identity development becomes stalled or the acquired gender is contrary to the child's birth-assigned sex, often leading to difficulties for the child, their family, and friends. Many trans people experience their first feelings of gender difference when they are young, so information about forming a trans identity is vital to their self-exploration.

The media, including the Internet, books, television, film, and video, have played an important role in helping people realize their trans identity. Scholarly books, Internet mailing lists and chat lines, book autobiographies, and television documentaries deliver a wealth of fact and fiction sources of interest to gender-diverse people. Some of these people are helped by reading novels with a gender-diverse theme. Visual media also play a significant role in allowing trans persons to gain a greater understanding of their new self-identity, especially when these people immerse themselves in its emotional, intellectual, and spiritual content.[4]

A trans person's identity is influenced by their self-image, especially their own body satisfaction. Many trans people are preoccupied with the aesthetics of their outward appearance, especially when in public and on social media. This obsession is centered on the shape of the body, secondary sex characteristics, and dress code. However, we should not ignore the possibility that a negative attitude toward one's own body, as indicated by discomfort when appearing in public, might result from problems in establishing relationships with other people. Many trans people who proceed to gender-affirming surgeries wish to ensure that the appearance of their physical self conforms to their inner sense of gender identity. By so doing they resolve the anxiety-provoking conflict between their own self-perception and their body representation as it is seen by others.

The body image of trans men and trans women has been studied using the Sensory Integration Body Imagery Test, which evaluates body-perception conflicts by measuring the time taken to perceive body parts. The neck area plays a prominent role in a trans woman's body image. However, there is less chance of a positive feeling toward the genital area in trans women and toward the chest area in trans men. As would be expected, there is a high investment of emotion in body parts that contribute to a trans person's gender comfort.[5]

5.3 PSYCHOLOGICAL CHARACTERISTICS OF TRANS PEOPLE

We now examine the psychological differences that have been observed between gender-diverse people and others. We will show how these differences can be assessed using commonly used psychological tests as well as by a few special tests that focus on matters of gender identity and incongruence. After a discussion of the important topic of mental health as it applies to gender-diverse people, we conclude with a review of research findings of people's own views about their gender diversity.

5.3.1 Diagnostic Tests

Psychological tests proposed for evaluating trans people, such as the Thematic Apperception Test (TAT), the Draw-a-Person Test, the Body Image Scale, the Symptom Checklist 90-revised (SCL-90-R), the Crown Crisp Experiential Index (CCEI), the Bem Sex Role Inventory (BSRI), the Minnesota Multiphasic Personality Inventory (MMPI), and the Rorschach Test have failed to discriminate reliably between those diagnosed with the obsolete medical condition of transsexualism and those who show no evidence of the condition. Psychiatric diagnostic tests such as the Interview for Dissociative Disorders, the Dissociative Experiences Scale, and the Childhood Trauma Questionnaire show no differences between trans people and others.

Nevertheless, as we saw in Chapter 2, there is some brain imaging evidence for the validity of trans people's dissociative experiences, impressions that their gender incongruence may result from a mismatch between their own ideal self-image and their perceived body prior to transition. However, there are no available psychological tests to adequately evaluate these feelings. As we will see, specialized tests focus almost exclusively on reports of gender dysphoria, likely to become an obsolete diagnosis in the next few years.

Personality differences can be measured by conventional question and answer tests as well as by projective tests such as the Rorschach, or inkblot, Test. Projective tests require the client to interpret ambiguous diagrams, the idea being that individual differences in interpretation reveal the operation of subconscious psychological processes that are not so evident in the results of paper-and-pencil tests. Rorschach scores tend to become more stable as people progress from adolescence to adulthood. However, the subjective nature of projective tests makes the prediction of a person's behavior based on their results unreliable.[6]

The personality profiles of trans people measured by the MMPI, a commonly used personality test, suggest that most trans people have few if any clinical symptoms. Only the *MF* scale that measures masculinity–femininity and the *PD* scale that measures personality exceed the expected range. Some trans women attracted to men differ from those attracted to women on some of the MMPI test scores, those attracted to women scoring higher on *Hypochondria*, *Depression,* and *Hysteria,* a combination of scores associated with possible neurotic symptoms.[7] When the MMPI was administered to young trans women seeking genital surgery, no psychopathology was evident. As expected, they scored higher than others on *Femininity*.

A special gender identity subscale, *Gd*, has been derived from items contained in the MMPI test. The scale was evaluated using clients at a gender clinic and a matched comparison group of male psychiatric outpatients, obviously an inappropriate comparison group. The diagnostically useful items, with the corresponding answer presumably reflecting a female gender identity indicated in brackets, were:

I have often wished I were a girl. (True)

I would like to be a private secretary. (True)

I like adventure stories better than romantic stories. (False)

I enjoy reading love stories. (True)

My judgment is better than it ever was. (True)

If I were a reporter I would very much like to report sporting news. (False)

I am very strongly attracted to members of my own sex. (True)

I would like to be a nurse. (True)[8]

Using an arbitrary cutoff score, 88 percent of the gender clinic clients were correctly classified as gender atypical and 92 percent of the mentally ill patients were classified as having a psychiatric condition. The key *Gd* items that identified gender atypicality in trans women were stereotypical feminine interests and denial of masculine interests, accompanied by excellent mental health. Comparing gender-affirming clients with other than a healthy comparison group is ill-advised and discriminatory.

The Utrecht Gender Dysphoria Scale was developed to measure distress in people identifying as transsexual, implying that they are seeking medical interventions such as hormones and surgeries. The trans female version of the scale contains items such as "My life would be meaningless if I would have to live as a boy/man"; "I feel unhappy because I have a male body"; "I hate myself because I am a boy/man"; "Only as a girl/woman my life would be worth living"; "I dislike urinating in a standing position," and so on. The trans male version of the scale contains items such as "I prefer to behave like a boy"; "Every time someone treats me like a girl I feel hurt"; "A boy's life is more attractive for me than a girl's life"; "I feel unhappy because I have to behave like a girl"; "I hate having breasts," and so forth.[9] The test has some validity for discriminating between gender-diverse people who identify as transsexual and cisgender people of the same birth-sex.

When they are assessed using the Draw-a-Person Test, trans women often produce drawings that are more female-typical than those drawn by others, including cisgender women. Drawings by trans women are rated higher on elaborateness and size but are similar to cisgender women's drawings in terms of their completeness. The overall quality of trans women's drawings is higher than those drawn by others, suggesting a potential use for the Draw-a-Person Test in the psychological assessment of gender incongruence.[10]

A few trans women tend to have a more pronounced female gender role and a poorer body image than do cisgender women. Nevertheless, there are no differences between the personality profiles of trans women and others on the more comprehensive and commonly used Big Five Personality Inventory (NEO-PI).[11] However, other studies have shown that trans women and cisgender men have higher scores on self-esteem and dynamic body-image than do cisgender women. Trans women differ from other people in their sex-role identification, 71 percent of trans women having high scores on both *Masculinity* and *Femininity*, a finding suggesting that these people might have an androgynous personality. These findings are consistent with these women's positive adjustment after genital surgery to their new lifestyle, which often involves a greater variety of flexible behaviors.[12]

As masculinity–femininity is an abstract personality characteristic, the psychological representation of gender may not correspond exactly with people's views about their own gender and that of others. From the psychological perspective, masculinity and femininity represent two separate personality characteristics rather than being at opposite ends of a single dimension. Masculinity, or *Instrumentality*, as it has been represented in personality assessment, is associated with dominance and independence, whereas femininity, or *Expressiveness*, is associated with warmth and compassion toward others. These personality traits are not limited exclusively to gender differences but are also associated with other personality variables that can be assessed using the Big Five Personality Inventory.

Gender diagnosticity distinguishes between masculine and feminine job interests by examining whether the job is more often performed by men or women. Women and feminine men are often more interested in people-oriented jobs such as personal care and counseling, whereas men and masculine women tend to be more interested in object-oriented jobs such as engineering and industrial trades.

Trans women historically differ from cisgender men in their career choice, their hobbies, and their self-rated femininity. Compared with cisgender men, trans women score lower in *Instrumentality* and higher in *Expressiveness*, so that in these respects they are more like cisgender women than cisgender men. When compared with cisgender women, trans men were more typically masculine on all personality measures except *Instrumentality* and *Expressiveness*. Although the *Instrumentality* and *Expressiveness* personality measures do not reliably distinguish between trans people and others, these people's gender-diagnostic job and hobby interests do. The gender-diagnostic scores for trans women are intermediate between those for cisgender men and women, whereas the gender-diagnostic scores for trans men are more like those of cisgender men.[13]

Despite the evidence presented so far, personality differences between trans people and others based on their gender incongruence are not so easy to find, except for expected differences in masculinity–femininity. Differences in depression and self-esteem most likely reflect adjustment difficulties resulting from the stress and stigma imposed by intolerance rather than from any fundamental differences in personality traits between trans people and others. Perhaps the most obvious difference lies in a reversal of gender role in the trans person's job interests. This is also likely to change as society's expectations evolve.

To summarize, trans people do not usually exhibit any serious personality difficulties. Trans women often differ from cisgender men by being closer to cisgender women in their personality profile. Some trans women's distress is indicated whenever their test scores suggest greater neuroticism and emotional disturbance, and perhaps a lower level of ego-strength. In general, trans women have occupational interests like those of cisgender women, and trans men prefer masculine occupations.

5.3.2 Mental Health

Gender-diverse people diagnosed without any proposed psychiatric condition related to their gender expression can comply with cultural stereotypes of their confirmed gender without any feeling of uneasiness or dysphoria. For example, trans women who are not diagnosed with a condition such as gender dysphoria belong to one of two groups, those with a vague sense of maladjustment linked to a pronounced feminine identity, and those with only a slight feminine tendency without significant adjustment problems.[14] There is no clear brain evidence for gender dysphoria or any of its related conditions that might reflect distress. Many trans people, however, have been pressured into reporting such feelings so that they can receive a diagnosis that will allow them to undergo desired medical interventions. Some of these people even know the script needed to convince mental health professionals of their distress and their need for a medical diagnosis so that they can progress to surgery and other positive outcomes.

One study reported that 9 percent of all trans people had been diagnosed with a serious psychiatric illness, mostly depression or borderline personality disorder.[15] Borderline personality disorder is characterized by problems associated with emotional control, sufferers experiencing intense episodes of anger, depression, and anxiety often accompanied by self-harm. Sufferers cannot easily change long-term goals, the disorder influencing friendships, career plans, and gender identity.[16] Some of these problems caused by anxiety and depression are most likely caused by discrimination from family and friends, and abuse and violence from others, rather than directly from any distress associated with the person's affirmed gender identity.

Of 82 clients tested at the Monash Medical Centre Gender Dysphoria Clinic in Australia, 48 were diagnosed with the now obsolete psychiatric labels of *transsexualism* or Gender Identity Disorder of Adolescence and Adulthood, non-transsexual type (GIDAANT) based on the old DSM-III diagnostic criteria proposed by the American Psychiatric Association. Those diagnosed with GIDAANT in this relatively small sample had all been married at some time in their lives. Both groups scored above average on *Femininity*, as well as on other scales assessing gender identity and gender-appropriate interests. Eighty-five percent of those diagnosed with transsexualism were rated as having a low level of psychiatric disorder, suggesting that these people were well adjusted despite being diagnosed with a mental illness. On the other hand, nearly half of those diagnosed with GIDAANT were classified in a higher psychiatric disorder category because they exhibited symptoms of depression, emotional distress, and chronic maladjustment. These people were generally older than those in the other diagnostic group and were more likely to have suffered distress from family separation, job loss, and discrimination.[17]

When compared with those who are psychologically well adjusted, trans women who experience more than their fair share of lifestyle difficulties tend to be more depressed, more sensitive to adverse events in their environment, and more apt to suffer from a greater number of health problems.[18] These problems are not necessarily related to any gender identity distress or diagnosed gender dysphoria. Rather, they might reflect how other people's responses to them impact on the trans person's mental health.

Transphobia and abuse are the major contributors to the onset of depression, especially in young trans people. Depression can sometimes be exacerbated by changes in hormone levels during the initial stages of transition. More often, the start of hormone therapy and living in one's affirmed gender can reduce depression in many trans people, compensating for any possible adverse physiological effects of hormone therapy.[19]

Evidence from several studies has shown that just three to six months of hormone therapy is effective in reducing any psychopathological symptoms such as anxiety and depression that might be present prior to treatment. However, none of these studies used any proper experimental controls nor did they follow the people for more than a year to evaluate long-term effects of the treatment on their subsequent mental health. Clearly, more research is needed that follows trans people's experiences over a long period of time.

5.3.3 People's Views of Gender

A test has been devised to measure *genderism*, the belief that one binary gender is in some sense superior to the other, as well as *transphobia*, the conscious effort some people make to demean and to treat with discrimination and violence anyone who appears to violate their society's gender norms. To evaluate the usefulness of the test, four different vignettes were composed involving, respectively, a masculine boy, a feminine girl, a feminine boy, and a masculine girl. For the feminine girl and the feminine boy, only the names and gender were changed, as shown in the following vignette that tells the story of a typically feminine boy:

> Your son, Timmy, is 6 years old and in his first year of kindergarten. He spends much of his time at school playing with his three best friends—Kimberly, Tiffany, and Lisa. Timmy and his three friends often play dress up. Timmy always insists on playing the fairy princess and wears a pink dress and a diamond crown. At school, Timmy excels in printing, reading, and painting. His teacher describes your son as sensitive, caring, and beautiful. After school, instead of going out to play with his older brother, Timmy always runs to his cousin Meghan's house to play. At his cousin's house, Timmy loves to have chocolate milk as an after-school snack and always visits the bathroom to wash up. Timmy sits on the toilet to urinate, rather than standing like dad does. Timmy often insists on playing "house" with Meghan where he plays the role of "mother" and Meghan plays the "father." Your son enjoys wearing Meghan's skirts and dresses and often speaks like a girl. He spends hours at Meghan's home, playing roles of mother, queen, Snow White, Sleeping Beauty, and Cinderella. When not role-playing with his cousin, Timmy enjoys playing with Meghan's Barbie toys. There are even times when Timmy likes to be called "Barbie." Your son dreams of growing up to be beautiful and successful, like Barbie.[20]

Scores on the scale show that cisgender men display more *Genderism, Transphobia,* and *Gender-bashing,* defined as targeting a person because of their gender expression, than do cisgender women, all three variables being significantly related so that people scoring highly on one variable also do so on the other two. People who had met a transgender person scored lower on the Genderism–Transphobia Scale than those who had not, indicating that knowing a trans person facilitates acceptance.

5.4 THE MENTAL HEALTH NEEDS OF TRANS PEOPLE

An important issue in transgender health is whether gender incongruence or gender dysphoria is a mental illness or a normal variation of gender experience. On the one hand, such gender variation may require a psychiatric diagnosis from a specialist clinic so that medical insurance in those countries where it is available can be obtained to pay for surgeries and other medical interventions. In this way, medical *gatekeepers* can select suitable candidates for surgery and these medical interventions can then proceed. On the other hand, client-centered gender affirmation makes a trans person's transition a basic human right, it removes stigma from a diagnosis, and it reflects the diversity of views in the trans community about a medical transition. Client-centered gender affirmation also reduces the need for large gender clinics with their associated services and personnel, and the intolerable delays in obtaining treatment. Most of the nonsurgical medical interventions can be performed by well-trained general practitioners.[21]

Young trans people who have been diagnosed with gender dysphoria according to DSM-5 criteria have fewer same-sex (relative to their birth-assigned sex) school friends and more opposite-sex school friends than do cisgender people of the same age and education. They also experience more bullying because of their gender identity.[22] A similar finding is also common among much older trans people.

Some of the obstacles to obtaining appropriate transgender health care include problems finding a trans-friendly doctor, the lack of transgender-appropriate training among most medical practitioners, and the occasional therapist who believes psychotherapy offers a "cure." Some untrained doctors have confused the trans person's situation inappropriately with sexual disorders such as transvestic fetishism and other sexual behaviors defined in the *Diagnostic and Statistical Manual.* Other health system barriers include an inability to properly accommodate trans people in binary sex medical wards and the imposition of excessive medical precautions to prevent unlikely instances of regret. All these prejudicial treatments and interventions jeopardize the trans person's good mental health and may lead to avoidance of general health care.

In 2014 the Behavioral Risk Factor Surveillance System reported transgender status in 19 U.S. states, thus allowing a comparison of trans people and cisgender people on a range of important health issues. Trans people reported poorer physical and mental health than their cisgender peers and were more likely to have problems performing their normal duties. Trans people in the United States were also less likely to have medical coverage and to consult their medical provider regularly.[23]

A recent review showed that trans people can benefit from more mental health nurses with prior training in transgender health care. Also, by encouraging clinicians to employ an affirmative approach in their care of trans clients while facilitating appropriate peer support, considerable improvements can be made in transgender health provision. Long-term studies are needed to follow trans people's progress through their various transition requirements, including studies that follow trans people from a young age. Partners of trans people need to be considered as deserving of special consideration and care, and mental health professionals need to stay up-to-date with new developments in transgender care.[24]

Many trans people have been able to live their lives successfully despite the impact on their welfare of discrimination and distress emanating from people and agencies that have as their goal the destruction of gender nonconformity as an acceptable lifestyle. An online survey of 629 trans women whose average age was 38 and 464 trans men with an average age of 26 conducted in the United States in 2003, but reported 10 years later in 2013, showed that 49 percent of the trans men and 37 percent of the trans women reported depression, with about a third of each reporting anxiety as mental health concern. These signs of mental distress were unrelated to scores on a test of gender dysphoria, suggesting that their source was the wider social environment rather than the trans person's gender affirmation. The sources of stigma in order of frequency of occurrence were verbal abuse, problems getting a job and dealing with health services, physical abuse, and assault. Most at risk from external sources of threat were those from minority ethnic groups, those on low incomes, and those who invested in passing and who were out and about often. However, a personal feeling of resilience was enhanced when trans women, especially, invested in their best presentation to the wider world, and when they had family and peer support.[25]

Resilience can be defined as a set of learned behaviors based on a person's beliefs that enhances their ability to cope in difficult circumstances. In an interview study of 21 trans people, resilience was enhanced when they stated ownership of their own gender feelings, when they embraced their own self-worth, and when they were aware of possible sources of discrimination and oppression. The trans people's greater resilience was associated with a supportive community and with their cultivating hope for the future. Other strategies mentioned by these trans people included engagement in trans activism and trying to be a positive role model for others in the transgender community. As one of those interviewed said:

> I think that there is a high level of survival instinct in trans culture in general. As transgender people, we have to be resilient. We have to be strong. Because when we say, "I am going ahead and making this transition," well, we know we could lose everything—our family, our children, our friends, our employment, our places of worship, our standing in the community. And even in some cases, we could lose our lives. —Christine (pseudonym)[26]

5.5 ADJUSTMENT PROBLEMS EXPERIENCED BY TRANS PEOPLE

Despite a potential diagnosis of gender incongruence being unrelated to the trans person's state of mental health, some trans people experience severe psychological distress. The following examples include cases of eating disorder concurrent with gender incongruence. Like other women, trans women are at a greater risk of developing eating disorders than are cisgender men. The prevalence of anorexia nervosa in adolescent and young adult cisgender women ranges from 0.5 percent to 1 percent. The prevalence of bulimia nervosa in similar cisgendered populations lies between 1 and 3 percent. Some cisgender men with eating disorders also report disturbed gender identity development. So, femininity is considered a risk factor for eating disorders in men and women of all affirmed genders.

Although not everyone's experience, the presence of an eating disorder can complicate gender expression. Hepp and Milos[27] provided case studies of two trans women with eating disorders, one aged 36, the other 22. Both women had severe body dissatisfaction leading to anorexia nervosa and bulimia nervosa, respectively. The third case was a 43-year-old trans man with anorexia nervosa complicated by a lack of menstruation that was evident prior to starting testosterone therapy.

There has been a rare case of anorexia nervosa in identical male twins, one of whom had early cross-gender yearnings but who was living primarily as a cisgender man. The other twin lived full-time as a woman after being referred to a gender clinic for possible genital surgery. Both twins had developmental delays in language and motor skills and were diagnosed as having an eating disorder.[28]

Anorexia nervosa has also been reported for a 24-year-old trans man following chest reconstruction surgery, as well as hystero-oophorectomy to remove the internal sex organs. Eating disorders are not uncommon in trans people, particularly when they desire to be sexually attractive. This client was unusual in having complications resulting from alcohol dependence, major depression, and borderline personality disorder. The MMPI personality test revealed difficulties in interpersonal relationships, impulsivity, low frustration tolerance, depression, and anxiety, as well as high suggestibility and immaturity.[29] Perhaps eating disorders are a risk for gender-diverse people that needs to be considered by their professional carers.

A 25-year-old trans woman suffering from bulimia nervosa, a rare condition in cisgender men, expressed her eating disorder by using excessive exercise to maintain a stable weight. She had done this to maintain an ideal feminine shape so that she could attract male attention. This woman was marginalized socially with no regular employment except for her involvement in escort services. She had been sexually abused as a child and was now living away from family and friends.[30]

Although personality and other psychological tests have been used to detect differences between trans people and others, there are no consistent findings. Nevertheless, there are some differences in scores on *Masculinity* and *Femininity* associated with occupational interests common to the opposite birth-assigned sex, as well as deviations from normal scores on tests indicating psychological disorders. Although current psychological tests may be of questionable value for assessing gender incongruence, psychological aspects of the trans lifestyle should be considered, especially when there are other health complications such as eating disorders.

5.6 GENDER INCONGRUENCE AS A MEDICAL CONDITION

The following sections provide a summary of psychological diagnostic procedures for people requesting help from gender services. For many years it was

common for all people seeking hormone therapy and gender-affirming surgeries to be assessed by a mental health professional, as if to think that anyone
would have to be *crazy* to want to adopt a gender role other than that corresponding to their birth-assigned sex.

Although many people presenting for medical transition are seeking hormone therapy and ultimately gender-affirming surgeries, the fear that doctors
have for their patient's welfare has meant that just about every one of them has
had to be assessed extensively and in many cases unnecessarily using lots of
psychological tests and interviews from mental health professionals. This is representative of the pathologization of gender diversity. Presently, according to
medical edict, anyone wanting hormone therapy must first be diagnosed with
either gender dysphoria or gender incongruence when that new classification
has been published in the International Classification of Diseases, Version 11.

Before 2013, the situation was even worse because people were then diagnosed with a clearly defined mental illness known as *gender identity disorder*.
Yes, indeed, to qualify for hormone therapy you had to be certified by a psychiatrist as having a mental health problem. But how can affirming your own
personal gender identity be a disease? Who is really suffering the dysphoria?
Is it the client or is it the mental health professional, desperately trying to
defend society's need to minimize the extent of gender diversity?

Save for medical complications, pregnancy is a natural variation of female
sexuality. Being pregnant is usually a joyful experience unless the pregnancy is
unwanted and abortion is not permitted because of cultural and religious
restrictions. In such circumstances, the distressed woman might experience
pregnancy dysphoria resulting from external pressures that are beyond her control.[31] Likewise, being trans is a normal variation of gendered behavior in
which there is a dissonance between the trans person's genitals and their
mindset regarding their affirmed gender. Any distress that might occur is most
likely due to other people's adverse response to the trans person's situation or
their inability to access the care they desire. Unless there are accompanying
psychological problems, there is no sense in which being trans is a mental illness. Yet, to obtain the desired medical treatment, most trans people must
sacrifice their sanity to the likes of psychiatrists and clinical psychologists who
are presumed to be experts in the diagnosis and treatment of gender identity
disorders. In many instances, these specialists are gatekeepers so that surgeons
who perform genital surgeries and other medical procedures for trans people
can be legally protected. Yet the ultimate outcome of pregnancy—childbirth—
is a much riskier medical procedure than any genital surgeries for trans folk!
A similar argument, also using pregnancy as a counterexample, has been made
by Christina Richards.[32]

Trying to diagnose any mental illness in otherwise healthy trans people may
be more challenging, especially when it is assumed that being trans is itself

sufficient. This is unfortunate as treating mental illness is vital for health and well-being. For one thing, some applicants consider that they have a right to hormone therapy and gender confirmation surgeries. They have learned to expect the various medical professionals involved in their treatment to act as gatekeepers whose primary role is to select candidates for medical or surgical therapy. Many applicants have mastered the scripts provided by successful peers who have managed to be approved for medical interventions. This, of course, is an undesirable situation that justifies the more widespread use of client-centered care for trans people who desire a medical transition.

A more enlightened approach to assisting gender-diverse people was sponsored by the Gender Identity Research and Educational Society (GIRES) in the United Kingdom in 2003 and coauthored by a group of international experts in the field chaired by Milton Diamond.[33] Advances based on these principles of humanity and concern for trans people's quality of life are evident in some current gender-affirming support procedures conducted at various gender centers throughout the world.

Many friends of the trans community deplore the unnecessary pathologization of gender-atypical behavior by the medical profession.[34] Such pathologization of their normal gender diversity can have devastating effects on trans people's self-esteem, especially if their medical records are shared with other professionals. Nevertheless, it is important to diagnose and treat psychiatric complications when they exist. The currently accepted medical prerequisites for transition are presented in Chapters 6 and 7.

5.7 PSYCHIATRIC COMPLICATIONS IN THE MEDICAL DIAGNOSIS OF GENDER INCONGRUENCE

Some trans people are offended by the medicalization of their situation, the implication being that they are mentally ill. Although their everyday lives are often complicated by accompanying medical conditions such as anxiety, post-traumatic stress, and depression, these afflictions are more likely the result of social isolation and relationship difficulties during transition rather than a consequence of these people's gender affirmation. People who are diagnosed with a mental illness, for example severe depression, are offered appropriate therapy leading to recovery. They can then progress more successfully through their transition treatment.

Often the client has read widely on hormone therapy and surgical procedures using Internet resources and books, as well as discussing the various procedures with people who have already undergone medical interventions. Perhaps the client has already self-diagnosed their condition and is seeking confirmation from medical consultants so that hormones can be prescribed. The diagnostician's task is difficult because clients might have learned the appropriate script for obtaining hormones after seeking advice from successful clients. As trans people try to present as disease-free as possible to obtain hormones and surgery, instances of depression may be underdiagnosed. This may lead to a missed opportunity to optimize mental health before or during transition.

Self-reference is rare in medical practice, most clients only seeking medical help when they are ill. With so much pressure placed on gender clinic personnel by eager aspirants for transition procedures, responsibility is required so that regret following surgery, a rare event, is minimized. This is undoubtedly the reason for gatekeeping and the maintenance of acceptable standards of care for those requesting medical assistance.[35]

Gender identity issues sometimes occur in people diagnosed with schizophrenia, some patients exhibiting delusional thought about proceeding with a sex change. These clients either should be excluded from medical transition or their progress should be delayed until the psychiatric problem has been reasonably well controlled. About 5 percent of those seeking genital surgeries have some symptoms of schizophrenia.[36] When a gender identity problem results from delusions accompanying undiagnosed schizophrenia, caution is required as, by the time antipsychotic medication has had its positive effects on the client's thought processes, they may regret hormonal and other treatments. However, such serious mental illnesses would be on a person's medical record before they request medical treatments to facilitate their transition. These problems are not usually associated with the transition process.

Delaying transition is not a neutral option. In their frustration, about 10 percent of preoperational trans women have attempted self-mutilation of the genitals, and 2 percent of trans men have attempted chest mutilation. A survey of 1,229 trans people from 48 states in the United States revealed a 32.4 percent lifetime attempted suicide rate and a 6.4 percent rate in the previous year. The attempted suicide rate was higher for trans men than for trans women, and for those who were nonwhite and without a college education. Internalized transphobia and living in an unsupportive social environment increased the suicide risk.[37] Genital surgery can be a life-saving procedure as the suicide rate in trans women is about 20 percent prior to the surgery and as low as 1 percent afterward. Quality of life, as measured by subjective reports, improves for most trans people following genital surgery.

The mental health of 180 twenty-year-old trans people from a community center in the United States that would attract mainly those who were poor and probably with inadequate educational experiences showed a twofold to threefold increase in depression, anxiety disorder, as well as self-harm incidents and suicide attempts prior to transition when compared with cisgender people of a similar age. There were no differences in any of these risks for those trans people who identified as either male or female.[38]

In a 2014 Australian survey of 189 young gender-diverse people aged 14 to 25 years, 73 percent of whom were birth-assigned females, most of those submitting the survey identified as genderqueer, boy/man, girl/woman, or genderfluid. The average age at which these young people started questioning their gender identity was 14 years. The most common pronouns used by these young people were *She*, *He*, and the singular *They*, and half of them were either queer or pansexual in their sexual orientation. Three-quarters of these young people had completed or were continuing a social transition and 26 percent were undertaking a medical transition. Forty percent were still unsure about whether they wanted a medical transition. These young people suffered the same kind of discrimination and bullying in school and elsewhere that other gender-diverse young people have had to endure. About 40 percent of the sample were suffering from anxiety and/or depression with around 30 percent having had suicidal thoughts at some previous time. Most of these young people avoided public toilets and changing rooms, and their involvement in other aspects of a normal social life was restricted in fear for their safety. In most cases, relief from this distress was obtained by chatting with friends either in person or online, including being engaged in activism, and partaking in activities by themselves such as listening to music, creating artwork, and reading. Sixty percent of those who reported that they were suffering depression did not feel supported by their family.[39]

The Trans Pathways online survey[40] of 859 young trans people aged 14 to 25 and 194 parents and guardians was conducted in Australia in 2017. About three-quarters of the gender-diverse young people who answered the survey were birth-assigned females; 58 percent of these had socially transitioned, 28 percent were on hormone therapy, and another 34 percent would like to be on hormone therapy at some later date. Six percent had undergone gender-affirming surgeries and 21 percent indicated that they would like to be offered surgical options in the future. In terms of their mental health, 75 percent of the trans people reported ever having been diagnosed with depression and anxiety. More serious mental illnesses suffered by around 20 percent of these young trans people were post-traumatic stress disorder, personality disorders, psychosis, neurodiversity on the autism spectrum, and an eating disorder. Alcohol and tobacco use was quite high, but the most disturbing finding was the 80 percent of young trans people who reported self-harming and the 48 percent who had attempted suicide at some time in the recent past. The report showed that 44 percent of parents realized that their child was trans when they were an adolescent, and 27 percent had realized that their child was trans much earlier when their child was five or younger. Most of the young trans people reported that they were pansexual, suggesting that their sexual and gender identifications were somewhat unconventional.

Of most concern to young people in the Trans Pathways survey were their distress with their body, peer rejection, discrimination and bullying, lack of family support, and homelessness, as well as sexual and physical abuse. The most frequent ways these young trans people could gain emotional and social support were being with friends and family, taking part in musical and artistic activities, and connecting with others using social media. When they were able to obtain medical help, about 57 percent of the young trans people were satisfied with what they received from their family doctor and a counselor, but only 43 percent were satisfied with the help they had received from a psychiatrist.

A Canadian study surveyed 323 trans people aged 14 to 18 years and an older group of 600 people aged 19 to 25. The younger group contained 11 percent trans women, 47 percent trans men, and 42 percent nonbinary people. In the older sample, 20 percent were trans women, 40 percent were trans men, and 40 percent were nonbinary. Mental health problems were evident in this survey, being significantly more likely in the younger group who were still at school. Having experienced stress was an issue for these young trans people as 65 percent of them had contemplated suicide. The suicidal thought rate was 74 percent for the older group, with mental health issues far exceeding those reported for cisgender people their age.[41] Compared with binary-gendered trans youth, nonbinary trans youth, who are mostly birth-assigned females, experienced a lower rated mental health and reported more incidents of self-harm. They were less likely to have a family doctor who understood their situation and with whom they could feel comfortable. Compared with binary-gendered trans youth, fewer nonbinary youth believed that hormone therapy was always necessary to live their lives the way they wanted.[42]

A 2012 study conducted by the Scottish Transgender Alliance received responses from 912 trans people, 60 percent of whom had a reasonably stable trans gender identity with 51 percent reporting their sexual orientation as either queer or bisexual. Whereas most of the respondents who had not transitioned were not satisfied with their life so far, those who had transitioned were mostly satisfied with how things were going. Slightly more than half of these trans people were on hormone therapy. Most of these people reported that hormone therapy had improved the appearance of their bodies and the quality of their lives. Almost 90 percent of these trans people thought that having surgeries would be beneficial.

Those with a nonbinary gender identity reported being the most nervous about social situations when compared with those who had a binary male or female identity. Most of these trans people had experienced hurt from family and some friends, but only a small number of them had experienced more serious instances of abuse and discrimination. Feelings of ill-ease were limited to their doctor's lack of knowledge about transgender care, and people referring to them by using the wrong pronoun. About 40 percent of these trans people had been prescribed antidepressants, 55 percent had been diagnosed with depression, and 38 percent had been diagnosed with anxiety.

About a quarter of those surveyed by the Scottish Transgender Alliance had had adverse experiences when consulting a mental health professional, such as being diagnosed unnecessarily with a mental illness and being asked uncomfortable questions about their sexual behavior. About half of them reported some type of abuse when they were younger than 16, including 19 percent reporting sexual abuse. The incidence of self-harm was lower following transition, while suicidal thoughts affected 63 percent of those surveyed before transition but only 3 percent following transition. Of considerable concern, 35 percent of those responding to the survey had made at least one suicide attempt. The proportion of people who were out to others regarding their trans status exceeded 50 percent for friends and close family members, but fewer than 50 percent of them had outed themselves to extended family, people in their workplace, and to members of some other social groups. The most supportive people were a spouse if they had one and their trans friends. Overall, transition produced a significant increase in life satisfaction, less avoidance of public spaces, reduced depression and a decreased use of mental health services, fewer thoughts of self-harm and suicide, and an improved sex life.[43]

Young trans people with good support from their family and others, including at school, were four times more likely to report good mental health and far less likely to contemplate suicide than trans people without such support. Poverty and hunger were issues for about 20 percent of these vulnerable young people and homelessness was a real risk. Most of them felt uncomfortable discussing their situation with a doctor, so much so that they did not raise their gender issues, especially if they did not want their parents to know about them. Those at school felt much safer in the library than they did in the washroom and changing room. Discrimination from others was an issue, especially with respect to their gender identity and physical appearance. What young trans people need most is support from their families, safer schools, and knowledgeable and accessible health care services.[44]

In an Australian study published in 2014, trans students who attended a single-sex school were unable to wear a uniform that reflected their gender identity, were subjected to transphobic violence, and were often forced to change schools. Thoughts of self-harm and suicide were important factors affecting the mental health of these young people.[45]

Disorders along the autistic spectrum have been observed in some young gender-diverse people. The prevalence of autistic spectrum disorders for cisgender children was estimated as 1.1 percent in the United Kingdom with slightly more than four times as many males as females being affected. A recent review suggests that the prevalence of autistic spectrum disorders in gender-diverse young people may be as high as 8 percent, but the sample sizes for these studies conducted by gender clinics are small.[46]

In a sample of 394 gender-diverse people 18 years and older, birth-assigned females scored higher on a test of autistic tendencies than did birth-assigned males, a finding that was opposite what has been observed in the cisgender population. The average autism score for those who identified as transsexual was 4.6, with an associated 95 percent confidence interval [4.2,5.0], and the average autism score for those identifying as genderqueer was 5.7, with an associated 95 percent confidence interval [5.2,6.3],[47] indicating that those identifying as genderqueer are more likely to lie on the autistic spectrum than those identifying as transsexual. Nevertheless, it is possible that the test used in this study to assess autistic spectrum disorder is more appropriately contrasting those who prefer an orderly object-based lifestyle to one that is more people-oriented and empathic, rather than it being useful for advancing our understanding of gender diversity.[48]

To summarize, evaluating the recently released ICD-11 diagnosis of gender incongruence using psychological criteria may be difficult because there are few individual difference characteristics that distinguish trans people reliably from others. For the few people who have been diagnosed with unrelated conditions such as schizophrenia and borderline personality disorder, those conditions should be controlled adequately before the client is offered hormone therapy or genital surgery.

SUMMARY

Providing affordable health care for trans people is important. Issues that require consideration include the problematic role of the gender professional as a gatekeeper, as many trans people feel they cannot always be honest in case they are excluded from a gender clinic program. A better alternative is a partnership approach in which the clinician assesses the client's capacity to provide informed consent after the trans person has been informed about the risks and benefits of medical interventions and understands the implications of these interventions for their future quality of life.

One of the problems faced by trans people is some medical practitioners' inexperience in transgender care. Patient information for both trans men and women should contain advice on medical aspects of their transition that empowers them to seek the care they need.

There is a dearth of scientific studies of the reliability and validity of the diagnostic criteria for gender incongruence and gender dysphoria, the two accepted diagnostic categories in 2019. Soon after starting cross-sex hormone treatment, trans people experience an improvement in their mental status, becoming less distressed and less anxious. With proper care and a satisfactory surgical result, postoperative regret among those proceeding to genital surgery is almost negligible.

Chapter 6

CHILDREN AND ADOLESCENTS

6.1 SUPPORT FOR GENDER-DIVERSE CHILDREN

Most children develop a gender identity that matches the sex that was assigned to them at birth, but transgender or gender-diverse children experience a difference or incongruence with this birth-assigned sex. A child may express or communicate their gender identity in an expansive way that does not fit with society's rigid expectations for someone of that birth-assigned sex, or they may be very clear and comfortable about their non-birth-assigned gender identity.

Gender identity develops progressively during childhood and adolescence, but gender forms part of self-identity very early, perhaps by the time the child is four. Early adolescence is another particularly important time, when young people begin to interact independently with their peers, society, and culture; this social interaction provides further insights and solidifies their emerging gender identity.[1] Gender diversity has always been part of the human experience and is not a disorder or disease.

Childhood Trajectory

Parents and families naturally want to know who their children will grow up to be, and this includes asking whether their gender-diverse child will grow up to be a gender-diverse adult. They may have concerns that society will expect their children to identify with the binary gender they were assigned at birth and that some people will consequently respond negatively. Studies that have followed children into adulthood have reported widely varying conclusions about this trajectory for a number of methodological reasons.[2] So, just as for other aspects of their child's life, parents are asked to exert patience around their child's gender identity. Winters et al. suggest that "changes and developments are to be expected (and celebrated) and not seen as destiny of their future identities."[3] Rather than predicting the future, the focus should be on whether young people are achieving their potential and whether they are getting the care they need.

Most of the available information about transgender health care has originated from the small group of young people attending specialist gender clinics. In the last decade, there have been four large studies from centers in Toronto, Canada,[4] and Amsterdam, The Netherlands.[5] These studies have followed the progress of gender-expansive children who were referred to specialist centers and who continued to attend the clinic for follow-up. Two important findings from these studies were that (a) children who communicate intense feelings of distress about their assigned gender are most likely to maintain their identified gender and (b) early puberty, around 10 to 13 years, is a critical period during which physical changes and romantic attachments make gender identity an important consideration for the young person.

Many children are able to communicate their gender identity at a young age;[6] the average age for transgender children was eight years in one U.S. study. However, it is important to recognize that for some people their trans experience is first expressed or understood later in adolescence or adulthood,[7] and for others their identity may change over their lifespan. There is not one story that can represent all trans narratives. All young people, gender expansive, trans, or gender diverse, should have their individual experiences respected by their family, community, and health care providers in order to support their well-being.

Mental Health Support for Families and Children

Being transgender or gender diverse is not a mental health condition, and there is little evidence that it causes distress in itself. Indeed, not all children require ongoing care from a mental health professional, but care should be easily accessible for those families who would benefit. Unfortunately, internalized stigma and discrimination commonly result in anxiety, depression, and isolation.[8] Family assessment by a mental health provider can identify any areas in which parents or children require psychological or social support. Therapy may relieve family conflict and increase individual resilience, while building the capacity of caregivers to provide effective support. Gender-diverse and gender-nonconforming young people who are supported by their family have much better levels of mental health.[9] Indeed, as noted by the World

Health Organization, "there are individuals who today present for gender reassignment who may be neither distressed nor impaired. This may be particularly true for young adolescents who are aware of the possibility of gender transition, live in an accepting environment, and who can have access to puberty suppressing treatments until they are able to take such a decision."[10]

Models of Supportive Care for Children

Children and parents may benefit from the support of medical professionals, although no medical interventions are needed in childhood. The optimal level of support depends on the family's circumstances. In some centers clinicians currently provide support as a "watchful waiting" approach, in which full social transition is delayed, but the child has space to explore their gender identity until early puberty[11] and parents are encouraged to keep all future outcomes open.[12]

However, clinicians, children, and their families increasingly prefer a *gender-affirming* approach, where the child is supported to live in the gender role that feels most comfortable to them.[13] This approach "is not about encouraging a child towards any particular path but removing the obstacles that have been preventing them from living fully and freely."[14] Children with *insistent, consistent,* and *persistent* communication of their gender incongruence have the right to assert their need for an early social transition to allow their gender role to become consistent with their identity. This allows the child to choose their preferred clothes and hairstyles, use the bathrooms and changing rooms that match their gender identity, and ask others to use their name and affirming pronouns such as *he, she,* or *they.* If the environment allows safe social transition, the child may choose to disclose their gender identity to their community.

Evidence shows that gender-affirming care is associated with improved well-being.[15] The North American TransYouth Project assessed a group of 63 binary-gender-identified trans children aged 6 to 14 years old and compared their mental health and self-worth with cis siblings and other children of the same age and gender. The trans children had socially transitioned in all contexts, such as in the home, at school, and in public. Both the children and their parents reported good mental health; levels of depression were no different from those found in the cis children, although slightly higher levels of anxiety were noted in the trans children. The authors comment that the findings were "in striking contrast to previous work with gender-nonconforming children who had not socially transitioned."[16]

Every child is unique and must of course be treated depending on their stage of gender development and their family context. Most importantly, children should not be discouraged or punished for demonstrating gender-variant behavior. It should be noted that any therapy aimed at altering gender identity, known as reparative or conversion therapy, is considered unethical and ineffective, and may cause long-term harm.[17] The ultimate goal should be to support a healthy, happy child.

Diagnostic Quandaries

The World Health Organization (WHO) has announced a revision of the International Classification of Diseases and Related Health Problems (ICD-11) to include a change in the classification of gender identity. They have moved to using the term *gender incongruence*, an acknowledgment that gender diversity is a normal human trait that also includes nonbinary individuals who may or may not wish to engage in medical or surgical intervention that personally affirms their gender. Unlike other classifications, such as in DSM-5, it does not require a person to suffer from any distress. In ICD-11, gender incongruence of adolescence and adulthood will not be placed in the chapter "Mental and Behavioral Disorders," where *transsexualism* was located, but will be placed in a new chapter titled "Conditions Related to Sexual Health." This is a positive paradigm shift in the way professionals view gender diversity.

A similarly placed diagnosis of *gender incongruence in childhood* has been proposed for the ICD-11 classification. This is contentious as it is questionable whether children should be labeled unnecessarily during a natural part of development, in a period where they need no medical intervention.[18] Conversely, it has been proposed that having a diagnosis can improve access to pediatric clinicians, provide protection from discrimination, and facilitate research.[19]

Children who identify as trans or gender-diverse should be referred to a pediatrician or pediatric endocrinologist promptly so that, if needed, they can pause puberty, as we will see in the next section, and avoid the development of body changes that conflict with their concept of self. It can be very distressing for children to experience or even anticipate body changes that do not align with their gender identity. There is strong evidence to suggest that mental health and well-being is improved for trans young people accessing puberty-blocking and gender-affirming care.

6.2 PHYSICAL AND HORMONAL ASPECTS OF PUBERTY

Puberty is the stage in a person's life during which they mature from childhood to adulthood. Hormones have a powerful effect on the physiological processes required for sexual development, growth, and metabolism. When puberty begins, a hormone called *gonadotrophin-releasing hormone* (GnRH) is

Table 6.1 The Stages of Breast Development

Tanner Stage	Breast Development
1	Prepubertal—no development
2	Breast and nipple elevated, with areola (the surrounding nipple) increased in diameter. On average this happens at 10.7 years.
3	Breast and areola enlarged, but without contour between the two
4	Nipple and areola form a mound with a contour with the breast
5	Mature breast with projecting nipple and an areola that is part of the breast contour

released in pulses from the hypothalamus into the hypophyseal circulation and acts on the anterior pituitary gland to release luteinizing hormone (LH) and follicle-stimulating hormone (FSH). These signals stimulate the synthesis and secretion of the sex hormones estrogen from the ovaries and testosterone from the testes. Estrogen and testosterone circulate around the body and bind to targets known as receptors on the cells of different organs. The physical changes of puberty develop as hormone levels rise, until eventually the person may become fertile and reproduce.

In young people assigned female at birth, the first sign of estrogen exposure is usually the development of breast buds that slowly progress toward a mature breast size and shape. The beginning of breast development coincides with a growth spurt and an increase in body fat. Hair develops gradually in the armpits and pubic region. The menstrual cycle indicated by monthly periods usually starts around two years later, after breast growth is well underway. During puberty, progesterone is not made until the ovaries have started to produce eggs, at a point when breast development has finished. The pubertal changes to chest, body shape, and height are irreversible once developed. The stages of breast development are described in Table 6.1.

The first change of puberty for those assigned male at birth is testicular growth. As shown in Table 6.2, a testes volume of 4 ml or more is considered to be evidence of puberty. When the testes volume reaches 10 ml, testosterone levels increase significantly and gradually result in an increase in penis size, a growth spurt, lowering of voice pitch, growth of facial hair, and increasing musculature. Mature sperm are usually not formed until the middle of puberty when the person is considered fertile. The lower voice pitch, Adam's apple, male hair pattern, final height, and change in bone structure in face, feet, and hands are irreversible once developed.

The age at which puberty takes place varies widely between individuals. In general, it usually happens between ages 8 and 16 years in people assigned

Table 6.2   The Development of Testicles and Penis in Adolescents

Tanner Stage	Testicles and Penis
1	Prepubertal—testicular size < 4 ml
2	Testicular size 4–6 ml; slight enlargement of penis and scrotum. On average this starts at around 11.5 years.
3	Testicular size 8–12 ml; penis lengthens
4	Testicular size 12–15 ml; penis lengthens/widens; scrotum darkens
5	Testicular size <15 ml; mature adult penis

female at birth and between ages 9 and 17 years in people assigned male at birth. The body changes are slow, and although sexual maturity is achieved in four to five years, the complete physical and mental changes may take longer.[20]

6.3 MEDICAL THERAPY IN ADOLESCENCE

Over the last decade, an increasing number of adolescents have been seeking medical therapy, perhaps because of a greater awareness of the availability of affirming care.[21] Gender-diverse youth are likely to seek initial support from their family doctor, mental health practitioners, or general pediatricians, so it is important that these professionals are ready to facilitate care. A recent study of 748 adolescents attending a specialist clinic in either Toronto or Amsterdam demonstrated a change in their referral patterns from 2006 to 2013. Previously more clinic attendees had people assigned male at birth, but recently people assigned female at birth had formed the majority.

Every individual's gender identity develops throughout infancy and childhood. During early puberty, gender identity becomes more concrete. The process of gender exploration at this age is influenced by many factors including the effect of physical changes during puberty, the experience of romantic attraction, and the influence of culture. Some individuals may have experienced long-standing gender incongruence from a young age, but for others, incongruence between their gender identity and assigned sex becomes apparent by the start of puberty or later. It is important to recognize that an adolescent may have taken years to develop their self-understanding, and only then feel prepared to disclose their gender identity to their family.

As the current generation is increasingly open to the concept of fluid expression, gender-diverse adolescents may not wish to seek medical intervention to change their body. However, for some the physical changes that happen at the start of puberty are distressing and need urgent intervention. At this point the young person and their family must consider the benefits and potential harms of medical therapy with the support of their clinical team.[22] This decision-making process usually starts with a psychological assessment, followed by discussion of reversible options such as GnRH blockers, partially reversible options using hormones, and irreversible options that include surgery. This stepwise approach seems to be safe and effective. Studies of adolescents in the Dutch specialist clinic that pioneered this model showed that all of the young people chose to proceed to gender-affirming surgery as adults, with a zero regret rate.[23] However, it is important to remember that these young people were part of the decision-making process and were well supported by their families and specialist team.

It may be difficult for trans youth to find competent gender-affirming health care. A U.S. study of 15 young people aged 14 to 22 years and 50 caregivers reported that they experienced many health care barriers including (a) only a few accessible trained pediatric providers; (b) a lack of culturally competent care, for example by misgendering and misnaming; (c) inconsistent use of medical protocols and guidelines; (d) uncoordinated care or gatekeeping; (e) limited or slow access to pubertal blockers and gender-affirming hormones; and (f) cost.[24]

The young person and their family deserve support and information when they do access services. A U.S. study showed that transgender and gender-nonconforming youth and their caregivers shared a number of common concerns.[25] Young people were most concerned about issues related to the transition, for example access to gender-affirming care and use of toilets and changing rooms, whereas caregivers were more concerned about safety and acceptance, as well as the problems caused by family rejection, bullying at school, and concerns about mental health.

Mental Health Support for Adolescents

An adolescent may live in an accepting and supportive environment or may have been rejected and stigmatized by their community. These external stresses may be extremely harmful. As is the case for anyone, their need for psychological care will be dependent on their individual resilience, emotional functioning, and support networks.[26] For trans youth, parental support is associated with better quality of life and protection against depression,[27] and unsurprisingly, the level of peer-group support is also an important predictor of mental health.[28]

For young people with a supportive family, an affirming environment (school and neighborhood), and an absence of mental health difficulties, a mental health provider may only need to provide an initial assessment or plan for medical transition. Other people may benefit from regular review with their mental health professional.

Resilience and positive coping strategies are particularly important for young people that live in intolerant communities.[29] Early puberty is a particularly vulnerable time for deterioration in mental health. A delay in providing gender-affirming treatment around this time is associated with a greater mental health burden[30] and an increase in self-medicating. Conversely, mental health usually improves with access to gender-affirming care,[31] perhaps because this avoids the emotional, social, and intellectual consequences of living in an incongruent gender role. Decisions about mental health care should be made collaboratively with the trans or gender-diverse young person.

Although the number of studies is not large, it is recognized that neurodiversity (autism spectrum) is more common among the transgender community.[32] Disordered eating behaviors are also more prevalent in people who identity as trans or gender-diverse.[33] People with autism or an eating disorder may benefit from mental health support. Guidelines have recently been developed for the care of people with co-occurring gender incongruence and neurodiversity.[34] Involving clinicians with the relevant diagnostic skills can be helpful for some people, as being able to identify as being on the autism spectrum can be helpful to understand behavior and learn strategies to manage any difficulties. Although some neurodiverse people may have difficulty in articulating their gender identity, this should not create an unnecessary barrier to accessing appropriate care. Instead, extra time and support may be helpful to navigate gender exploration and social, medical, and surgical transition.

There may be few mental health concerns for young people who access care and receive support. One study of consecutive referrals to the VU clinic in the Netherlands compared 86 adolescents aged 13 to 18 years and 293 trans adults aged 18 to 65 years using a Minnesota Multiphasic Personality Inventory questionnaire.[35] Most of the adolescents (68%) showed little or no evidence of any psychological dysfunction, an outcome that contrasted with the adult group. Thus, "early coming out and seeking care in adolescence (versus adulthood) might prevent some of the psychological burden that transgender individuals experience during their lives,"[36] perhaps because of access to puberty blockers that minimize the distress resulting from the physical changes of adolescence.

Models of Supportive Care for Adolescents

Some health services offer a coordinated multidisciplinary clinic in which the young person can access endocrinology, nursing care, psychiatry, psychology, and allied services in one place. Other health services deliver care using a network of clinicians coordinated by a primary care physician. A medical appointment is an opportunity to identify risk factors for future health including being overweight and obese, physical activity levels, smoking, and drug use. If

Table 6.3 Common Steps in Gender Affirmation

Step	Possible Actions	Usual Age	Reversibility
Social transition	Gender-affirming clothes, hairstyles, name, and pronouns	Any age	Reversible
Legal transition	School records and identity documents	Any age*	Reversible
Puberty blockers	GnRH analogs	Young adolescents	Reversible
Hormone therapy	Testosterone and estrogen	Adolescents and adults	Partly reversible
Surgery	Chest, genital, facial	Adults (and some older adolescents)	Permanent

* Changes to some documents, e.g., birth certificates, will depend on local law.

a young person wants to start puberty blockers or gender-affirming hormones, they can discuss their options with the clinical team.[37] Individual goals for social and medical transition should be discussed and a plan made to meet these needs, as shown in Table 6.3.

6.3.1 Puberty Suppression (Stage 1 Treatment)

Puberty blockers are injectable gonadotrophin-releasing hormone (GnRH) analogs, a synthetic mimic of the hormone that controls sex hormones. This medication acts by overstimulating and desensitizing the GnRH receptors in the pituitary gland to stop hormone signaling to the ovaries and testicles by luteinizing hormone (LH) and follicle-stimulating hormone (FSH), as shown in Figure 6.1. This causes a gradual fall in estrogen and testosterone levels over several weeks and stops the further development of secondary sexual characteristics.

Puberty suppression is a relatively recent innovation, first used as a treatment for trans adolescents in 1998.[38] Prior to that, GnRH analogs had also been used to treat people in whom puberty has started too early, a condition known as precocious puberty. For trans young people, GnRH analogs can be commenced early in puberty at Tanner stage 2. This stage corresponds to the start of early breast development with breast bud formation and widening of the areola or enlargement of the testes to be greater than 4 ml. There is a wide normal range for the timing for this stage of puberty, but to be most effective the intervention should start quickly once the initial changes commence.

The effects of GnRH analogs are entirely reversible; if the injections are ever stopped, then the signals from the hypothalamus become reactivated. This

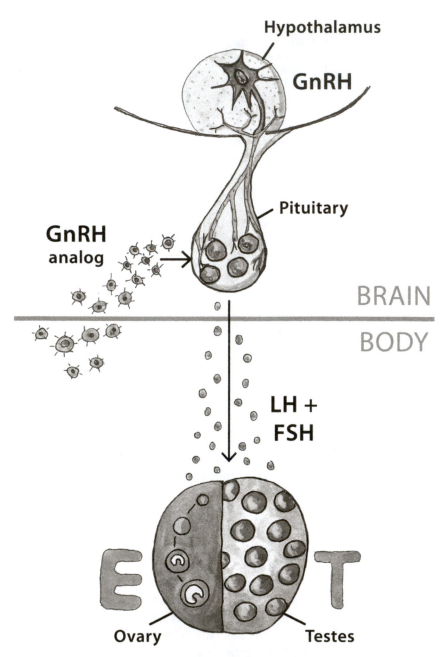

Figure 6.1 **The production of estrogen (E) and testosterone (T).** The hypothalamus produces gonadotropin-releasing hormone (GnRH), which signals the pituitary gland to produce luteinizing hormone (LH) and follicle-stimulating hormone (FSH). These hormones stimulate the production of estrogen from the ovary (granulosa cells) or testosterone from the testes (Leydig cells). GnRH analogs attach instead of native GnRH to desensitize the pituitary gland. This results in dampening down of the hormone signals and the eventual reduction in estrogen and testosterone levels.

potential for reversibility may allow the young person time to develop the capacity to consent before starting gender-affirming hormone therapy.[39] Guidelines recommend that adolescents wanting puberty suppression, and who meet criteria for diagnosis and treatment, should be given GnRH analogs. In general, the criteria include:

1. Persistent and well-documented gender incongruence.

2. Evidence of the physical changes of puberty: Tanner stage 2 or above (breast buds or testicular volume greater than 4 ml and biochemical evidence of puberty, e.g., luteinizing hormone ≥ 0.5 IU/l).

3. A consensus that treatment is appropriate.

GnRH analogs are designed to prevent further development of unwanted physical characteristics of the birth-assigned sex. If the injections are started early, it may cause certain features to regress, resulting, for example, in a slight reduction in testicular size or breast tissue volume.[40] In later puberty beyond Tanner stage 2, GnRH analogs can still prevent progressive testosterone-induced masculinization of the face and stop periods, a condition known as amenorrhea. Although the changes of puberty cease, the other modalities of growth and development continue, including the expected increases in weight and height.

GnRH analogs can be given in a variety of formulations, for example a Goserelin 10.8 mg subcutaneous implant administered every 10 to 12 weeks; a Leuprorelin 22.5 mg or 30 mg intramuscular injection administered every three to four months; and a Triptorelin 22.5 mg intramuscular injection administered every five to six months. Puberty blockade is extremely effective for people in whom the physical changes of puberty are causing distress. Puberty suppression may also reduce the need for or invasiveness of future surgical procedures, for example chest surgery for men and facial feminization surgery for women. Puberty suppression can also enhance the effectiveness of gender-affirming hormones to produce the desired physical changes when these begin at a later stage.

Long-term outcome studies of puberty suppression are not available as GnRH analogs have only been available over the last 20 years. However, available evidence from the Netherlands suggests that therapy improves symptoms of depression and enhances psychological functioning.[41] A follow-up study of 201 young people referred to a U.K. clinic also showed better psychological functioning after starting GnRH therapy.[42]

There are a number of potential adverse effects that should be weighed against the benefits when starting GnRH analogs. The therapy is usually well tolerated. However, a chart review of 27 Canadian young people aged 14.7 years who were prescribed GnRH analogs in a Vancouver clinic showed that one person had a noninfected sterile abscess at the injection site; one reported self-limiting leg pains and headaches; and one overweight person gained 19 kg weight. Only one person needed to cease therapy, in this case because of emotional lability.[43] Depletion of estrogen may increase blood pressure; three separate cases have been reported of GnRH analog therapy causing hypertension.[44]

Final Height

GnRH analogs can affect height and make a person slightly taller if administered before the onset of the pubertal growth spurt, unless stage 2 gender-affirming hormones are commenced. This is because the bones do not stop growing until the growth plates are exposed to estrogen or testosterone. The most important factor for final height, apart from parental height, will be the timing of the commencement of these gender-affirming hormones. Growth measurements, including height, weight, and pubertal or Tanner stage, are usually measured at clinic visits. Measurement of skeletal age, using an annual hand X-ray, can indicate how much growth potential remains. Timely treatment with estrogen results in a final height in a female reference range. Administration of androgens can result in a growth spurt and then fusion of the growth plates to produce a height consistent with a male reference range. After hormonal treatment, body proportions, as measured by sitting height and sitting height/height ratios, remain in the normal ranges.

Bone Health

One potential concern with the use of GnRH analogs in early puberty is their potential impact on bone mineralization, a predictor of future bone health, osteoporosis, and fracture. Adolescence and young adulthood is a key time for building up bone minerals as 85 to 90 percent of total bone mass will have been acquired at the end of puberty. Sex hormones have a pivotal role in the accumulation of this bone mass. Indeed, estrogen and testosterone are important for bone mineralization across the whole lifespan.

One study of 34 trans boys and 22 trans girls followed bone health using densitometry measurement during GnRH analog therapy with Triptorelin subcutaneous injections every four weeks started from early puberty onward, and then hormone therapy with incremental doses of testosterone as Sustanon or estrogen as 17β estradiol commenced at age 16 years.[45] During puberty suppression, there was an initial slowing of bone turnover and a slight reduction in the bone mineral density of the lower lumbar spine when compared with a U.K. reference population using matched age and sex assigned at birth. This finding was most evident for the younger trans women with a bone age less than 14 years. Once estrogen therapy was started, there was an increase in bone mineral density, particularly in the lumbar spine for trans women. After 24 months of hormone therapy the bone mineral density of the group had recovered, but not quite to the relative pretreatment level when compared with their peers.

The long-term effect of puberty blockade on bone health and fracture risk is unknown. Reassuringly, a report of one 35-year-old trans man, who commenced GnRH analogs aged 13 years and testosterone therapy aged 17 years, showed that after 22 years of therapy his bone density was in the normal range.[46]

Current guidelines recommend monitoring of bone density, adequate calcium and vitamin D supplementation if needed, and encouragement of weight-bearing exercise. Clinicians should consider early commencement of gender-affirming hormones in adolescents with evidence of reduced bone mineral density. There are no data available on the lifetime risk of bone fractures.

Brain Development

Puberty is a time in which the brain develops rapidly and reorganizes, providing improved skills for complex decision-making, a process that resides in the prefrontal cortex and relies on what is known as executive functioning. There are theoretical concerns that GnRH analogs could influence these developmental changes, as sex hormones are known to be important in the development of executive functioning. One study of 20 trans young people taking GnRH analogs compared their ability to complete the "Tower of London" task, one that requires adequate executive functioning, with 45 cis young people.[47] There was no evidence of detrimental effects of GnRH analogs on this task in either trans boys or trans girls. Similarly, the trans man described above who had taken GnRH analogs followed by 22 years of testosterone therapy showed no negative effects on brain function.

Fertility

Fertility counseling should be provided to all adolescents before commencing puberty suppression or gender-affirming hormones. The information should be communicated in a way consistent with their developmental stage and understanding of reproduction; this may be difficult in the younger age group.[48] This topic is discussed comprehensively in Chapter 8.

Alternatives to GnRH Analogs

Recently, GnRH antagonists such as elagolix and degarelix have been developed. These are nonpeptide molecules that can be taken as oral tablets. The use of this medication has not been assessed specifically as puberty suppression for trans young people. However, it has been successfully used to lower testosterone in men with prostate cancer[49] and estrogen in women with endometriosis.[50]

Therapies not based upon GnRH should be discussed with adolescents who have reached later puberty in Tanner stage 3 or greater. The benefits of GnRH analogs are fewer if many of the physical changes of puberty have already taken place, and the higher cost of GnRH analogs may not be covered by the local health services. Therefore, in trans girls, anti-androgens such as spirono-lactone and cyproterone acetate may be used, whereas in trans boys, progester-one as medroxyprogesterone, lynestrenol, or norethisterone can be used to suppress menstrual cycles; the combined oral contraception pill is less success-ful for this purpose as it contains estrogen.

One study of 45 Belgian trans boys in late puberty during Tanner stages 4 and 5 used lynestrenol as a progestin therapy. Pubertal hormones, such as endogenous gonadotrophins, were partly suppressed as intended, but irregular menstrual bleeding was common.[51] The same research group used cyproterone acetate as the only therapy in 27 trans girls at a similar stage of puberty, but who were unable to commence estrogen for at least six months. They had a successful reduction in hair growth, and some mild breast development equiv-alent to Tanner stages 2 and 3 occurred in 30 percent of users, which was appreciated as a significant positive for them.[52]

Nonmedical therapies may also be helpful interventions for many trans and gender-diverse young people. Chest binding in trans men and padding of the hips, buttocks, or breasts in trans women are often part of social transition. Safe chest binding practices should be encouraged and include using a prop-erly fitted binder, ensuring occasional days without binding, and using tape that does not cause skin irritation or difficulty in breathing.[53] Genital tucking for trans women or packing by use of a penile prosthesis for trans men may also support socially affirming gender.

6.3.2 Gender-Affirming Hormonal Therapy (Stage 2 Therapy)

Masculinizing therapy using testosterone and feminizing therapy with estro-gen can be given as synthetic versions of the natural hormones. These gender-affirming hormone therapies reduce the levels of the person's own sex hormones, if present, and replace them with hormones consistent with their gender identity. These hormones promote the development of secondary sex-ual characteristics such as facial hair, voice pitch, fat distribution, and muscle mass. The physical changes are gradual and occur over a similar duration and order as the changes seen in spontaneous puberty.

Hormonal treatment can be started when the young person wants to and the prescribing physician gains their informed consent. This capacity may be determined by the legal age of majority, which varies in different countries, or it may be based on *Gillick competency* when the individual can make their own decisions. As hormone therapy is only partially reversible, it is usual for there to be:

1. Persistent and well-documented gender incongruence.
2. A fully informed decision and consent to treatment.
3. Good physical and mental health (or appropriately managed health conditions).
4. A consensus that treatment is appropriate.

There is a well-established body of evidence for those aged 16 years and older showing that gender-affirming hormones reduce distress, increase comfort with physical appearance, and, importantly, improve mental health and well-being outcomes. This does not mean hormone therapy should necessarily be delayed until the young person is 16 years old. Many clinics are starting to provide gender-affirming hormonal treatment from the age of 14 years,[54] driven partly by clinician concern that delays increase the chances of mental health problems for the young people awaiting therapy. For those on GnRH analog therapy, the delay in hormone therapy may have a further psychological cost as their physical changes lag behind those of their peers, and there is a potential physical cost to their bone mineralization and final height. Prolonged pubertal suppression for more than four years is not recommended, which could certainly occur if a young person started puberty early and their hormone therapy was delayed until later in adolescence. Some authors have argued that commencing hormones at the age of 14 years is still late, as by this age most people have completed puberty. Currently, there is minimal published experience of the safety or benefit of starting hormone therapy before 14 years of age.

The aim of gender-affirming hormone therapy is to achieve the physiological levels measurable in cisgender people of the affirmed gender. Without ongoing lifelong hormone therapy, most physical changes will regress over one to two years. Some changes are permanent, particularly testosterone-induced facial hair growth and estrogen-induced breast development.

Testosterone

Testosterone can be given topically through the skin as a cream or gel, as a tablet, or as a short-acting injection administered every 1 to 4 weeks or as a long-acting injection administered every 10 to 14 weeks. The availability of preparations often differs according to the local health system. Trans boys in early to mid-puberty during Tanner stages 2 to 3 or who have received puberty suppression should be commenced on an initial low dose of testosterone, for example, 0.5 ml or 125 mg intramuscular testosterone enanthate every 2 to

4 weeks. Alternative dosing by body surface area, calculated from height and weight (using: www.rch.org.au/genmed/clinical_resources/Body_Surface_Area _BSA_Calculator), is a 25 mg/m² intramuscular injection every 2 weeks, increasing by 25 mg/m² every 3 to 6 months up to a dose of 100 mg/m², or depending on size, up to 250 mg intramuscularly every 2 to 4 weeks, increasing to these full doses over 1 to 2 years. Transdermal testosterone preparations can also be used to increase the levels of testosterone gradually. For example, testosterone 1% (12.5 mg per actuation) as a gel pump can be increased every 3 to 6 months from a single actuation, to two actuations, then up to a full dose of four actuations; similarly testosterone 5% (50 g/ml) cream can be increased every 3 to 6 months from 1 ml on alternate days to 1 ml each day, then 2 mls daily. As an alternative, patients may then choose to change to a longer-acting injectable preparation of testosterone undecanoate. Trans men who have almost completed puberty by Tanner stages 4 and 5 may similarly start on these initial low doses or commence a full physiological dose from the start of therapy depending on their preference and the clinical situation.

The physiological effects of testosterone start at different times. An increase in skin oiliness, acne, and a redistribution of body fat may be apparent in the first few months, but takes several years to reach maximum. Menses generally cease within six months of testosterone treatment. The clitoris begins to elongate but does not develop to the same size as a penis in a birth-assigned male. Other physical changes, such as a lowering of voice pitch, increasing muscle strength, and facial and body hair growth, start after several months and continue to develop over years. These changes are described in detail in Chapter 7. The effects of testosterone therapy on facial and body hair growth, scalp hair loss, voice change, clitoral enlargement, and vaginal atrophy are unlikely to be reversible if testosterone is ceased.

At the beginning of therapy, testosterone levels are not high enough to suppress puberty alone. GnRH analogs should be continued for at least six months after starting testosterone. Likewise, if norethisterone is being used to prevent menstruation, it should be continued for a similar duration. If the combined oral contraceptive has been used, although this is not recommended, it should be ceased, as the estrogen will oppose the effects of testosterone. As testosterone does not necessarily cause infertility, trans boys should be counseled to use adequate contraception if their sexual behavior puts them at risk of pregnancy, particularly as testosterone is harmful or teratogenic to a fetus.

Estrogen

Estrogen should be administered as estradiol or 17β-estradiol. Estrogen can be given, for example, as a tablet of estradiol valerate, or it can be delivered topically through the skin as a daily gel or in the form of transdermal patches changed twice a week. Like testosterone, the available preparations differ according to the local health system. Estrogen therapy is initially given at low doses, for example 6.25 mcg or a quarter of a 25 mcg/day estrogen patch or oral tablets starting at 5mcg/kg/day. An increase in dose can be made every 3 to 6 months by doubling the patch, or by increasing the dose by 5 mcg/kg/day up to 20 mcg/kg/day. Once a dose of 25 mcg/day is reached, this can then be switched to a full dose of 2 mg oral daily and titrated until target physiological levels of estrogen are achieved. This gradual approach replicates the incremental changes in spontaneous puberty and has been found in cisgender girls to produce optimal breast development. A rapid exposure to high levels of estrogen can result in a conical breast shape. There are no available studies at the current time that demonstrate that any one of the possible approaches to prescribing estrogen is preferable to any other for trans girls.

The physiological effects of estrogen therapy begin in the first few months of treatment. These early effects often include a reduced libido and decreased spontaneous erections. This is followed by softening of the skin and reduced oiliness. Over several months and years a range of other physical changes become increasingly noticeable. These include decreased muscle mass and redistribution of body fat, a reduction in testicular volume, and gradual breast growth. The effect of estrogen on breast growth reaches maximum over one to two years and is not reversible. The physical effects of estrogen are discussed in detail in Chapter 7.

Estrogen alone is usually not always sufficient to suppress testosterone to a female reference range level. If GnRH analogs have been used for puberty blocking, they should be continued if possible. If GnRH analogs are not being taken or are not funded, then a testosterone or androgen blocker, for example spironolactone 50 to 200 mg daily or cyproterone acetate 12.5 to 50 mg daily, should be used in conjunction with the estrogen therapy. Estrogen usually impairs spermatogenesis, but its effect is unpredictable and so consideration of contraception may be relevant depending on the sexual behavior of the adolescent.

6.3.3 Hormone Regimens for Nonbinary People

There has been little exploration of specific hormonal treatment regimens for nonbinary people. As it is almost impossible to forecast the exact nature and timing of physiological changes associated with hormone therapy, it can be difficult to best support the physical changes sometimes desired by nonbinary people while controlling for those that are not desired. For example, there is no way to lower voice pitch without increasing body hair growth. Hormones are important for health, so prolonged GnRH analog therapy without gender-affirming hormones or providing androgen blockers without an estrogen replacement may lead to osteoporosis and early-onset heart disease, as has been suggested by studies of cis people lacking hormone production. As there are no data on the outcomes of nonbinary hormone therapy, it is "extremely important to understand the person's expectations of physical changes to make sure they are realistic and accurate, and that they address the actual mind-body discrepancy that is causing distress to the person."[55] This may enable the prescribing physician to design the safest and most effective regimen for the individual. This issue is discussed in some detail in Chapter 7.

6.3.4 Monitoring

Hormone therapy should be regularly monitored in order to reduce the risk of potential side effects. In general, a clinical review including assessment of puberty in terms of Tanner stage should be undertaken every 3 to 6 months with a blood sample every 6 to 12 months. During puberty suppression, regular three-monthly monitoring of height, weight, and blood pressure and documentation of physical changes is helpful. A blood test can be taken that includes assays of gonadotrophin levels prior to the third dose of GnRH analog to confirm puberty suppression. If puberty is not adequately blocked, the interval of GnRH analog therapy can be decreased, or the dose increased. A laboratory measurement that includes a full blood count, as well as tests of renal and liver function, lipid, glucose, LH, FSH, estradiol, and testosterone should be taken annually. A bone mineral density measurement should be performed every one to two years, and an X-ray for bone age should be performed as appropriate to indicate whether the bone structure is typical for a person of that age.

The available evidence suggests that the use of GnRH analogs and gender-affirming hormones is very safe and effective. The main concern with estrogen is the slightly increased risk of a blood clot developing in a vessel. This is referred to as thromboembolism: deep vein thrombosis or pulmonary embolus. Testosterone can sometimes contribute to erythrocytosis, the development of too many red blood cells, which is routinely monitored on the laboratory profile. Further research is being undertaken to investigate the outcomes of long-term use of GnRH blockers and the use of gender-affirming hormones, particularly when they are started at a younger age. Although these medical therapies are commonly used in other conditions, they remain unlicensed in many health systems for use in transgender health care. The ongoing monitoring and available longer-term data from adults are discussed in Chapter 7.

6.4 SURGICAL INTERVENTIONS FOR ADOLESCENTS

Surgical interventions are usually only considered once an individual reaches the age of consent in a given country. Surgery is irreversible, so a careful assessment is needed to determine the benefits and explain the potential risks. Some large clinics have provided surgery to younger people under the age of 18 years.[56] The most common surgical procedure undertaken by trans boys is chest reconstruction or *top* surgery.[57] Chest reconstructive surgery is regularly performed for people aged 16 years and older in countries where this is the age of majority for medical procedures. Guidelines recommend but do not mandate a year of testosterone therapy for adolescents before undergoing surgery.

A U.S. study reported the outcomes of 14 trans males aged 13.4 to 19.7 years who had chest surgery between 2013 and 2017. They had a high rate of satisfaction and five people had minor complications. These were not uncommon issues related to surgery, such as a temporary collection of fluid, a seroma, or blood, a hematoma, or the development of abnormal or keloid scar tissue. Most men reported reduced or complete loss of sensation in the nipple area. Notably, the young people reported a reduced level of anxiety and depression after surgery.

Genital or *bottom* surgery is sometimes performed under the age of 18 years. Completion of at least a year of hormone therapy is recommended, as it is for adults. As this is major surgery that can result in permanent infertility and changes to sexual function, it requires careful decision-making beforehand. For young people who have received GnRH analogs in early puberty before Tanner stage 4, it may be more challenging to form a vagina using the surgical technique of vaginoplasty because of the reduced amount of skin available from the penis and scrotum. If this is the case, tissue expanders, such as a graft from the skin or if necessary, ileum or sigmoid intestine can be used to create the new vagina known as the neovagina.[58] Similarly, forming a penis using the surgical technique known as phalloplasty may be easier after having been exposed to estrogen, due to the hormonal effect on the structural integrity of the vagina and epithelial tissue.

If genital surgery is performed for a young trans adult, lifelong estrogen or testosterone therapy will still be needed. However, if the testes have been removed using orchidectomy, there is no further need for GnRH analogs or androgen blockers. The follow-up studies of adults who have accessed hormonal and surgical treatment show good longer-term outcomes, and very few have any regrets about surgery. In a Dutch clinic, no young people dropped out of the program or regretted their transition.[59]

6.5 FROM PEDIATRICS TO ADULT CARE

Transition to adult services can be difficult for any adolescent. They may have forged a therapeutic relationship with their pediatric team over many years. In particular, trans or gender-diverse adolescents may have only just begun gender-affirming hormones when they meet a new clinical team. Many young trans or gender-diverse people report challenges in their educational environment, and entry to adulthood is a time when they may need outside advocacy with their college or workplace. A competent clinician should coordinate the effective handover of care.

Most young people succeed and grow into healthy and productive adults, and trans or gender-diverse people are no different. A prospective study from the Netherlands[60] reported the mental health outcomes of 22 trans women and 33 trans men who had accessed GnRH therapy in early to middle puberty at Tanner stages 2 and 3 when they were 14.8 years old, hormone therapy at 16.7 years, and gender-affirming surgery at 20.7 years. When the group had started GnRH analogs, they had been assessed to ensure they were well supported. With access to transition care, health and well-being outcomes improved, and distress ceased. As adults, their measures of well-being, satisfaction, and happiness were similar or better than those observed in cis adults of the same age.

SUMMARY

The experience of accessing gender-affirming health care for trans or gender-diverse children and their families should be supportive and center the human rights of the child. The young person should feel able to express their identity as they grow into adulthood. There is no test that can predict the future gender identity of a child. There are observed gender differences in the toys and playmates chosen by young children, but there is a wide and normal variation in behavior for both trans, gender-diverse, and cis children. By early adolescence gender identity is usually well established. Therefore, the best and only test of gender identity is to ask the young person.

Medical therapy is not required until early adolescence. At that point, young people may need GnRH analogs to prevent the irreversible changes of puberty. Sex hormones can then be given to gradually change the body so that it is congruent with the young person's gender identity. Some surgical interventions are available in late adolescence when the individual can consent to treatment. Trans or gender-diverse young people who are supported and have access to gender-affirming health care have the best health and outcomes.

Chapter 7

HORMONE AND SURGICAL THERAPIES FOR ADULTS

7.1 MEDICAL ASSESSMENT

The social, medical, and surgical goals of therapy should be individualized for each trans or gender-diverse (TGD) person planning transition. Rather than considering whether the person is a trans man, trans woman, or a nonbinary individual and assuming their needs, each person's own goals should be addressed in terms of their aspiration for feminization, masculinization, or desire to move toward androgyny. Social transition with changes in clothing, cosmetics, and behavior may be sufficient to affirm gender. However, many people desire medical transition with hormone therapy and/or surgical intervention to alter their physical appearance to match their gender identity. There is no predetermined sequence for this transition, and surgery may be desired without hormonal intervention, or hormones may be offered without social transition, and so on.

International standards of care are available to guide clinicians when providing care to the TGD community.[1] A variety of health professionals may be included in the facilitating team, including a general practitioner, nurse specialist, endocrinologist, sexual health physician, speech therapist, urologist, gynecologist, counselor, psychologist, or psychiatrist, as needed. Mental health review may be helpful, as TGD people experience a disproportionate burden of mental health conditions, including anxiety and depression resulting from their experience of societal stigma and discrimination. It is important that culturally competent mental health services are available and accessible to those who can benefit from their care, but that this approach is not mandated as it may act as a barrier to transgender health services.

It is important to recognize that TGD people may avoid or delay accessing clinical care because they perceive, or have experienced, discrimination by health providers.[2] It is not surprising that people who have a poor experience of health providers have worse medical outcomes. It is encouraging that an increasing number of health services are starting to deliver a respectful and safe environment. For the individual, it is important to find a supportive clinical environment in which to receive care.

People may decide to socially transition before or after initiating hormone therapy. Often, the decision to start hormone therapy is the precipitant for a first consultation with a health professional. There are different models for the initiation of hormone therapy. In the context of a specialist gender service, a comprehensive assessment may occur in a multidisciplinary clinic including a therapeutic plan from a mental health professional to provide support during the transition process. Alternatively, the TGD individual may start hormonal treatment with an experienced physician, such as a GP, endocrinologist, sexual health consultant, or some other specialist as part of an informed consent process without necessarily meeting a mental health professional. Community health centers in the United States, for example Callen Lorde, New York, or Fenway Community Health, Boston, and Equinox in Melbourne, Australia, are examples of this model in which TGD people identity their own needs and choose their own care options.[3] The Endocrine Society Guidelines recommends, but does not demand, a mental health assessment to provide support for TGD adults undergoing medical transition. The WPATH Guidelines support both approaches. These guidelines provide a clear clinical framework for the delivery of transgender health care, but the management of gender incongruence still varies substantially around the world with respect to individual eligibility, funding, access, hormonal regimens, and service delivery.[4]

7.2 MEDICAL THERAPY

Hormone therapy is often the first medical step for people who seek to masculinize or feminize their body to align with their gender identity. A person starting on hormone therapy should understand the expected physical changes and approximately how long those changes take to develop, as explained later in this chapter. A clinician should discuss[5] the potential adverse effects in the context of the individual's medical history and the irreversible nature of some of the changes resulting from hormone therapy, such as voice-lowering with testosterone or breast development with estrogen. The clinical team may use written information to support this process. There are very few reasons why hormonal treatment needs to be delayed. These reasons include uncontrolled serious medical conditions, current or imminently planned pregnancy, or the presence of a hormone-sensitive cancer such as breast cancer.

The initial medical appointment for transition care usually includes an assessment of the person's general health and provides an opportunity to identify any modifiable health risks, such as being overweight or obese, smoking, high blood pressure, or high cholesterol. It is also an opportunity to ensure appropriate management for those with relevant medical problems including thrombosis, diabetes mellitus, liver disease, or vitamin D deficiency. A bone mineral density test may be conducted using a special X-ray; this test may be useful for older people or for those with a personal or family history of osteoporosis.

Evidence shows that there is a high prevalence of depression, anxiety, and suicidal ideation among TGD people who want to transition but either have not been able to or cannot access care. Treatment of any concurrent mental health conditions improves health outcomes after transition. There are data suggesting that commencement of hormone therapy itself improves mental health, psychological functioning, and quality of life. A systematic review published in 2016[6] identified three studies that measured psychological functioning and quality of life in 180 trans women and 67 trans men who were accessing hormone therapy. Two of these studies showed improved psychological functioning, as indicated by reduced depression, somatization, interpersonal sensitivity, anxiety, hostility, phobic anxiety, and agoraphobia after 3 to 6 months and after 12 months of therapy.[7] The third study[8] showed an improvement in quality of life after 12 months, an effect that was most clear for trans women and less so for trans men. The team from the Netherlands reported one trans women who regretted transition out of 162 adults who had accessed hormone treatment. She indicated that "professional guidance regarding adverse consequences (i.e. intolerance from society, family and her own children) would have made transition more endurable." This suggests that some trans people benefit from ongoing counseling and support during and after transition.[9]

The types of hormone therapy vary widely in different health systems due to cost and availability. As yet there are no data that suggest a particular type or route of therapy, whether it be oral, by injection, or by skin absorption, that is better at achieving masculinizing or feminizing physical changes. Therefore, the available patient safety data and personal preference of the individual are the key factors that guide the therapeutic plan. In terms of evidence of safety, estradiol or 17β estradiol, a synthetic estrogen, is generally used in preference to either conjugated equine estrogen or ethinyl estradiol, as these medications are both associated with an increased risk of thrombosis and cardiovascular disease, and they cannot be measured in blood samples to help guide doses.

In general, the aim of feminizing and masculinizing therapy is to adjust the dose of hormone medication until the blood levels are in the physiological range of the affirmed gender or for nonbinary individuals according to their goals, as is discussed further in Section 7.2.4. However, it should be remembered that the clinical affects and well-being of the person are the most important factors. Similar hormone levels can have dissimilar biological effects, due to the individual characteristics of the cellular structures that respond to hormonal signals, that is, the receptors, in different people.[10]

7.2.1 Physical Effects of Hormone Therapy

The aim of hormonal treatment is to reduce the production and/or effect of the hormones produced by the individual's own body and replace them with the hormones aligned with their gender identity. For example, someone who is assigned female at birth and who now identifies as a trans man will start testosterone and gradually develop male physical characteristics. Conversely, a birth-assigned male identifying as a trans woman will start estrogen and gradually develop female physical characteristics. Some TGD people will not identify with a binary gender and may not wish to maximally masculinize or feminize their bodies. Currently, there is little research on how best to provide nonbinary care. The clinician and nonbinary person may agree on a plan that ensures sufficient hormones are available to prevent any adverse effects of hormone deficiency.

Once the levels of testosterone or estrogen begin to increase, physical changes will take place over a time course similar to that of puberty. For each TGD person, the final effect of taking gender-affirming hormones will depend partly on their genetically predetermined individual response.

To start hormone therapy a TGD individual usually has:

1. A persistent need to alter their body to align with their gender identity.

2. A medical assessment and explanation of the benefits and potential risks of therapy.

3. The capacity to consent.

4. Well-controlled medical or mental health issues, if any are present.

Hormone treatment results in some permanent physical changes, and it follows that if for some reason hormone therapy is suspended, not all of the physical effects will regress. The specific effects of masculinizing and feminizing therapy are discussed later in this chapter.

7.2.2 Masculinizing Therapy

Testosterone results in the development of masculine features slowly over a period of two to five years. If a person desires maximal masculinization, the

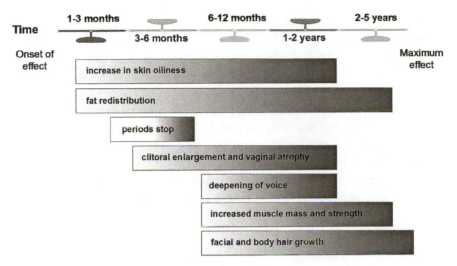

Figure 7.1 Testosterone results in physiological changes that develop gradually over several years. Many physical changes become evident in the first six months after testosterone commences, and the effects become maximal over months and years. The estimated timings shown here for the development of these changes are adapted from the Standards of Care, Version 7 and the Endocrine Society Guidelines, but may vary widely for each individual.

goal of therapy is to reach a physiological range of testosterone that allows the development of their desired physical changes. In general, the target testosterone levels are between 320 and 1,000 ng/dL, or 11 to 34 nmol/l, with a trough level toward the lower end of this range; but these levels will depend on the individual and perhaps the type of testosterone. The expected timing of physical changes is shown in Figure 7.1. However, it should be remembered that this information comes from studies of relatively small numbers of people and could be different for any individual.

Facial and Body Hair

The development of masculine facial and body hair generally begins after six to nine months of testosterone therapy and reaches maximum growth over a period of two to five years. There is a noticeable increase in overall body hair on the face, chest, abdomen, lower back, and inner thighs, and a change of genital hair toward a masculine pattern.[11] Hair growth is generally accompanied by a roughening of skin texture. One study of 17 trans men showed an increase in the rate of hair growth and skin oil or sebum production within the first few months of therapy. However, even by 12 months the men's facial and abdominal hair was still changing and had not yet reached the wider hair shaft diameter found in cisgender males.[12] This rate of beard growth is not unexpected as it is similar to the pubertal development of facial hair in testosterone-driven puberty. There is similarly a wide variation in the final amount and distribution of hair growth. Susceptible individuals may develop thinning of their hair over the temples and crown if they are prone to male-pattern baldness. Should this occur, it usually develops gradually over several years.[13] In a prospective study over just one year, only 1 in 20 people on testosterone developed hair loss in the frontotemporal regions of the scalp. A cross-sectional study of 50 trans men who had taken testosterone for around 10 years showed mild frontotemporal hair loss in a third (16) of participants and moderate to severe balding in almost as many (15),[14] suggesting that testosterone may take 1 to 10 years to have this effect.

Body Composition and Strength

Testosterone results in an increase in lean body mass and upper body strength, with a decrease in body fat. Studies have shown an average 1.7 to 6.0 kg increase in muscle weight, known as lean mass, and a 2.3 to 4.0 kg reduction in fat weight, known as adipose mass. These changes do not tend to occur until the testosterone levels reach the physiological range for adult cisgender men.

Genital Changes

A noticeable increase in the length of the clitoris begins from three to six months after initiation of testosterone treatment and is complete by around one year. In a 12-month prospective study of transgender men taking intramuscular testosterone in the form of undecanoate, a final clitoral length of 4.6 cm was recorded.[15] Penetrative intercourse is not usually possible despite this change in appearance.

Menstrual Cycle

Testosterone levels in the target range are usually sufficient to suppress the hormone signals from the pituitary gland that control the menstrual cycle. The cessation of regular periods, a state known as amenorrhea, is often one of the most desirable effects of testosterone therapy. Menstruation usually stops within two to six months of starting testosterone therapy, or else in two to six cycles if the interval between periods is shorter or longer than a month. However, in some people it takes significantly longer before menstruation stops.[16] If menstruation does not stop and is causing distress, then the dose of testosterone can be altered so that testosterone levels are increased further toward the upper end of the physiological range. Alternatively, a progestogen can be given to further suppress the pituitary gonadotrophins. Among the available proges-togens are medroxyprogesterone acetate given with a dose of 10 mg three times daily or via a 150 mg intramuscular depot and norethisterone given at 5 mg three times daily. GnRH analogs can also be used in this context, if funding is available. Other options include the insertion of a progestin-releasing intra-uterine device, such as Mirena©, or referral to a gynecologist for consideration of surgical options such as endometrial ablation or hysterectomy.

Sexual Health, Mood, and Cognition

Testosterone is known to have effects on behavior. Aggression, levels of moti-vation, and libido may increase during testosterone therapy. Although, as dis-cussed in previous chapters, there are few measurable differences in the way male and female brains behave during psychological testing, it is notable that testosterone treatment does cause a minor change in visual and spatial aware-ness.[17] Testosterone therapy is also associated with increased sexual desire. In a study that reviewed 45 trans men retrospectively, 74 percent reported an increase in sexual desire.[18] Similarly, a one-year prospective study that fol-lowed 50 trans men from the start of testosterone therapy demonstrated an increased frequency of self-reported sexual desire and fantasy, and of arousal and masturbation.[19]

Voice

Testosterone irreversibly deepens the voice to a lower pitch. This change occurs by causing vocal cord thickening and enlargement of the larynx. A noticeable deepening in voice usually begins 6 to 12 months after the commencement of testosterone treatment but can take up to one or two years to reach its maxi-mum extent. A cross-sectional study comparing trans men on long-term tes-tosterone therapy showed that 90 percent had voices that were indistinguishable from those of a group of cisgender men.[20] Although hormone therapy has a potent effect on voice, speech therapy may still be useful for trans men to assist with vocal fatigue, instability, and projection, as well as for other forms of communication.

Types of Testosterone Therapy

As testosterone is commonly used as hormone-replacement therapy for cis-gender men with underproduction of testosterone, a condition known as hypogonadism, its use as a medication is well understood. For TGD individu-als who seek masculinization, there are no data comparing the different medi-cation regimens to determine which one produces the best outcomes. Many specialists start testosterone at a full standard hormone replacement dose for adults, as is done for people with hypogonadism, whereas others start with a lower dose of testosterone and gradually increase the dose as described in Chapter 6, aiming to reach the same final target testosterone level by 6 to 12 months. At present, there is no evidence that one approach is better than the other, so both options should be discussed with the person starting therapy. It may be that a gradual increase in testosterone dose is preferable for patients who have used puberty blockers and who are therefore prepubertal.[21] A gradual increase in dosage can also allow dose adjustment if side effects, such as chest discomfort, develop early in therapy.

Testosterone can be given in a variety of forms including by injection and via skin absorption using a transdermal approach. Testosterone is available in short-acting or long-acting injectable forms. For example, testosterone enanthate 250 mg injected intramuscularly (i.e., into the muscle) can be given every two to three weeks; or alternatively a partial dose, usually 75 to 80 mg, can be given under the skin (i.e., subcutaneously) each week. Subcutaneous weekly administration may be the preferred method as it can be given by self-injection and may provide a more consistent testosterone level.[22] Testosterone undecanoate 1,000 mg is given intramuscularly and forms a reservoir or depot under the skin. The first two doses are given six weeks apart and thereafter at intervals of around 12 weeks. There are several forms of transdermal testosterone available as both gels and creams. These include testosterone 1% (50 mg to 5 g) gel sachets, a testosterone 1% (12.5 mg per actuation) gel pump pack, and testosterone 5% (50 mg per ml) applied daily. In some health systems, formulations absorbed through the skin of the mouth, the buccal approach, nasal sprays, and subcutaneous implants are available. However, these methods have not been widely studied and are therefore generally not a first choice. Anabolic or alkylated oral testosterone, otherwise known as anabolic steroids, are associated with liver failure due to their hepatotoxicity and are certainly not recommended.[23]

7.2.3 Feminizing Therapy

Feminizing therapy gradually alters the hormonal balance so that estradiol levels increase and testosterone levels fall toward or into the female physiological range. The U.S. Endocrine Society suggests aiming for estradiol levels of 100 to 200 pg/mL or 367 to 734 pmol/l and testosterone levels less than 50 ng/dL or less than 2 nmol/l. Australian practice suggests an estradiol target of 250 to 600 pmol/l, with a similarly suppressed testosterone level. There have been no robust studies that have directly assessed these targets. The optimal duration over which estrogen therapy should be titrated, that is, measured and adjusted, before reaching these target levels is not known. However, it is

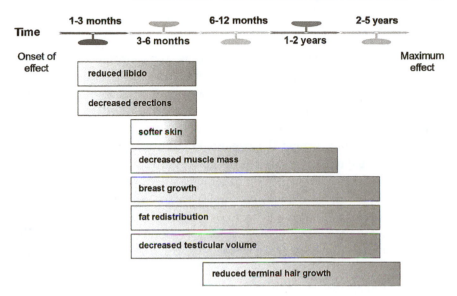

Figure 7.2   The effects of estrogen start in the first few months of therapy and continue to develop over months and years. These physical changes may vary between individuals, but average timings are shown here (adapted from the Standards of Care, Version 7 and the Endocrine Society Guidelines).

thought that replicating the timing of estrogen-driven puberty in cisgender females with a gradual increase in estrogen dosage every two to three months, aiming for physiological levels by six to nine months may result in the best physical outcome, particularly in breast development. A gradual approach to increasing the doses of estrogen may be especially important for those who have previously used GnRH puberty blockers and who are have not previously experienced puberty.

In contrast to masculinizing therapy, the effect of estrogen is often insufficient to suppress the production of testosterone when given alone. Therefore, an additional medication is usually used to suppress or block testosterone. This can either be a GnRH analog or an anti-androgen such as spironolactone or cyproterone acetate. The GnRH analog or anti-androgen may be started before estrogen, at the same time as estrogen, or after estrogen, and perhaps included in the medication only if testosterone has not been adequately suppressed. As GnRH analogs can induce a rapid and profound reduction in testosterone, perhaps in this case it is preferable to commence with estrogen and then add the GnRH analog, otherwise there could be a protracted period with both very low estrogen and low testosterone that could affect bone health. The physical changes and expected timings, though variable, are shown in Figure 7.2.

Breast Development

Breast development begins three to six months after estrogen is initiated and reaches a maximum over a period of two to three years. As in cisgender women, the final outcome is dependent on the person's genetically predetermined response to estrogen stimulation. Breast size and shape also depends on the length of time estrogen has been taken. It may help to be of a younger age at the start of hormone therapy. The extent of breast development does not seem to depend on the type of estrogen or the dose used. Indirect evidence suggests that the speed at which the body is exposed to full-dose estrogen is a critical factor. Studies of cis females who have not spontaneously entered puberty and who are started on estrogen therapy to induce puberty have shown that rapid exposure to full doses of estrogen leads to early fusion of the breast buds. This sometimes results in poor breast development and small, conically shaped breasts.[24]

There are few studies specifically investigating breast size or shape as an outcome, despite it being one of the most important considerations for TGD individuals requesting feminizing therapy. Up to 70 percent of trans women proceed to surgical breast augmentation, suggesting possible discontent with the outcome of hormone therapy alone. However, other more difficult to measure factors such as personal satisfaction with body image and baseline physique, perhaps due to the proportions of the bony skeleton and lateral nipple positioning following previous testosterone exposure, may contribute to an individual's decision to have breast augmentation surgery.

It has been reported that the average final breast size for transgender women is close to that of cisgender females, who themselves show a large variation in breast size and shape. However, as mentioned, it is not uncommon for trans women to consider the final outcome from estrogen therapy to be suboptimal. The only study to prospectively measure breast size was a recent study by the ENIGI group from Amsterdam, Florence, Ghent, and Oslo that followed breast development in 229 trans women taking hormone therapy.[25] The hormone regimens used were oral or transdermal estradiol valerate with spironolactone or cyproterone acetate used to block their testosterone. The estradiol levels achieved were slightly lower than those recommended by the Endocrine Society (an average value of 184 to 206 pmol per liter), as a relatively fixed dose of estrogen was used in the study. Breast growth was measured as the difference between circumferences measured at the fullest part of the breast, the *breast circumference*, and at the chest wall, the so-called *infra-mammary thoracic circumference*. The breast–chest difference increased by 3.7 cm over 12 months, from 4.1 cm at the start to 7.9 cm after a year of therapy, with most of the increase, 3.2 cm, occurring in the first six months. This meant that almost half the women had a European bra size of less than a AAA cup, and only 11 percent gained an A cup bra size or larger. The authors note this may be an underestimate as cup size may be based upon shape as well as the measurements used in this method for estimating breast size. Cup sizes are different depending on the country and are not standardized across the world. Using the data from this study, and assuming that the chest measurement did not change over the 12 months, gives an Australia/New Zealand/U.K./U.S. cup size of C using an average frame size of 88.8 cm and final bust size of 96.7 cm (calculated using the calculator found at http://www.calculator.net/bra -size-calculator). In this study, age, weight change, smoking status, body-mass index, estradiol levels, and the way estrogen was administered, either oral or transdermal, did not predict breast development after 12 months. Another recent study showed breast development had not fully matured to Tanner stage 3 after two years of hormone therapy,[26] indicating that well-designed studies with longer follow-up periods may be needed to provide the best advice regarding likely final outcomes.

One retrospective study compared 165 transgender women requesting U.K. National Health Service–funded augmentation mammoplasty with an age-matched transgender group who had not requested surgery.[27] All those included in the study had well-developed breasts to at least Tanner stage 4 out of a maximum of 5 and had completed over two years of estrogen treatment. Interestingly, for these trans women, previous self-medication with estrogen was associated with a higher likelihood of surgery, perhaps because of "too large a dose at initiation to promote appropriate subsequent breast growth, resulting in a poorer final breast outcome." Indeed, these women did have significantly higher estradiol levels at their first clinic appointment. The type of estrogen prescribed, estrogen valerate (17β estradiol), ethinyl estradiol, or conjugated equine estrogen, did not affect whether surgery was requested. For those women using 17β estradiol, which can be measured in blood samples, the level of estradiol was not related to breast growth, and lower estrogen levels did not increase the likelihood of a request for surgery.

Progesterone is not involved in breast development in cisgender females. The levels of progesterone only increase late in puberty when breast development is complete.[28] Progesterone is therefore not included in the initiating hormonal regimens for young cisgender women who have not spontaneously entered puberty.[29] Neither does the current available evidence suggest that progestins enhance breast development for transgender women. However, there is insufficient high-quality evidence to form an absolute conclusion regarding the usefulness of progestins, and some Internet resources and clinical services still recommend their use. Progestins, administered for example as medroxyprogesterone acetate with a dose of 5 to 10 mg/daily, is sometimes useful as a short-duration supplement to hormone therapy to reduce the estrogen dose needed to suppress testosterone levels. However, concerns about adverse effects in the short term, such as thromboembolism, bloating, nausea, and weight gain, and longer-term risks, such as an increased risk of breast cancer and cardiovascular disease that have been observed in cisgender women,[30] mean that progestins are not generally recommended. There is emerging evidence that micronized progesterone, say a daily oral dosage of 100 mg, has a lower breast cancer risk than traditional progestins and does not appear to attenuate the cardiovascular benefits of estrogen.[31] This preparation is more similar in structure to natural progesterone and has been available in Europe for 20 years. It is now available more widely, including in Australia.

Body Shape

The distribution of body fat and muscle alters during the first months of feminizing therapy and continues to develop over several years. One prospective study of 37 transgender women with a normal body-mass index showed that combined ethinyl estradiol (100 mcg/day) and cyproterone acetate (100 mg/day) therapy resulted in an increase in both subcutaneous and internal or visceral fat.[32] After 12 months of therapy, there was an accompanying 3.8 kg weight gain, with fat being redistributed to the hip and buttock regions. Once the body has been exposed to testosterone, it is not possible to change the effect of androgen exposure on the skeleton. The greater average height, size and shape of hands, feet, jaw, pelvis and Adam's apple, otherwise known as the laryngeal prominence, remain unaltered by hormone therapy.

Skin and Hair

Sex hormones play an important role in determining body hair characteristics and distribution. The sebaceous glands that are responsible for the secretion of skin oils or sebum, and the developing cells of the hair follicle both contain testosterone receptors. All hair locations except the upper arm and back of the forearm are considered androgen-dependent. When feminizing therapy is started, testosterone levels fall and the growth of androgen-dependent hair on the lip, chin, chest, upper back, lower back, abdomen, and front of the forearm decreases.

The effect of sex steroids on hair growth can be measured in a standard way by the assessment of a variety of skin areas using the Ferriman–Gallwey score. After four months of estrogen therapy, the hair is already observed to be much finer due to a reduction in the diameter of the hair shaft, which does not change much more with continuing hormone treatment. The speed at which hair grows and its density reduce more gradually, particularly on the face and abdomen. After 12 months, one study showed that androgen-dependent hair growth had decreased significantly, but 85 percent of trans women still had a Ferriman–Gallwey score consistent with the excess hair condition of hirsutism that can occur in cisgender women.[33]

Although somewhat effective, hormone therapy alone is often insufficient to control facial hair, perhaps because of its greater density and hair shaft diameter. Other methods such as shaving, applying eflornithine topical cream, waxing, electrolysis, and laser therapy are all commonly used to reduce facial hair. Electrolysis involves the insertion of a fine needle into each individual follicle, which is then destroyed by passage of an electric current. This technique is useful for small areas such as the chin or lip but is dependent on the skill of the operator. Laser therapy destroys the follicle as the melanin or pigment in the hair absorbs light energy and converts it to heat. Several follicles can be treated simultaneously but, like electrolysis, repeated treatments may be needed. Although cosmetic specialists make an individual assessment, laser therapy is usually ineffective for people with blond, red, or gray hair, as these hairs contain less melanin.

For those who have experienced androgen-dependent hair loss, this thinning of scalp hair can slow and stabilize in response to hormone therapy, but hair does not normally regrow in the affected areas. Finasteride, a 5-alpha reductase inhibitor that reduces the conversion of testosterone to active dihydrotestosterone, may be useful, as it is the latter that mediates much of the effect of testosterone on hair.[34] More information about hair removal is contained in Chapter 9.

Genital Changes and Libido

Estrogen therapy is known to lead to a reduction in sex drive or libido. Trans women often experience a loss of spontaneous erections and the strength of these erections when aroused. This effect may be considered desirable or viewed as an adverse effect. Some trans women prefer to maintain erectile function and therefore aim for partial suppression of testosterone levels to above 5 nmol per liter, although this strategy limits the feminizing effects of estrogen. As feminizing therapy suppresses the pituitary gonadotrophins that actively send messages to the testes, testicular size may reduce gradually over time.

Sexual Health, Mood, and Cognition

Estrogen therapy influences mood and can cause a mildly low mood early in treatment. However, in the medium term, estrogen therapy has a positive effect on mood for most trans women.[35] There are few studies on sexual function in trans women who have started hormone therapy but have not had genital surgery. However, available evidence suggests that low levels of free testosterone via the effect of estrogen to increase sex-hormone binding globulin may lead to a reduced sexual drive or libido.[36]

Types of Estrogen Therapy

Various formulations of estrogen are available in different countries. However, many clinicians agree that compounds of 17β estradiol have the lowest side effect profile, and this type of estrogen can helpfully be measured in blood samples. This is therefore the preferred type of estrogen for both oral and transdermal treatment. A common approach to the initiation of therapy is to start at a low dose of 17β estradiol, for example 2 mg oral daily with an increase over the course of six to eight months to a full dose, aiming for a similar level to that measured in cisgender women. The typical doses required to achieve this target level depend on the delivery route, for example oral estradiol valerate 2 to 8 mg daily, transdermal estradiol patches 100 to 150 mcg/day, or estradiol gel sachet 1 to 2 mg/day.

In one study from New York, it was noted that over 70 percent of 156 trans women achieved their target estradiol levels with an oral 17β estradiol dose of 4 mg daily or more. However, there was wide individual variation in the amount of estrogen required.[37] Other formulations, such as injectable estradiol valerate delivered 2 to 10 mg weekly into the muscle, and sublingual estrogen absorbed under the tongue may result in more rapid peaks accompanied by larger fluctuations in blood levels that are more difficult to monitor.[38] There is no clear evidence that these estrogen delivery routes are overtly harmful, although they are generally not preferred. Preliminary observations suggest that the different formulations of estrogen all produce similar outcomes with no difference in breast development, body fat distribution, or bone health.

The transdermal route may be most beneficial for some women, as this form of estrogen does not expose the liver to high estradiol concentrations, unlike the oral formulations that are absorbed through the gastrointestinal tract and then pass through the portal circulation directly to the liver. This avoidance of the first-pass metabolism in the liver decreases the risk of these women developing abnormal lipid levels and an increase in clotting factors that can lead to thrombosis.[39] The transdermal route is often used for women over 40 years old, for smokers, or for those with other risk factors. If transdermal administration is the preferred route, the gel formulation may be better than patches for hot, humid climates where the adhesive can fail to stick adequately to the skin.

Estradiol implants are an alternative form of transdermal estrogen. They are not widely available commercially as they are no longer on the list of regulated medications in many countries. Some clinicians can access implants from compounding pharmacies. Implants have a unknown rate of estrogen absorption, and compounding may produce a variable estrogen content on either the low or high side that could predispose to adverse effects. Although there is no clear evidence of harm from these potentially higher levels, rarely, extremely high estrogen levels have been reported to cause fluid retention, bloating, and swelling. For some trans women this is as close as they can get to the normal delivery of estrogen cisgender women obtain via their ovaries. Estrogen implants may therefore be an option in selected cases if this decision has been made between the individual and their health provider with discussion of potential risks. Estrogen implants are given as 50 mg or 100 mg pellets replaced every 6 to 24 months depending on individual response, although there is little data to guide practice. The implant is inserted under the skin using local anesthetic; this procedure can result in bleeding, bruising, infection, and occasional pellet extrusion when the implant comes back out of the skin.

Ethinyl estradiol causes higher incidences of blood clots in the form of venous thromboembolism.[40] There are currently no carefully controlled randomized trials studies that directly compare 17β estradiol with ethinyl estradiol, but when higher-dose ethinyl estradiol of 100 mcg daily was used before the 1990s, a significant, almost 50 times risk of venous thromboembolism was observed.[41] This serious side effect may be caused by the particular molecular structure of ethinyl estradiol.[42] Low doses of the oral contraceptive pill containing ethinyl estradiol and progesterone as the combined oral contraceptive pill, usually administered with a dose of 2 to 50 mcg daily, have been used effectively and may be the only form available for some TGD people. However, it is important to recognize that blood sampling cannot measure either ethinyl estradiol or conjugated estrogens. Therefore, monitoring is limited to clinician observation of physical changes and the magnitude of testosterone suppression. This may theoretically result in a higher side effect risk.

GnRH Analogs and Anti-Androgens

GnRH analogs such as goserelin are often used to block puberty in adolescents but can also be used for adults.[43] This medication is given as long-acting monthly or three-monthly injections to induce profound testosterone suppression. GnRH analogs have few side effects as they only work on the pathway that controls the production of the sex hormones, for example, testosterone. Although GnRH analogs have been observed to cause short-term flushing and longer-term osteoporosis when used in fertility medicine and in the treatment of prostate cancer, this is not a problem for TGD people undergoing feminization as the simultaneous use of estrogen prevents these symptoms.[44] Unfortunately, they are expensive therapies that are not funded for adults in many health systems. For adolescent patients who are transitioning to adult services, GnRH analogs are sometimes changed to androgen blockers such as spironolactone or cyproterone acetate. However, these anti-androgens are associated with a higher rate of depression in users when compared with GnRH analogs. GnRH analog therapy can usually be ceased in TGD people who are undergoing masculinizing therapy once target levels of testosterone have been achieved and are stable for several weeks or months.

Spironolactone is an aldosterone receptor antagonist drug used commonly for blood pressure management and heart failure. It blocks the effect of testosterone at the receptor, and at doses of 100 to 200 mg it also has a weak estrogen-like action. Spironolactone can occasionally produce elevated levels of potassium that can affect the heart rhythm in susceptible individuals, although with normal kidney function this risk is very low and can be easily monitored by testing blood levels. A population-based cohort study of 3,653 people taking spironolactone for various medical conditions surprisingly demonstrated an increased 2.7 times risk of gastrointestinal bleeding, a risk that was 5.4 times higher in people taking doses of 100 mg or more that are commonly used in the treatment of TGD people for blocking the effect of androgens.[45] This undesirable effect of spironolactone was particularly notable in older people for whom there was a 13.1 times increased risk of gastrointestinal bleeding for people aged between 55 and 74. The risk did not change if the person had been using the medication for a shorter or longer time and was unchanged whether or not they were also taking aspirin or nonsteroidal therapy, drugs that can predispose to gastrointestinal bleeding. This effect on gastrointestinal bleeding has not been reported in the longitudinal studies of trans women, but perhaps caution should still be applied for the older age group. There is limited evidence from a reduced analysis of data of 24 participants from a retrospective study that spironolactone was associated with an increase in the number of trans women requesting augmentation mammoplasty (4.8% compared with 18%). The authors postulate that this effect could be a consequence of the weak additional estrogen-like effect of spironolactone resulting in early estrogen overexposure at the start of treatment.[46] Further research is needed to determine the optimal drug dosage regimen. However, if spironolactone is used, it may be preferable to start with the anti-androgen and follow after 6 to 12 weeks with estrogen therapy or vice versa to ensure gradual hormone rebalancing and perhaps promote maximal breast development. Some clinicians start both androgen blockade and estrogen therapy concurrently, and this is an equally reasonable approach.

Cyproterone acetate is a progestin medication that as a receptor antagonist blocks the effect of testosterone and also reduces the stimulating signals, the gonadotrophins, LH and FSH, to the testes, causing reduced testosterone release. Cyproterone acetate is commonly used at low doses of 12.5 to 25 mg daily for trans women and, like spironolactone, is effective and safe. Cyproterone acetate is not available in the United States but is commonly used in Europe. In other countries, such as Australia, it can be more expensive than spironolactone. Cyproterone acetate is associated with depression in up to 60 percent of transgender women. However, it is unclear whether this change in mood is a direct effect of the medication, a result of suppressing testosterone levels, or the effect of cyproterone on stress hormones as it interacts with the glucocorticoid receptor.[47] Adverse effects on mood and liver function tests, as cyproterone acetate is metabolized by the liver, have been found in cisgender women treated for polycystic ovarian syndrome.[48]

A large study involving 2,474 men and women who were on a higher dose of 50 mg or more of cyproterone acetate looked for less common adverse effects by gathering data over a long duration of 6,333 person-years, calculated by multiplying the number of people by the number of years they were in the study. This analysis revealed a slight increase in the risk of meningioma, a benign tumor of the lining of the brain, associated with a year or more of treatment. The relative risk was increased by 11.4 times, but the absolute risk remained small, 60 occurrences per 100,000 person-years.[49] Although there are no data for trans women, this finding could be important because of the possible need for long-term therapy. These data suggest that the lowest effective dose of cyproterone acetate should be used.

Finasteride dosed at 2.5 to 5 mg daily may be useful if excess hair growth and acne are of concern. Finasteride only blocks one of the two 5-alpha reductase enzymes and therefore only has mild anti-androgen effects and is not used as the first-choice androgen blocker. As is the case for cyproterone acetate, it can be associated with low mood and abnormal liver function.

7.2.4 Hormone Regimens for Nonbinary and Genderqueer People

People who identify as nonbinary or genderqueer may have diverse goals for transition. Some people may prefer a gender-neutral appearance, whereas others may wish to combine both a feminine and masculine appearance, or present as binary masculine or feminine.[50] These goals may be achieved using nonmedical means or by taking advantage of hormone therapy and/or surgery. As the experience of being transgender becomes depathologized and self-determined, and moves away from clinician-led diagnosis, it is more likely that nonbinary or genderqueer people will become more visible in health care.

A recent online survey examining the needs of trans people identified a significant minority (18.3%) of nonbinary and genderqueer among a group of 415 trans people.[51] The nonbinary group was less likely to have accessed health care, but also perceived that fewer treatments would be required to complete their transition when compared with the trans binary group. The authors suggest that "traditional binary-focused treatment practice could have hindered [nonbinary or genderqueer] individuals from accessing trans health care or sufficiently articulating their needs."

It is possible to achieve testosterone and estrogen hormone levels that are between the male and female ranges. However, at this point, there is little evidence for this practice as most research only considers binary gender options. Hormonal decisions are therefore based upon our understanding of cisgender puberty and the minimal available literature assessing therapy for trans binary people. It is difficult to tailor therapy to achieve the development of some secondary sexual characteristics but not others. These characteristics develop gradually once a threshold level of hormone is reached. Increasing the hormone level above this threshold does not generally result in a greater magnitude of effect. For example, once breast growth has started, increasingly higher levels of estrogen would not lead to larger breasts. The exception is testosterone-driven development of muscle mass in trans men, for whom higher levels continue to exert an incremental effect.[52]

There are no studies specifically designed to test the consequences of achieving different estrogen and testosterone thresholds. However, some observed principles might provide useful information, despite this lack of data.

a. Estrogen treatment: In estrogen-driven puberty, as was discussed in Chapter 6, breast development occurs even at lower levels of estrogen. For example, in stage two of puberty, an estradiol level as low as 25 pg/ml or 90 pmol/l may be sufficient to initiate breast growth. This means that other later changes such as feminizing of the body shape and skin softening are difficult to achieve without some concurrent breast growth.

b. Testosterone reduction: If a reduction in the production of testosterone is desired, there are some predictable symptoms that could be anticipated from those observed in cisgender men after a reduction in testosterone levels.[53] In one study, loss of libido was seen first when the testosterone level dropped below 430 ng/dl or 15 nmol/l. Low mood, obesity, and diabetes were more common when testosterone levels fell below the adult reference range, less than 300 ng/dl or 10 nmol/l. Erectile dysfunction and hot flashes were seen at lower levels of testosterone below 230 ng/dl or 8 nmol/l. These thresholds are not absolute and some studies have not shown similar effects at these reported testosterone thresholds and have instead attributed the observed symptoms to the aging of the participants, rather than their hormone insufficiency.[54] Other studies have indicated different testosterone thresholds; for example, in another study erectile dysfunction only seemed to occur when testosterone was below 145 ng/dl or 5 nmol/l.[55] Perhaps if erectile function is desired, the testosterone level could be maintained somewhere between 5 and 8 nmol/l. It should be noted that medication that blocks the action of testosterone, such as spironolactone, would not necessarily reduce the measured level of testosterone, just its effect. Therefore, symptoms could occur with higher, but ineffective, testosterone levels. If a birth-assigned male does not wish to develop breasts, then GnRH analogs or finasteride may be better choices for androgen blockage, as both cyproterone acetate and spironolactone cause breast tissue growth and gynecomastia.

c. Testosterone treatment: In testosterone-driven puberty, even the low testosterone levels of stage 3 puberty below 130 ng/dl or 4.5 nmol/l are likely to result in clitoral enlargement and breaking of the voice, although perhaps not full deepening of pitch until a later stage 4 of puberty when the testosterone level reaches around 200 ng/dl or 7 nmol/l. If facial hair or a masculine body shape is desired, then complete masculinization is necessary. The adult testosterone levels of Tanner stage 5 puberty, within the range 300 to 700 ng/dl or 10 to 24 nmol/l, need to be reached before these physical changes occur.

It is well understood in the general population that a failure to supply sufficient hormone therapy or the use of hormone suppression without replacement can lead to adverse effects on health. For example, lower testosterone levels are associated with a higher death rate in cisgender males,[56] and cisgender women are at higher risk of cardiovascular disease after loss of estrogen at menopause, particularly if menopause is surgically induced by oophorectomy in women under 50 years.[57] Perhaps this supports consideration of alternative methods of achieving transition goals for nonbinary and genderqueer people, beyond that of suppressing both estrogen and testosterone. Nonmedical interventions such as speech therapy and laser hair removal could be of benefit. Progestins or micronized progesterone can be used to stop the menstrual cycle, and preventive osteoporosis treatment could be used for bone protection in people with low hormone levels. Indeed, estrogen seems particularly important in the maintenance of strong bones in both sexes. Testosterone is converted to estrogen by aromatase enzymes and provides bone protection indirectly. For cisgender men with prostate cancer who have their hormones suppressed by GnRH analogs without replacement hormones, it seems probably safe to give up to four 3-month doses (over a year) without there being a significant impact on bone health.[58]

Reassuringly, it also seems that any observed bone density loss during GnRH analog therapy can recover in trans youth once hormonal therapy commences.[59] Even low levels of estradiol above 10 pg/ml or 37 pmol/l and/ or testosterone levels above 200 ng/dL or 7.0 nmol/l may be sufficient to prevent a reduction in bone density in cisgender men.[60] The administration of ultra-low doses of 17β estradiol, say 0.5 mg daily, has been shown to protect bones over two years in postmenopausal cisgender women.[61] Perhaps combined treatment with low-dose estrogen and testosterone would give even better bone protection than estrogen or testosterone alone.[62]

More studies are awaited before a formal guideline or protocol can be developed for nonbinary or genderqueer people. Combinations of estrogen, testosterone, and perhaps progesterone should be studied for efficacy and adverse events. At present, a bespoke plan is created for each person with their endocrinologist and negotiated with them depending on the physical changes requested and their own personal preferences.

7.2.5 Potential Adverse Effects and Monitoring

In the first year of hormone therapy, it is recommended that clinical review occur at two- to three-month intervals. At this appointment the physician can assess body changes, measure hormone levels, and look for potential complications such as changes in mood. Clinical practice varies somewhat, as there are no clear data to support any particular approach. Hormonal treatment can be adjusted at these visits depending on the rate of the person's physical changes and/or their hormone levels on blood sampling. Clinic visits usually become less frequent over time, often at intervals of 6 to 12 months. At these visits, the clinician and client will discuss the adequacy of treatment and any adverse effects that may have developed, and use the opportunity to update preventive health screening.

Available research indicates that hormone therapy is safe and effective. A systematic review of all studies performed up to 2014 showed, importantly, that hormone therapy does not increase the risk of cancer or early death.[63] The authors conclude that "hormone therapy for transgender individuals is safe without a large risk of adverse events when followed carefully for a few well-documented medical concerns." Further medical research is under-way to understand the long-term effects of hormone therapies in TGD people, for example the ENIGI study in Europe,[64] the STRONG study in the United States,[65] and a large study using Veterans Health Administration[66] participants.

Masculinizing Therapy

The currently available long-term studies suggest that testosterone treatment does not increase either the risk of future cardiovascular disease or overall mortality. A Dutch study of 365 trans men who had been on testosterone for an average of 19 years noted their death rates were no different from those of the general population.[67] A study from Sweden using data gathered from 1973 to 2003 showed a mortality rate for transgender men in the first 10 years after hormone treatment and genital surgery, similar to that observed for 1,330 age-matched people.[68] After 10 years there was a very slight increase in mortality, attributed to an increased suicide rate. It should be noted that most of the published data on the outcomes for trans men were obtained from a small number of specialist multidisciplinary clinics in high-income locations and therefore may not be widely applicable to the broader population that receive care in other contexts.[69] There have not been any prospective studies to date that have selected participants at the start of therapy and followed them over their entire lifespan.

Testosterone and Erythrocytosis

One of the more common consequences of testosterone therapy is the increased production of red blood cells, a process known as erythrocytosis. However, the development of erythrocytosis is uncommon when the level of testosterone achieved lies within the physiological target range[70] and may be less common for those on testosterone undecanoate due to the stability of testosterone levels.[71] Hemoglobin, as indicated by red blood cell concentration, and hematocrit levels should be compared with the male reference range and not the lower female reference range that may appear on pathology reports. Testosterone increases the level of the hormone erythropoietin in blood that then increases red cell production from bone marrow. If the increase is extreme, the concern is that there will be thickening or an increase in the viscosity of blood with the possible risk of clot development and stroke.[72] However, there is no direct evidence to conclude that testosterone-induced erythrocytosis, as opposed to erythrocytosis from bone marrow disorders, causes these serious complications.[73] A full blood count can be used for monitoring, and if hemoglobin remains above the male reference range or hematocrit is above 0.50 L/L (or 50 percent), a reduction in the testosterone dose or an increase in dose interval should occur. An underlying cause for erythrocytosis such as cigarette smoking, obstructive sleep apnea, or blood cancer due to myeloproliferative neoplasms should always be considered.

Testosterone and Acne

Acne is a common complaint of those receiving testosterone therapy as oil or sebum production by the sebaceous glands increases. Acne tends to be most prominent during the first six months of treatment, and then gradually improves and resolves over the following one to two years. In one study, most people had acne on the face (94%) and back (88%) after four months of testosterone therapy.[74] For mild to moderate acne, topical treatments containing retinoids, retinoid/benzoyl peroxide combinations, and azelaic acid or salicylic acid are recommended. If these treatments are not effective, then referral to a dermatologist should be sought.[75]

Testosterone and Cardiovascular Risk

There is no evidence that testosterone directly increases the risk of cardiovascular disease leading to heart attacks and strokes. The rate of myocardial infarction in trans men is lower than in the general male population. A review has been performed combining the results of 16 studies to include 1,471 participants using what is known as meta-analysis. This study showed that testosterone therapy is associated with unfavorable changes in fat or lipid profiles, including a minor increase in triglyceride levels and a decrease in beneficial HDL cholesterol levels, but without an adverse increase in total or LDL cholesterol.[76] Another review that included the 29 studies undertaken prior to 2015 showed similar results and also demonstrated an increase in LDL cholesterol.[77] There is some evidence that the risk of pre-diabetes or diabetes may be increased by testosterone therapy in TGD people.[78] Abnormalities in lipids and glucose levels are known to contribute to cardiovascular disease, but an actual change in the rates of cardiovascular events has not been consistently shown in the studies reported so far with a sample of TGD people.

Testosterone and Bone Health

Sex hormones are important determinants of the amount of bone acquisition during puberty and of bone health in adults. Studies suggest that testosterone therapy maintains bone strength, even when estrogen is suppressed, likely a result of aromatization that converts testosterone to estrogen.[79] One cross-sectional study demonstrated that trans men had a more masculine bone composition after about a decade of treatment and had larger bones than cisgender women.[80] The increased muscle mass that occurs during testosterone therapy causes a greater mechanical loading on bone that may consequently increase the thickness of the cortical long bones of the skeleton.

A review of available studies up to 2015 that followed the progress of 247 trans men over two years of testosterone therapy showed no deterioration in bone mineral density, a diagnostic tool used to detect osteoporosis and estimate future fracture risk.[81] Although these effects seem reassuring, monitoring of bone health should be considered as bone health can be compromised in people who have received insufficient testosterone.[82] However, the actual effect of masculinizing therapy on bone fracture risk remains uncertain.

Testosterone and Breast Cancer

Trans men have lower rates of breast cancer compared with cisgender women. Testosterone, produced inside the body or given as hormonal treatment, is, as we know, partially transformed by a process of aromatization to estrogen in the form of estradiol. Therefore, trans males receiving testosterone may still have some circulating estrogen, particularly if they are overweight or obese, as fat tissue is an aromatizer that converts testosterone into estrogen.

It is well established that prolonged exposure to estrogen increases the risk of breast cancer in cisgender women.[83] However, for TGD people taking testosterone, the risk of breast cancer seems to be low, as it also is for cisgender men with a prevalence of about one in a thousand. In a study of 795 Dutch trans men on testosterone therapy yielding data for 15,974 person-years, only one case of breast cancer was diagnosed. This translated to a rate of 5.9 per 100,000 person-years, similar to the rate observed in the cisgender male population. Similarly, no cases of breast cancer were observed in a group of 133 trans men who attended a Swedish clinic. The Veterans Health Administration data set, collected from 1996 to 2013, identified 7 cases of breast cancer in veterans on testosterone, bringing the total number of cases reported world-wide at that time to 12. The researchers concluded that the rate of breast cancer was not increased by testosterone treatment.[84]

Testosterone decreases the amount of glandular tissue in the breast, which may reduce the cancer risk. In addition, many trans men elect to undergo chest reconstruction. This procedure may also reduce the risk of breast cancer as usually only a small amount of glandular tissue remains. However, it is notable that one case of breast cancer identified in the Veterans study did occur in residual breast tissue in the armpit or axilla that remained after chest reconstruction. Guidelines recommend that trans men have breast screening according to local protocols, but more evidence is needed to show that screening clearly improves the breast cancer outcome for TGD individuals on testosterone.

Testosterone and Ovarian Cancer

A study of 112 trans men who had received testosterone for at least six months before genital surgery with removal of the uterus, fallopian tubes, and ovaries using hystero-salpingo-oophorectomy surgery showed that by the time of surgical removal, 80 percent of ovaries contained multiple cysts as indicated by a polycystic histology.[85] At the time, this study raised some concerns that testosterone could cause precancerous changes to the ovaries. However, later studies have not shown the same changes to ovary structure.[86] Furthermore, the observed ovarian cancer risk is extremely low, with only a few cases having been reported.[87]

Testosterone and Endometrial Cancer

As already discussed, testosterone can be aromatized to produce estradiol. When there is no progesterone present to counteract estradiol, the uterine lining or endometrium can thicken to produce hyperplasia. In cisgender women this thickening has been found to lead to an increased risk of endometrial cancer. A small early study of the effect of testosterone demonstrated endometrial hyperplasia in 3 of 19 people treated with androgen therapy, leading to concerns that this could increase the cancer risk.[88] However, this did not seem to be the case as a subsequent larger study showed the opposite result, that the endometrial lining thinned or regressed in 45 percent of people who had undergone testosterone therapy.[89] Indeed, like ovarian cancer, observed cases of endometrial cancer are rare in trans men, suggesting that the overall risk is low. Current guidelines recommend ongoing endometrial surveillance by ultrasound or an elective hysterectomy after two years of testosterone therapy.[90] However, it is likely that surveillance will become less stringent, as it has not been shown that these precautions reduce the risk of cancer or improve the outcome should such cancer occur.

Testosterone and Cervical Cancer

Trans men retain cervical tissue unless a hysterectomy has been performed. One study from Kaiser Permanente reported 6 cases of cervical cancer in a group of 2,098 trans men, or 80 cases of cancer per 100,000 person-years.[91] Cervical screening is recommended for trans men on testosterone therapy. However, trans men have poor uptake of traditional pap smear testing, and sometimes the microscopic cytology analysis of this test is technically challenging for the laboratory assessor. In one study, trans men had a report of *inadequate* or *unsatisfactory* cytology results 10 times more often than did cisgender women. This difficulty in providing a definitive negative or positive result is likely due to an effect of testosterone on the physical appearance of cervical cells and patient or provider difficulty in performing the procedure successfully.[92] Many places now test for human papilloma virus (HPV type 16–18), the virus that leads to almost all cervical cancer. If this test is negative, further investigation may not be warranted. New data suggest that self-collected swabs for human papilloma virus using DNA testing may be the most acceptable and effective method of cervical cancer screening for trans men.[93]

Feminizing Therapy

The available studies following people taking 17β estradiol suggest that estrogen therapy is safe and effective. However, one long-term study of feminizing therapy suggests a slightly higher death rate compared with the general population.[94] This increased risk was attributed to a slightly higher rate of suicide and cardiovascular disease. This increase in cardiovascular risk may be due to the historical use of higher-dose ethinyl estradiol and cyproterone acetate 100 mg per day in older trans women. Other studies have not shown this difference between death rates in trans women and the general population.

Estrogen and Blood Clotting

Venous thromboembolism is the most serious complication for people treated with estrogen. Estrogen affects blood clotting and can increase the chance of developing blood clots in veins, particularly over the first 12 months of therapy.[95] The rates of venous thromboembolism have fallen over time with changes in practice. A sustained high dose of estrogen, oral administration, the use of ethinyl estradiol and conjugated equine estrogen, and concurrent use of progestins have now been identified as important contributors to the risk of venous thromboembolism. Modifiable lifestyle factors are very important when considering this risk. In a large case-control study of cisgender women taking the oral contraceptive pill, the risk of venous thromboembolism increased moderately in current smokers by a factor of 1.4 when compared with nonsmokers and was also higher in women with a body-mass index greater than 35 kg/m^2.[96]

As discussed, the older estrogen preparations, conjugated equine estrogen and ethinyl estradiol that are used in the oral contraceptive pill, are associated with a higher incidence of venous thromboembolism. An early retrospective study in the Netherlands, which followed people for over four years with an average time period of 4.4 years, showed that a combination of ethinyl estradiol (100 mcg/day) and cyproterone acetate (100 mcg/day) resulted in a 45-fold increased risk, 1,140 events per 100,000 exposure years, of venous thromboembolism when compared with the general population's 30 events per 100,000 exposure years.[97] This was a level even higher than that observed in oral contraceptive users of the same era, 300 events per 100,000 exposure years.[98] Importantly, the rate of venous thromboembolism varied according to the age of the ethinyl estradiol user. Venous thromboembolism was more common at 12 percent in the over 40 years group, with a much lower rate of 1.2 percent for those under 40 years. This Dutch group subsequently switched to using 17β estradiol in the form of estradiol valerate or transdermal estrogen and found that the incidence of venous thromboembolism fell to 2.6 percent, much lower but still a 20-times risk compared with the general population. Venous thromboembolism was most common over the first 24 months of treatment, with a much lower risk of 0.4 percent per year occurring after the first two years of estrogen therapy.[99] The rate of venous thromboembolism was also found to be lower at 0.6 percent for oral 17β estradiol than the 4.4 percent recorded for oral conjugated equine estrogen in a U.K. study.[100] This provides evidence that it is the type of estrogen, as well as how it is administered, that is important in determining the risk of venous thromboembolism.

Ethinyl estradiol alters the levels of the clotting agents, proteins S, C, and prothrombin, that predispose a person to venous thromboembolism. However, 17β estradiol and transdermal estradiol are not found to have these adverse effects on clotting factors. Estrogen that is delivered by absorption through the skin may therefore be the best option for feminizing therapy for people older than 40. In the Dutch study, most of the venous thromboembolism incidents were found in women who were on oral ethinyl estradiol and cyproterone acetate, the single exception being a case of a trans woman on transdermal estrogen who had a previous venous thromboembolism and had discontinued oral anticoagulation medication.

Guidelines for starting hormone replacement therapy do not recommend screening women for a genetic or acquired condition in which the blood clots more easily, a condition known as thrombophilia.[101] Women with a high risk of venous thromboembolism for any reason, such as smoking, obesity, a previous blood clot, or known thrombophilia, should be commenced on transdermal estrogen.[102] An analysis of available data for postmenopausal cisgender women suggested that there was no risk of venous thromboembolism with transdermal preparations, even in women with a prior history of thrombosis. However, it may be that the actual dose of transdermal estrogen is also relevant. An analysis of data from a large U.K. GP research database showed almost a doubling of the risk of stroke in cisgender women aged 50 to 79 years who are on transdermal estrogen at doses of more than 50 mcg per day.[103]

If a thrombosis occurs in trans women on estrogen, hormone therapy does not need to be discontinued, but anticoagulant medication that increases the time it takes blood to clot should be started and a switch to transdermal therapy strongly considered. The risk of a recurrent thrombosis is low while on anticoagulant medication. However, as was the case for the single case from the Netherlands, indirect evidence from cisgender women suggests that the risk of recurrent thrombosis is high if the anticoagulant is stopped while estrogen therapy is continued. So, in such people, anticoagulant medication should be continued indefinitely.

Estrogen and Cardiovascular Risk

In the general population, sex hormones are known to alter the risk of a person developing diabetes, as well as cardiovascular disease with its life-threatening complications such as heart attacks and strokes. For example, men are more susceptible to cardiovascular disease than are women of a similar age, until this protective effect is lost after menopause.

During feminization therapy, there is an increase in both the body-mass index and the amount of body fat. A study using magnetic resonance imaging in 20 trans women who had been taking ethinyl estradiol and cyproterone acetate over a 12-month period showed an increase in both subcutaneous and internal or visceral fat.[104] This site of fat accumulation is important. If fat accumulates in organs, known as visceral fat, a person has a higher risk of cardiovascular disease, compared with when there is accumulation of subcutaneous fat. This may be the reason why trans women are more susceptible to cardiovascular disease.[105] Although this change in body composition is mainly an effect of estrogen, some of the cardiovascular disease risk might occur because of lifestyle, as it has been shown that trans women perform less sports-related activity compared with the general population.[106]

The relationship between hormone treatment and cardiovascular risk factors is complex. Estrogen therapy has been shown to both improve and impair metabolic measures such as fasting glucose and insulin levels, plasma docosahexaenoic acid or omega-3 fatty acid levels, adipokines, and C-reactive protein. One review of 16 cohort studies[107] and another of 29 studies[108] reported that estrogen increased triglyceride levels but had no effect on cholesterol levels. Blood pressure and arterial stiffness increase slightly during treatment with estrogen and an anti-androgen.[109]

A long-term study from the Netherlands suggests that feminizing hormone therapy using historical high-dose estrogen and cyproterone acetate does increase cardiovascular risk. In this cohort study, the current use of ethinyl estradiol was associated with a threefold increase in the risk of cardiovascular death. However, a meta-analysis suggested the data linking estrogen therapy and cardiovascular disease in the transgender community are still inconclusive.[110] Large multicenter studies are needed to assess cardiovascular risk with modern estrogen treatment regimens. However, these long-term studies will take some time, as usually several decades of usage must occur before any potential effects of hormone therapy on heart attack or stroke become evident.

Estrogen and Bone Health

Estrogen can maintain bone strength despite testosterone suppression. Bone biopsies taken after treatment with a combination of ethinyl estradiol (10 mcg per day) and cyproterone acetate (100 mg per day) over 8 to 41 months showed a possible reduction in bone turnover, an important requirement for bone health, but reassuringly without any change in bone mineral density.[111] A study of the effects of a combination of 10 mg intramuscular estradiol valerate administered every 10 days and a four-week GnRH blocker also showed maintenance of bone mineral density over a two-year period.[112]

In a small study of 20 trans women, there was an inverse relationship between bone mineral density and the levels of luteinizing hormone, the signal from the pituitary gland that is suppressed by estrogen therapy, suggesting that if the estrogen dose is too low it is more likely to be associated with a decline in bone density.[113] A review of 392 trans women included in mostly observational studies up to 2015 showed an increase in lumbar spine bone-mass density over a one- to two-year period of estrogen therapy but no change in hip bone-mass density. It is not known if this type of therapy changes the risk of fractures.[114] Importantly, it seems that trans women have a high incidence of osteoporosis *before* commencing medical transition, potentially due to reduced vitamin D levels or perhaps reduced weight-bearing activity.[115] Current guidelines suggest that doctors should ensure that modifiable risk factors for osteoporosis such as low calcium intake or low serum vitamin D level are addressed. A bone mineral density scan should be performed on people at risk for osteoporosis, or who have a history of inadequate hormone replacement, elevated luteinizing hormone, or who are over 60 years.

Estrogen and Hyperprolactinemia

The lactotroph cells in the pituitary gland make prolactin. Prolactin is released into circulation and can be measured using a blood sample. Prolactin has a role in lactation by signaling breast cells to produce milk during pregnancy. The pituitary lactotroph cells have estrogen receptors, so estrogen may increase prolactin levels, particularly if estradiol levels are high.

In some cases, high levels of prolactin in excess of, say, 50 µg/L or 1,000 mU/l can result in galactorrhea, secretion of milk from the nipple ducts, and a reduced sex drive or libido. The proportion of individuals with high prolactin or hyperprolactinemia was 2.3 percent in one study that employed a combination of estradiol and GnRH analog treatment.[116] In people taking a combination of ethinyl estradiol and cyproterone acetate the incidence was found to be higher at 3.7 to 7.2 percent per treatment year.[117] This may be a higher proportion than is normally found in the general population as progestins such as cyproterone acetate also increase prolactin levels. A reduction in estrogen dose or cessation of cyproterone acetate can allow prolactin levels to fall back toward the reference range. In those patients demonstrating persistent hyperprolactinemia, up to a third may have evidence of pituitary enlargement on computerized tomography scanning. Reassuringly, there are few published cases of raised prolactin levels being caused by the development of a prolactinoma, a benign tumor of the lactotroph cells in the pituitary gland,[118] despite this being a common condition for many people. Patients with a prolactinoma generally have higher prolactin levels, over 150 µg/L or 3,000 mU/l.[119] Pituitary magnetic resonance imaging is recommended for assessment if prolactin levels do not normalize with a reduction in estrogen dose.

Estrogen and Breast Cancer Risk

Breast cancer risk does not seem to be increased for trans women[120] and remains similar to the low rate of one in every 1,000 for cisgender males.[121] A large Dutch cohort study of 2,307 trans women on long-term hormone therapy that involved 52,370 person-years of exposure to estrogen reported only one case of breast cancer, this being the equivalent of 4.1 to 5.9 cases of breast cancer per 100,000 patient-years of therapy.[122] In this reported case of breast cancer, the tissue had estrogen receptors, suggesting that exposure to estrogen may have contributed to cancer growth.

A U.S. study of 1,112 transgender women taking estrogen therapy involving 9,057 person-years obtained from Veterans Health Administration data collected from 1997 to 2013 reported two cases of breast cancer, which equated to 20 cases of breast cancer per 100,000 patient years. The rate observed in the U.S. study was higher than in the European study; however, this was not unexpected as the rates of breast cancer are higher in the U.S. population as a whole.[123]

The risk of breast cancer for trans women may be higher if they carry a gene that predisposes them to breast cancer. There is no direct evidence for trans women, but it is notable that the risk is significantly increased in cisgender males with abnormalities such as germline mutations in the BRCA1 or BRCA2 gene.[124] In practice, it is useful to ask about a family history of breast cancer to determine whether someone falls into a higher risk category.

Overall, the studies are reassuring. However, it should be noted that the data collected for trans women is not as extensive as that for cisgender women. Therefore, it is possible that a slightly increased risk of breast cancer exists but has not yet been detected. Indeed, the risk of breast cancer is slightly increased in cisgender women with prolonged exposure to estrogen, and this risk is higher when estrogen is used in combination with progestins. Therefore, although the risk of developing breast cancer in trans women is low, guidelines recommend screening in line with the national guidelines for all women.

Estrogen and Prostate Cancer Risk

Trans women retain a prostate gland even after genital reconstruction surgery. However, if testosterone levels are persistently low, this gland tends to shrink in size. A study has demonstrated the effect of hormone therapy by showing that cisgender men who underwent removal of the testicles by means of orchidectomy that produces a testosterone deficiency and then took estrogen were found to have small prostate glands with no evidence of premalignant cells.[125]

Commensurate with this low-risk appearance, there are very few reported cases of prostate cancer in transgender females[126] despite it being a very common cancer. A review of 2,306 Dutch trans women treated from 1975 to 2006 demonstrated only one case of prostate cancer over a follow-up duration of 21.4 years and a total of 51,173 person–years of therapy.[127]

An epidemiological case-control study by Kaiser Permanente, a large U.S. health insurer, confirmed a much lower risk of prostate cancer when compared with the risk observed in cisgender men.[128] These authors noted that although prostate cancer is rare, the cancers that develop tend to be aggressive and, unsurprisingly, they do not respond to anti-androgens, a feature that indicates a poorer prognosis. Women who have had genital reconstruction surgery can have a prostate examination preformed vaginally as necessary. It has been proposed that in countries that screen for prostate cancer, prostate monitoring should be performed according to these guidelines.

7.3 SURGICAL INTERVENTIONS FOR ADULTS

The presence or absence of breast tissue is one of the characteristics that may identify a person to others as male or female. Therefore, many trans people seek chest surgery to help achieve their goals. Others desire genital surgery that encompasses a number of procedures that can align genital anatomy with a person's gender identity. This may involve the surgical construction of penis, testes, and scrotum for trans men; a vagina, vulva, and clitoris for trans women; or for nonbinary people a variation that may include the removal of reproductive organs or construction of a smooth contour to the genitals.[129] Often but not always this is the last step in a long transition process after social transition and hormone therapy. For many, it is a prerequisite for sexual health and fulfillment of a life-long dream.

The most recent Standards of Care of the World Professional Association for Transgender Health (WPATH) set out the current prerequisites for surgery, which include letters of recommendation from experienced health professionals. WPATH still recommends one letter in support of chest surgery and two letters in support of genital surgery. Guidelines also stipulate 12 months of continuous hormone therapy and living in a role concordant with gender identity before genital surgery is considered, unless hormonal therapy is not desired or medically contraindicated. These requirements are different from those for cisgender people who wish to undergo similarly irreversible surgeries that remove reproductive capacity, and therefore these requirements are discriminatory.[130] It is hoped that this position may be altered in newer guidelines to enable clinicians to change their practice and support patient choice.

An online survey of 280 trans people in the United States reported that of the trans men, 26 percent had undergone mastectomy, with 65 percent planning surgery. None had undergone genital surgery, but 30 percent of them were planning to pursue an operation. Of the trans women, 5 percent had undergone breast augmentation, with 38 percent planning such surgery. Five percent had already undergone genital surgery, while 43 percent were planning to pursue this surgery.[131] Treatment cost was identified as a reason for not having surgery for 29 percent of trans men and 23 percent of trans women. The lack of a qualified provider was the primary reason not to seek surgery for 41 percent of trans men and 2 percent of trans women. These data are helpful to build a picture of common practices, but it should be recognized that the numbers of people accessing different interventions vary widely depending on socioeconomic and cultural factors.

Surgical techniques for women have advanced over the last two decades, yielding results that are almost indistinguishable in appearance, and to some extent function, from the genitals of cisgender women. The surgical techniques for men are not quite so impressive due to the complexity of constructing a functional penis. Nevertheless, technical advances continue so that improvement in the surgical outcomes for men can be expected. The procedures are safe and recovery from surgery is usually complete. Those people who have managed well during the transition before surgery tend to manage well afterward. Caution is required for people with significant medical and psychological problems prior to surgery as their adjustment may be more challenging.

Surgical procedures are generally performed in private practice, the U.K. National Health Service being one exception, and so are unfortunately expensive if not covered by medical insurance. A review of 6,973 records in the Amsterdam Clinic from 1972 to 2015 showed that only 0.6 percent of trans women and 0.3 percent of trans men who underwent *bottom surgery* were identified as experiencing regret. Some of this regret was related to surgical complications. This result shows that surgery is a positive experience for almost all trans people when delivered in a system that provides multidisciplinary support.[132]

7.3.1 Masculinizing Chest Surgery

Testosterone therapy is effective in masculinizing a trans man's external appearance, but will not remove breast tissue if someone has already been exposed to estrogen. Many people choose chest binding to conceal the appearance of their breasts prior to surgery. This can lead to skin irritation, pain, bruising, and respiratory problems if done incorrectly. It is recommended that trans men or nonbinary people identifying on the masculine spectrum purchase a specifically designed binder that fits well. The use of elastic bandages, duct tape, or plastic wrap should be avoided. Binders should be removed when sleeping and be used for no longer than 8 to 12 hours a day.[133]

The presence of breasts may be a source of distress, so many trans men choose to have chest reconstruction, or *top surgery*, performed by a specialist surgeon. Discussions about surgery usually take place after hormone therapy has started, although this may not be the case for those who do not wish to, or cannot, have hormone therapy, including some nonbinary people. The goals of this surgery are to flatten the chest and to reduce and reshape the nipple so that it has a male appearance. This surgery is performed as a day procedure or it may include an overnight stay in the hospital. Several different techniques for subcutaneous mastectomy or breast removal have been described.[134]

The chosen surgical technique is usually based upon the amount of breast tissue, its shape or ptosis, and skin elasticity. The location and extent of any postsurgical scarring will depend on the surgical procedure that was used. People with a small amount of breast tissue can often have a mastectomy performed in a circumareolar fashion through a small incision around the nipple. For other people, a more extensive reduction is required with the breast removed in the form of an ellipse and the scar concealed in a groove under the chest, with the nipple relocated using a skin graft. This procedure is known as double mastectomy with free nipple grafting. The breast shape and skin elasticity are often affected by long-term chest binding. This may mean a nipple graft technique is recommended, even when there is only a small amount of glandular tissue present. The surgical team will assess the best procedure for each person, based upon their personal preference and these clinical considerations.

The potential complications of surgery include bleeding, infection, and breakdown or necrosis of the nipple. One study of 295 trans men undergoing surgery between 2006 and 2015 showed that 37 percent of men underwent a circumareolar approach and 63 percent had a nipple graft technique.[135] In this study, the overall complication rate was 18 percent, with a collection of blood or hematoma occurring in 7 percent of cases and a further 5 percent of cases having a collection of clear fluid or seroma. Infections occurred in 2 percent and partial nipple necrosis occurred after 3 percent of operations. There was no difference in complications between the two types of surgery, the circumareolar approach or nipple graft technique. For those who had a follow-up consultation more than 180 days after surgery, 39 percent had needed some minor revisions performed to improve their aesthetic appearance. Trans men were more likely to require surgical revision if they began with a medium amount of breast tissue but were considered still able to have circumareolar surgery. Although only one person needed to convert to the nipple graft technique, the authors suggested it would be wise to consider this more extensive technique in all but those with minimal to moderate glandular tissue, good skin elasticity, and a nipple position that sits above the inframammary fold.

7.3.2 Feminizing Chest Surgery

Estrogen therapy results in growth of breast tissue that reaches its maximum extent after two to three years. If a trans woman feels her breast growth is unacceptable, she may opt to have breast augmentation or *top surgery*. Maximal breast growth with hormone therapy takes two to three years, although the greatest change in breast size generally may occur in the first six months. It has been suggested that at least two years of estrogen therapy should be completed before a trans woman considers breast augmentation surgery.

The surgical techniques used are similar to those used for cisgender women. Usually surgery takes place as a day case performed under general anesthetic. A submammary incision can be placed under the breast or an axillary incision can be made in the armpit. Saline or silicone gel prostheses are inserted under a muscle, or under the developed breast tissue if there has been a good response to estrogen. If breast augmentation is occurring after a testosterone-driven puberty, the nipple will lie more laterally on the chest wall.

In a study of 359 trans women seen in a clinic from 1979 to 1996, of the 56 percent who underwent augmentation mammoplasty, the average size of implanted prostheses was 254 ml, leading to an increase in breast size from an A cup to a B cup, with 75 percent of trans women being satisfied with their new breast size.[136] However, the desired implant size may have increased more recently to a C or D cup or even larger.[137] This surgery is rarely covered by health insurance and remains expensive. Some people elect out of desperation to use injections of silicone or mineral oil to aid the feminization of their chest, which leads to serious complications including infection and deformity.[138]

7.3.3 Masculinizing Genital Surgery

Since gender-affirmation surgery for trans men is complicated and expensive, many men are content to experience the secondary sex characteristics induced by testosterone therapy. Financial considerations and reports from others of poor surgical outcomes have been the greatest reported deterrents to surgery.[139] However, more recent studies have shown that trans men report a good quality of life and satisfactory sexual function after genital surgery.[140]

The most straightforward genital surgery is removal of the uterus via hysterectomy with or without oophorectomy, the surgical removal of the ovaries, a common procedure performed by a gynecologist. This procedure can be useful for those people experiencing ongoing unwanted periods or menses despite adequate testosterone therapy, but it does result in complete infertility, unless ovarian tissue is frozen and preserved as described in Chapter 8. There is no clear evidence to recommend performing hysterectomy and oophorectomy just to prevent cancer in these organs.

The goals of genital surgery for trans men have been proposed by others as threefold: the creation of a penis that provides erotic sensation, the ability to have penetrative sexual intercourse, and the ability to urinate while standing. Surgical procedures include phalloplasty, the creation of a penis using other tissue, and metoidioplasty, the release of the clitoris from surrounding structures. These types of surgery are colloquially known as *bottom surgery*. Urologists with a special interest in reconstructive surgery usually perform these procedures. They are major operations with a moderate risk of complications and a recovery time of several months or longer. For this reason, some patients opt to simplify their surgery by avoiding construction of a urethra and instead choose to urinate sitting down.

The most common surgical technique for constructing a penis uses a skin and muscle flap from the nondominant forearm, also known as a *radial flap*. This procedure is performed as either a multiple-step operation to allow recovery following each procedure or, in some centers, in one long operation lasting from 6 to 12 hours. Classically, the operation usually starts with removal of the uterus and ovaries using a keyhole or laparoscopic approach. This is followed by removal of the vagina using vaginectomy and construction of a urethra from the skin of the forearm or other tissues to make a tube to transport urine from the bladder. A penis is formed by making another tube from the forearm flap with connection of the arteries, veins, and nerves. This is combined with the new urethra to form a *tube in tube* structure. The clitoris is preserved and left underneath or above the new penis to preserve erotic sensation, and a scrotum is constructed from the labia majora. The forearm graft site is covered with skin from the abdomen, but scarring of this site remains a major disadvantage of the radial flap approach.

In a third stage, often up to a year later, testicular prostheses are implanted and a glans at the head of the penis can be formed to improve the aesthetic appearance of the reconstructed genitals. The shaft of the penis is usually wide enough to incorporate a permanent semirigid erectile prosthesis to facilitate sexual intercourse if desired. Alternatively, a silicon implant can be placed inside the penis to achieve continuous rigidity while also providing sufficient flexibility to permit the wearing of shorts and swimming costumes. A review of available studies in 2016 showed that 70 percent of trans men reported that they were pleased with their genital appearance using this technique, and a similar percentage had erotic sensation. Penetrative sexual intercourse was possible for 40 percent, and standing urination could be achieved by 90 percent of men.

An alternative procedure involves using skin from the anterior thigh on a vascular pedicle, combined with the formation of a urethra made from the skin of the forearm to allow standing urination. This produces a less conspicuous forearm scar, which for the radial flap method can be as large as two-thirds of the circumference of the forearm. Although this technique can cause a similarly large scar on one thigh, clothing can more easily conceal it. Using this *anterior thigh flap* technique has potential cosmetic benefit, as the skin of the thigh is more likely to match the skin of the genital region in color and texture.[141]

Metoidioplasty is a somewhat less complex technique that involves exposing the enlarged clitoris that has grown as a result of testosterone therapy. It exploits the similar distribution and course of the nerves and vessels, the neurovascular bundle, in the clitoris and penis, so that the clitoris becomes the head of the penis and retains its sensitivity. Metoidioplasty releases, straightens, and appears to lengthen the hormonally enlarged clitoris by detaching its suspensory ligament. If standing urination is desired, then a urethra can be formed using genital skin or tissue from inside the cheek. The new phallus is shorter and smaller (3 to 8 cm) after metoidioplasty than with phalloplasty. This procedure is often performed in a single operation lasting from two to five hours. Alternatively, the labia majora can be joined to form a scrotum into which testicular implants are placed during a second-stage procedure.

Metoidioplasty does not require a flap harvested from another body location, and the new penis has sufficient erectile function not to need implantation of prostheses. The operation therefore usually has a shorter recovery time.

A review of studies showed that almost 90 percent of trans men were pleased with the appearance of their genitals after metoidioplasty, all had erotic sensation, half achieved penetrative intercourse, and 90 percent were able to urinate standing up.[142]

Any surgical procedure may have complications such as hemorrhage or bleeding, hematoma or bruising, and infection. In both metoidioplasty and phalloplasty, the most important complication relates to the newly formed urethra. Such complications include leakage of urine from the urethra directly on to the skin via a urethra-cutaneous fistula, observed in from 10 to 70 percent of cases, or urethral stenosis or narrowing that can occur in from 15 to 35 percent of cases. The risk of this complication seems to be similar in both types of surgery. After phalloplasty, there is also a chance that there can be a loss of blood supply and death of the penis due to radial flap failure, a risk in from 1 to 5 percent of surgeries. Problems may also occur with the donor site on the forearm.

Despite the potential risks and complications, satisfaction rates are reasonably high for those who are motivated sufficiently to endure these surgical procedures. The available studies make it difficult to directly compare the different procedures to aid decision-making at the time of choosing an operation. This choice should therefore be based on personal goals and discussion with the surgeon.

7.3.4 Feminizing Genital Surgery

The simplest surgical option for trans women is removal of the testes, or orchidectomy, which stops the production of testosterone. This often allows lower doses of estrogen to be used and allows cessation of anti-androgen therapy and progesterone, if used for testosterone suppression. A change to the appearance of a person's genitals can be achieved by constructing a vagina using vaginoplasty with or without orchidectomy, colloquially known as *bottom surgery*. There are many similarities between male and female genitals that provide a useful starting point for this type of surgery.

Penile Inversion Vaginoplasty

Penile inversion vaginoplasty is the most commonly performed and researched form of feminizing genital reconstruction surgery. The surgeon usually takes between two and four hours to construct a vagina using the skin of the penis and scrotum, and to make a sensate clitoris and labia majora.[143] Different surgeons may have their own preferred techniques and may suggest a single-step or two-step procedure. Generally, the operation begins by removal of both testicles, if a prior orchidectomy has not been performed, followed by separation of the penis into its component parts, the erectile tissue or corpora cavernosa, the head or glans, opening of the tube for urine or urethra, the nerves and vessels or neurovascular bundle, together with the skin and its blood supply. The corpora cavernosa is removed to where it meets the pelvic bones.

To create the vagina, the skin of the penis is inverted and used to line a new cavity formed in the pelvis. The urethra is shortened and the opening repositioned to the anatomical position of cisgender females. Part of the urethral tube can be flattened and included in the vaginal cavity to create a self-lubricating section. If necessary, skin from the abdomen or scrotum can also be used in the new vagina to provide additional depth and width. It is important that hair removal occurs at these sites before the skin is used to improve the appearance and reduce the chance of complications.

The most sensitive part of the original glans of the penis, the dorsum or rear, is used to form a clitoris and the remainder, the ventrum or front, can be relocated to form a cervix. The prostate gland remains in position. The external genitals, the labia minora and labia majora, are constructed from the remaining penile and scrotal skin. In the final stage of the surgery a temporary drain, a urinary catheter, and vaginal packing are placed and left for the first few days. After these are removed, a vaginal dilator, often of increasing size, must be used regularly to maintain depth and shape. Hygiene and regular dilation, initially several times a day, are critical aspects of postoperative care. A good support network is also crucial during the recovery period and it is important to avoid heavy lifting for several weeks. The surgeon should provide clear instructions for postoperative care and a list of potential complications of which those undergoing the procedure should be aware.

Intestinal Vaginoplasty

The surgical construction of a vagina can be performed using other techniques. An intestinal vaginoplasty uses a 15- to 20- cm segment of ileum or sigmoid colon that is removed through an incision in the abdomen, after which the rest of the bowel is reconnected. Similar to penile inversion surgery, the testicles and penis are removed and a clitoris and labia formed. However, in intestinal vaginoplasty the segment of bowel, rather than skin, is used to form the new vaginal cavity.

Although this technique usually produces a self-lubricating vagina with a reduced requirement for dilatation, the production of mucus by the bowel segment can cause excess discharge, particularly over the first few months. Intestinal vaginoplasty is also a more complex operation and usually takes the surgeon six to eight hours to complete. This may be a particularly useful technique for trans women who have insufficient penile skin, for example in those who have immature genitalia because of GnRH analog therapy, or when a trans woman requests a second rescue procedure if penile inversion was unsuccessful.

The improved quality of life reported after gender reconstruction surgery is closely associated with the appearance and function of the person's new anatomy.[144] A review of the surgical outcomes of vaginoplasty in 2015 collated the results of 13 studies of penile inversion and 9 studies of intestinal vaginoplasty.[145] The penile inversion technique was studied in 1,461 patients. The average vaginal depth was between 10 and 13.5 cm, and vaginal width, although not often reported, was 3 to 4 cm. After surgery, 75 percent of the women were having vaginal sexual intercourse. The women experienced few problems with only a minority of them reporting discomfort (up to 6%) or bleeding (up to 3%). Patient satisfaction with sexual function was rated 7.8 out of 10 points, and 70 to 85 percent of the women were able to achieve orgasm. Narrowing or shortening of the vagina caused by stricture or stenosis occurred in 1 to 12 percent of women. Failure or necrosis of the new vagina, usually due to loss of blood supply, occurred after up to 4 percent of surgeries, and collapse or prolapse of the vaginal cavity occurred in up to 2 percent of cases.

The intestinal vaginoplasty technique was studied in a total of 102 patients. The average vaginal depth was 12 to 18 cm and its width was 2.5 to 4.5 cm. Almost 80 percent of patients were sexually active, and a similar proportion reported satisfactory sexual function. Vaginal discharge or an unpleasant odor was mentioned as an adverse outcome in 1 to 10 percent of women. There was a variable rate of stricture or stenosis from between 1 and 50 percent. This wide range of results probably represents the small patient numbers in some studies and the different surgical techniques used. The rate of vaginal prolapse was 8 percent, and vaginal necrosis and bowel complications were rare.

Penile inversion and intestinal vaginoplasty resulted in comparable outcomes in this review. Although there are no studies directly comparing the procedures by allocating patients to one or the other technique at random, it is fair to say that intestinal vaginoplasty does not seem inferior to penile inversion vaginoplasty. Narrowing and shortening of the vagina were the most common complications after both procedures. Changes to the urine stream and the development of a urine infection also occurred in up to a third of women. There are less common but potentially serious adverse consequences of these surgeries, for example damage to the rectum, venous thromboembolism, or the development of abnormal channels or fistula, for example from rectum to vagina or from urethra to vagina. Although postsurgical complications can be distressing, they are rarely life threatening provided appropriate medical intervention can be obtained.

Vulvuloplasty

Vulvuloplasty or shallow depth vaginoplasty is an alternative surgical option in which the testicles and penis are removed, and labia and clitoris are made by repositioning the urethra, but a vaginal cavity is not created. Many people choose to form a shallow dimple without depth at the site of the vaginal entrance. This results in a similar outward appearance as vaginoplasty, but a vagina is not present so penetrative sexual intercourse is not possible. This option may be a positive choice that represents a person's gender identity or goals. It is also a less complex form of surgery that may come with a reduced chance of complications for women who have a higher surgical risk. The procedure also makes dilation unnecessary, which is important for some people.

A study from Portland, United States of 486 transfeminine people accessing gender reconstruction surgery showed that 396 had vaginoplasty and 39 had vulvuloplasty.[146] The majority, 63 percent, of those requesting vulvuloplasty did so by choice without having a medical reason that might have prevented vaginoplasty. Almost all (93%) women who underwent vulvuloplasty were satisfied with both their decision and the surgical outcome.

It should be noted there is some uncertainty whether estrogen therapy needs to be stopped before elective planned surgery. The surgeon may be concerned that continuing estrogen therapy will increase the risk of thromboembolism beyond that of the surgery itself and the immobility that often occurs afterward. Evidence from cisgender women on the oral contraceptive pill suggests that two to eight weeks are needed before estrogen-induced alterations in clotting, or hemostatic, factors reverse. Based on such data, cessation of the oral contraceptive pill therapy is often recommended at least four weeks prior to any major elective surgery.[147]

However, it should be remembered that hormonal therapy confers only a small risk compared with the larger risk of the surgery itself, and therefore continuing estrogen may not add significantly to a person's overall risk if continued. This is evident for hormone replacement therapy provided to postmenopausal women for whom there is a two or three times increased risk for thromboembolism in users of hormone replacement compared with nonusers, whereas there is a 40- to 50-fold increased risk of deep vein thrombosis in patients undergoing orthopedic surgery.[148] Postoperative thrombosis is a serious complication of surgery and is certainly a risk for trans women undergoing genital reconstruction surgery. This has led to the common recommendation to cease estrogen several weeks before the operation, and to resume hormone therapy only once mobility is back to normal. However, extrapolating the available information from the general population to trans women suggests that by far the most important precaution is the use of anticlotting medications, such as injectable heparin, and mechanical devices to improve circulation after the operation when it may be difficult to move around normally for several days. Further research in this area would be helpful to avoid unnecessary hormone cessation, while ensuring the safest management after surgery.

SUMMARY

The medical and surgical options for transition are safe and effective in the short and medium to long term. Several larger studies are underway to determine the lifelong health implications of therapy. The optimal types and doses of hormones are under investigation, and there is still a paucity of research regarding the best therapy for nonbinary people. As the understanding of trans health improves, clinicians will become better at individualizing hormone treatment to meet the goals of the TGD community. At the current time, the desire for top and bottom surgery is often thwarted by its high cost and lack of insurance coverage for these procedures. Perhaps over the next decade there will be increased recognition of the medical need for access to appropriate care to enable TGD people to achieve their optimal health and well-being.

Chapter 8

FERTILITY

8.1 THE POTENTIAL IMPACT OF TRANSITION ON FERTILITY

The desire of transgender and gender-diverse (TGD) people to have children is no different from that of the general population. Two studies from Belgium have reported that around half of trans women[1] and trans men[2] wished to have children at the time of the interview. The potential to have biologically related children may be compromised by gender-affirming hormonal or surgical therapies. These treatments can impair long-term fertility, and the effect of some types of surgery is permanent. For many members of the trans community, gender transition and reproduction have been mutually exclusive choices.[3] This is no longer necessarily the case, and artificial fertility techniques have advanced rapidly over the past decade. Unfortunately, in some countries, trans people still have to forego their reproductive rights to obtain transition care.[4]

Children may or may not be genetically related to their parents, and there are many ways to build a family. Communicating the potential impact of treatment and the available options to start a family informs this individual choice. Regardless of whether a person desires genetically related biological children, the majority of trans people agree that fertility preservation should be discussed and offered before starting transition. Therefore, clinicians should be willing and able to discuss (a) the effects of GnRH blockers; (b) the partially reversible effects of hormones; (c) the permanent consequences of some types of surgery; and (d) the locally available methods to preserve future reproductive potential if desired.[5]

The removal of reproductive organs, testicles or ovaries, causes absolute and permanent infertility, unless eggs or sperm can be stored at this time. Also, the removal of the womb or uterus will prevent carrying a baby during pregnancy. For this reason, these surgeries are usually delayed until the person is over the age of majority in their country. Other procedures such as metoidioplasty, scrotoplasty, or phalloplasty would not necessarily impede pregnancy. It is unclear what effect they would have on birth.[6]

Estrogen may reduce fertility, particularly if higher doses are taken over an extended period. Prolonged hormonal therapy with estrogen reduces the quality of semen and decreases sperm concentration, shape, and function.[7] This eventually leads to a lack of sperm in the semen and subsequent infertility that may be reversible if estrogen is stopped.[8] If sperm is preserved but it is of low quality, artificial fertility techniques can be used to directly inject sperm into an egg using intracytoplasmic sperm injection to achieve fertilization.

Hormonal therapy with testosterone usually causes the menstrual cycle to stop; this amenorrhea generally occurs within two to six months of starting therapy, although in some people it can take longer.[9] Unlike the effect of estrogen on sperm, treatment with testosterone does not reduce the quality or number of eggs in the ovary. However, testosterone does prevent ovulation, which occurs when the fully mature eggs are released. Testosterone also reduces the thickness of the endometrium, the lining of the womb.[10] This process is not absolute, so testosterone should not be considered as a contraceptive.[11] This is important to understand as testosterone can cause birth defects if a trans man conceives unexpectedly.

Contraceptive options for trans men that will not interfere with hormonal transition include barrier methods, progesterone-based oral contraceptive tablets, or a progesterone-based intrauterine device; these latter two options also prevent endometrial hyperplasia, an abnormal thickening of the lining of the uterus. If testosterone is ceased, a person's eggs can begin to grow and mature again, and the effect on fertility may reverse. There are no definitive recommendations about how long testosterone should be ceased before attempting to conceive. Expert opinion generally recommends at least three months.

This chapter describes the current knowledge about fertility preservation for trans or gender-diverse people. Much of the evidence for artificial fertility techniques comes not from research in this context, but from research with people about to undergo chemotherapy for cancer. Fertility preservation does not guarantee having biological children. At the time of starting a family, success will depend on the quality of eggs and sperm, the success rate of the fertility technique, and the partner's health. Notably, a younger age at the time of fertility preservation is often the most significant factor. The establishment of international registers to provide data for the short- and long-term outcomes of these techniques in the general population has been recommended.[12] Some of the available data has been reported in this chapter, but it is important to remember that success rates are entirely dependent on the individual's circumstances.

Research is needed to further study the consequences of hormones and surgery on fertility, fertility preservation, and the outcomes of artificial fertility techniques in trans people. Although some techniques are well established, there remains much uncertainty regarding future technologies, particularly related to maturation of immature eggs and sperm. The available information on pregnancy and chestfeeding and breastfeeding from the trans and gender-diverse community is discussed.

8.1.1 Younger Adolescents

Young trans people may choose to take GnRH blockers in early puberty to prevent the permanent consequences of progressing further through puberty in their birth-assigned sex. Puberty suppression is entirely reversible and does not directly affect long-term fertility.[13] Ceasing GnRH blockers at any stage will restart puberty, but having reached this point, many young people would not contemplate stopping therapy as an option. While GnRH blockers are continued, this pause in early puberty means the person's body will not begin to make mature eggs or sperm.

With today's medical technology it is not yet possible to have genetically related children using immature eggs or sperm, but the future holds a number of possibilities that are discussed further later in this chapter. With these emerging techniques, discussions about fertility are being held with families of young adolescents before or soon after they start GnRH blockers. Their parents may be concerned that by allowing their child to transition at an early age they may be depriving them of the option to have biological children and provide grandchildren. This raises some ethical concerns, as parents could attempt to make decisions on behalf of their child, despite holding opposing views. As a working group has recently commented, "[F]or example, parent's wishes may differ from those of their child or may differ between parents sharing legal decision-making rights."[14]

It may be challenging to discuss fertility options with the young person themselves at an age when reproductive wishes are not well defined. However, postponing decision-making until the young person develops greater capacity for decision-making may cause them to miss the optimal time for fertility preservation. Family therapy and/or fertility counseling may provide an essential opportunity to discuss these options in a way that preserves the young person's right to decide.

It is recommended that clinicians inform young people about their options in a way that is consistent with their developmental stage and understanding of reproduction.[15] However, a study from Chicago between 2013 and 2016 showed that only 13 (12.4%) of 105 transgender adolescents aged 16.5 years had a review with a fertility specialist before starting treatment.[16] Only five patients (4.8%) subsequently chose to freeze their sperm or eggs, citing cost and the invasiveness of the procedures as reasons not to proceed. Interestingly, this team noted anecdotally that some young people felt that after hormonal treatment they became more comfortable in their body and were therefore able to better consider future parenthood. This suggests that it may be important to check back with the young person regarding fertility options early after hormone treatment is initiated.

The other large study of U.S. adolescents that accessed clients from a pediatric gender clinic, who were aged 15.2 years at their first visit and had been attending the clinic from 2014 to 2016, showed that 72 of 73 young people (98.6%) were counseled about fertility. However, despite this discussion, only two attempted fertility preservation by sperm banking.[17] As is the case for the general population, attitudes toward fertility may alter when young trans or gender-diverse people reach adulthood.

A recent innovation is the *Transgender Youth Fertility Attitudes Questionnaire* that aims to support the conversation around fertility preservation with trans youth and their families.[18] This allows the young person to consider statements such as *I am aware that hormone treatment could cause issues with my ability to have my own biological children; I want to have kids someday (this could be either your own biological kids or adopted kids); my feelings about my wanting my own biological child might change when I'm older; I am aware that there are options that would allow me to have my own biological child even if I'm on hormones; I would feel that I'm disappointing my family if I could not have my own biological child; and I would consider medical procedures that would allow me to preserve my eggs or sperm in order to have my own biological children in the future.*

Interestingly, using this tool the majority of young trans or gender-diverse people expressed a wish to have children at some point in their lives. The importance of having their own biological child was not said to be particularly important, but half the respondents also indicated that this feeling might change in the future. The questionnaire may prove useful in starting a discussion about fertility preservation and can be downloaded at https://children snational.org/TYFAQ.

We now consider the experimental techniques for ovarian and testicular tissue banking using freezing or cryopreservation. This is the only currently available option for a young person in early puberty. It may not be available in all centers, as it is usually done in academic hospitals where scientists support fertility research. Immature tissue is frozen with the hope that medical science will have progressed by the time fertility is desired.[19] The alternative option is to delay or discontinue GnRH blockers to allow the eggs or sperm to mature.

This would be an appropriate option if the distress caused by potential infertility is greater than the distress caused by progression of puberty.

There is no research with young trans or gender-diverse people to help estimate how long it would take for the development of maturity after stopping GnRH blockers and/or starting treatment to stimulate puberty with gonadotropin analogs. However, when people treated for abnormally early or precocious puberty ceased their GnRH blockers, sperm production restarted between eight months and three years.[20] It should be noted that stopping treatment to wait for sperm to mature allows testosterone levels to rise and most of the physical changes of puberty progress to reach Tanner stages 3 and 4. There is no information on how long it usually takes to restart ovulation after cessation of GnRH blockers.

Young people who are partway through puberty at Tanner stages 3 or 4 may already have some mature eggs or sperm present. Those that have reached maturity have preservation options similar to those available to older adolescents and adults.

8.1.2 Older Adolescents and Adults

People who have reached late puberty at Tanner stages 3 or 4, or who have completed puberty are able to produce mature eggs and sperm. There are a number of options available for fertility preservation,[21] as shown in Figure 8.1. These techniques are the same as those provided to cisgender people.

People may choose to preserve mature eggs after hormone stimulation or sperm after ejaculation or surgical extraction using cryogenic freezing. Ideally this would be performed before starting hormones. The chances of having a successful birth using these procedures should be discussed for each person, as the outcome will vary greatly as a result of individual factors and may also depend on the partner or any future partner. Assessment by a fertility specialist is recommended, particularly as some options remain experimental and access may be limited. Egg, sperm, or embryo cryopreservations are the first options for fertility preservation and are discussed in detail below.

8.2 ARTIFICIAL REPRODUCTIVE TECHNIQUES

8.2.1 Egg or Oocyte Banking

The ovary consists of clusters of cells called follicles, each of which contains a single immature egg or oocyte. This oocyte contains genetic material in the form of DNA. The follicles release hormones, estrogen and progesterone, that control the menstrual cycle. Some of the eggs develop to maturity and are released once each cycle during ovulation.

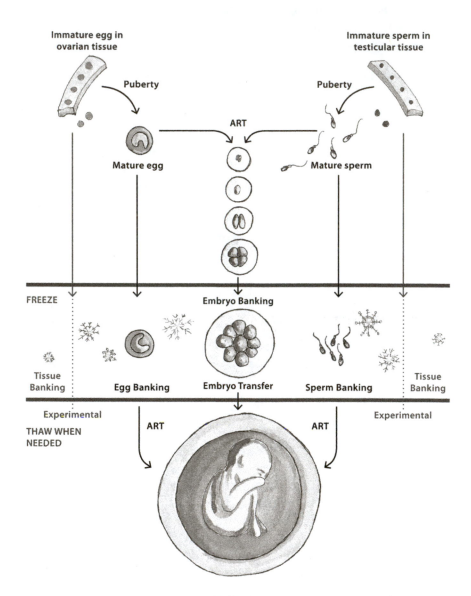

Figure 8.1 Fertility preservation and artificial reproductive technology (ART).
People may choose to collect eggs or sperm and cryogenically freeze or bank these
gametes to preserve their fertility. Alternatively, an egg and sperm can be used to
produce an embryo that can be similarly stored. These can be thawed at the time
fertility is desired and a pregnancy achieved using artificial reproductive technology (ART). The fertility techniques that use immature eggs and sperm are still
under investigation, but many children have been born with the established techniques using stored mature eggs, mature sperm, or embryos.

Egg banking, known as egg cryopreservation, is a process in which the egg is collected, frozen, and stored. To do this, the person is given artificial hormones to stimulate the ovaries so that the egg can be collected under controlled circumstances. The stages of egg maturation can be monitored using vaginal ultrasound scans. Once the egg cell has matured, it can be collected by a surgical procedure that gains access to the ovary through the vagina. For trans men this may be a challenging procedure both physically and mentally. Many centers would recommend that this procedure be undertaken before commencing testosterone, or after medication has been stopped. However, it may be possible to harvest eggs while on testosterone therapy, as cisgender women with elevated testosterone levels successfully achieve live births without complication. Egg banking can be performed without the need for a partner or donor at the time of fertility preservation.

A person's eggs can be reliably frozen until they are needed. After thawing, either a partner's or donor sperm can be used for fertilization. The resulting embryo is transferred to the womb of the person who wishes to carry the pregnancy, the gestational carrier. This may be the trans man who has banked the eggs, if they have not had a hysterectomy and have stopped testosterone, a female partner, or a surrogate. The need for assisted reproductive technologies will depend on the trans man's desire to carry the pregnancy, the method of combining sperm and egg, and the presence of a regular hormone cycle.

There can be no absolute assurance that a successful pregnancy will result from this process. Not all eggs survive the freezing and thawing process. Although there are no data for the trans population, for comparison, in one study an overall birth rate of 50 percent was reported for younger women who are 35 years and under, and 23 percent for older women when eggs were preserved for either delayed childbearing or medical conditions unrelated to cancer.[22]

A recent publication[23] reported the stories of two American trans men who decided to bank eggs and then went on to start a family. These stories provide a helpful insight into the process. One person was a 30-year-old single transgender man who preserved their eggs before starting testosterone therapy. He received hormonal stimulation using low-dose leuprolide acetate; 45 eggs were retrieved and then frozen. After eight years of testosterone therapy, he decided to create an embryo with his partner using donor sperm. Twenty eggs were thawed, 18 (90%) survived this process, and 17 (84%) were successfully fertilized after injection of sperm into the eggs using intracytoplasmic sperm injection. The embryos were allowed to develop in the laboratory for five to six days. After testing for genetic defects, one embryo was transferred into the womb of his cisgender female partner with accompanying hormonal support. A pregnancy with monozygotic-diamniotic twins resulted, and healthy babies were born at 34 weeks gestation.

The second person was a 32-year-old single trans man who had already proceeded with chest reconstruction and was planning to start testosterone therapy. He similarly underwent ovarian stimulation; 13 mature and 6 immature eggs were retrieved for banking. Five years later he decided to create an embryo with his cis female partner and donor sperm. Nineteen eggs were thawed, with a 95 percent survival rate. Fourteen were mature and 11 of those were fertilized after intracytoplasmic sperm injection. A day 5 embryo was transferred to his partner's womb but did not achieve ongoing pregnancy. A further two stored embryos were transferred, resulting in a pregnancy with dichorionic-diamniotic twins, each embryo having its own chorionic and amniotic sacs. Healthy twins were delivered at 35 weeks gestation.

8.2.2 Ovarian Tissue Banking

Ovarian tissue banking may only be available in research institutions that have established a protocol within their fertility laboratory. This method involves the removal and freezing of tissue from the ovary using a surgical procedure. The tissue is obtained by surgical biopsy or can be collected if the ovaries are removed using a surgical technique known as oophorectomy. Eggs are still present in the ovaries even after prolonged treatment with testosterone. It is therefore also possible to preserve ovarian tissue as part of genital reconstruction surgery, even if testosterone has been used for a prolonged period. This technique can be used for both prepubertal and postpubertal trans men. Unlike egg cryopreservation, this process does not require the person to have artificial hormone stimulation of their ovaries.

So far, over a hundred births have been achieved in the general population by re-implanting banked ovarian tissue into the woman's pelvic cavity using an orthotopic or in-place procedure or elsewhere in the woman's body using a heterotopic procedure. These babies were born to adult women who had banked mature eggs to preserve their fertility before cancer treatment. There has also been one report of success with banked immature ovarian tissue that was reimplanted in adulthood; the ovarian tissue was able to then mature and release eggs.[24]

Although retransplantation of ovarian tissue may restore fertility, it may have potential issues for trans men. This technique requires discontinuation of testosterone therapy and leads to an increase in estrogen levels as the ovarian tissue produces hormones. For trans men who have undergone ovarian removal via oophorectomy, the transplanted ovarian tissue would need to be placed away from the ovarian surface, say in the peritoneal region, a site that may be associated with diminished pregnancy success. A further increase in estrogen levels occurs if ovarian stimulation is needed to collect eggs from the transplanted tissue before using artificial fertility techniques. After ovarian tissue reimplantation, natural spontaneous conception is possible, without use of further artificial fertility techniques, if the person still has a womb or uterus.

An alternative for immature ovarian tissue is to trigger the maturation process in the laboratory in vitro to develop a mature egg. At present, these techniques are entirely experimental[25] and are not yet available in clinical practice.[26] There has been one report of a successful birth after artificially triggering the in vitro maturation process and then re-implanting the tissue, a process that seemed to accelerate the woman's ability to produce mature eggs.

Other innovative techniques that would allow maturation in the laboratory, such as a three-dimensional culture or the creation of artificial ovaries, appear to be promising possibilities for the future. As with other techniques, if mature eggs were produced in the laboratory, the partner's or donor sperm could then be used for fertilization. The resulting embryo could be transferred to the womb of the person who wishes to carry the pregnancy.

As reasonably positive outcomes have been observed in women undergoing chemotherapy, it has been proposed that ovarian tissue banking is now ready for use in routine clinical practice. In the general population, a 30 percent live birth rate was reported in 111 women who had their mature ovarian tissue preserved prior to cancer treatment.[27] Ovarian tissue banking does show potential for those trans men with mature tissue, but much research is needed to make it a realistic option for those who have not gone through puberty. This makes the discussion with young people complex, as little certainty can be provided. This is an important consideration for trans men who have used GnRH blockers. To date, there have been no cases to demonstrate that ovarian tissue preservation can lead to successful fertility for this group.

8.2.3 Sperm Banking

The freezing of mature sperm by cryopreservation allows the preservation of genetic material or DNA for reproduction. This is the simplest and most reliable method of fertility preservation. When the time is right to start a family, the samples can be used to fertilize an egg. There is good evidence that sperm banking is effective, even when the sperm is kept frozen for a long time. Indeed, this is a well-established fertility technique, with the longest reported successful storage time being 40 years.[28] It may be distressing for a trans women or girl to obtain sperm through self-stimulation.[29] As an alternative, surgical sperm extraction can be used. This involves placing a needle through scrotal skin into the testicle to extract mature sperm.

The type of artificial fertility techniques used to conceive will depend on the quality of the sperm samples. If the sperm count remains high after freezing and thawing, there is a good chance that a pregnancy can be achieved by placing the sperm at the neck of the womb by insemination of a partner with ovaries and a womb or of a surrogate at the time of ovulation. If the sperm is of lower quality, a pregnancy can still be achieved, although the chance is reduced. In this case, ovarian stimulation and collection of the partner's or donor egg is needed before the sperm can be used to fertilize the egg in the laboratory using in vitro fertilization, with insertion of the sperm into the egg using intracytoplasmic sperm injection if needed. The resulting embryo can then be implanted into the womb of a partner or surrogate. Although there is no specific data for trans women, for comparison, a live birth rate of 62 percent was noted using intracytoplasmic sperm injection using stored sperm from a group of 272 men who had undergone treatment for cancer.[30]

8.2.4 Testicular Tissue Banking

Testicular tissue banking involves removal and freezing of testicular tissue using a surgical biopsy or a procedure performed at the time of genital surgery if the testicles are removed using orchidectomy. This technique can be performed for both postpubertal and prepubertal trans women.

Like ovarian tissue banking, testicular tissue banking remains experimental. Indeed, this science is not nearly as developed as it is for ovarian tissue banking. Although researchers can develop mature sperm in animal models, testicular tissue banking has not been performed in humans. In future, in vitro laboratory maturation of testicular tissue or isolated immature sperm cells with or without a reimplantation procedure may be possible. However, it is not known if this would be safe in humans, and so the procedure remains untested. If reimplantation is performed, the testicular tissue would start producing testosterone again. Therefore, for trans women who do not wish to be masculinized, it would be ideal if laboratory techniques could be developed to allow fertilization of an embryo by sperm that is matured in vitro using artificial fertility techniques.

8.2.5 Embryo Banking

Embryo banking is a well-established method of fertility preservation that may be a feasible option for people who have a partner with ovaries if they have sperm, or vice versa. Alternatively, an individual may be able to access a donor sperm or egg, giving them the option to create an embryo and still delay the timing of any pregnancy. It should be noted that there could be legal implications if partners separate after creation of an embryo together.

Embryo banking begins in a similar way as egg banking. Ovaries are stimulated to produce eggs using hormones, and eggs are collected using a surgical procedure. However, to proceed with embryo banking, the eggs are fertilized with sperm *before* storage. An embryo is allowed to develop for a short time, usually to blastocyst stage, five days after fertilization, and is then frozen. At the right time, the embryo can be thawed and transferred to the womb of the gestational carrier. This may be the trans man, if they have a womb and are not on testosterone, a partner, or a surrogate.

Embryo banking has high pregnancy success rates in the general population. Compared with other techniques, a more accurate estimate of the chance of live birth may be possible, as many of the required steps have already taken place. As for other fertility preservation techniques, data for the trans population is not available. For comparison, a live birth rate of 22 to 45 percent for each embryo transfer has been reported in groups of cisgender women who have been treated for cancer.[31]

8.3 THE CURRENT REALITY FOR FERTILITY PRESERVATION

The American Society for Reproductive Medicine has stated that fertility programs should "treat all requests for assisted reproduction without regard to gender identity status."[32] Similarly, the American Congress of Obstetricians and Gynecologists states that they oppose discrimination based on gender identity.[33] These statements are underpinned by a range of evidence confirming that children of families with a transgender parent are healthy and well adjusted, and show a normal secure attachment to their parents.

Despite this more equitable approach to fertility preservation and a desire for children, many people choose not to preserve their fertility as it may delay their transition. It can sometimes take several weeks to move ahead with fertility procedures, particularly for those who require hormone stimulation. Also, hormonal stimulation and egg retrieval can be an unwanted procedure for many trans men. Perhaps in the future, ovarian tissue banking may solve this issue.

At one center, one in three adult trans women and one in eight adult trans men chose to freeze their sperm and eggs. There may be many reasons for these low rates of fertility preservation. It may be extremely challenging to access fertility care in what is commonly a highly gender-specific environment. People may also be unwilling to discontinue hormone therapy because of its possible impact on their well-being. There may be inadequate knowledge among members of the clinical team delivering care, so that fertility options are not explained well to the individual. Cost and access are other deterrents, as fertility preservation is rarely covered by public health care or private health insurance. Fees are usually charged for medical consultations, the retrieval of eggs and sperm, and any necessary hormonal treatment, and an annual payment may be required for processing and potentially long-term storage. When discussing the opportunity for fertility preservation with trans people, are we always offering them truly feasible options?

There is little research on trans or gender-diverse people, so it is difficult to quantify the fertility benefits when weighing the cost. As discussed, most of the science is based on the experience of people undergoing treatments such as chemotherapy in what is called oncofertility research. The birth rates reported from each assisted reproductive technology procedure may be different for the trans population. To add to this uncertainty, different centers have variable success rates with each technique, for example a better outcome from embryo banking compared with egg banking. Indeed, people considering fertility preservation should be informed that the short-term fertility outcomes from these procedures are not clearly known, and there is a lack of data describing the long-term reproductive and psychosocial consequences. For people who have not progressed through puberty in their assigned gender, it has been proposed that we should use the term *cryopotential* rather than cryo-preservation when discussing the freezing of immature eggs and sperm as at this stage achieving a successful pregnancy is theoretical.

Transgender health care and fertility medicine are rapidly evolving fields promising a brighter future for gender-diverse people and their loved ones.[34] The next step for artificial fertility techniques may be to allow the maturation of egg and sperm to occur in the laboratory so that opportunities are opened for young trans or gender-diverse people who have used GnRH blockers in early puberty to forestall the development of undesired secondary sex characteristics. In the future, it may even be possible to generate artificial eggs or sperm derived from other stem cells or by nuclear cell transfer. This would increase the reproductive options for people who have not preserved their fertility.

8.4 PREGNANCY

8.4.1 Trans Men

Some trans men who retain their womb, that is, uterus, choose to become pregnant and give birth. The struggles of Thomas Beatie, the first legally recognized man in the United States to give birth, have highlighted some of the challenges that face the trans community when starting a family.[35] Since that time, social change and empowerment have led to an increased frequency of, and openness around, trans men's need for pregnancy and childbearing.

There are clear barriers in obstetric health care that can disempower trans men at this important life stage. Health care workers may project a lack of understanding that someone could be *male and pregnant,* and they may have little knowledge or capacity to provide appropriate care. Conversely, if people encounter health care workers who respect privacy, affirm gender, and normalize their pregnancy, they will have a more positive experience.

The participants in the study by Hoffkling (see note 6) spoke highly of providers that "did not expect the patient to teach them, but listened and learned when the patient did teach" and those who were able to discuss areas of uncertainty in situations where good evidence was not available. In another study, trans men suggested that clinicians ensure that they call body parts the names that the person themselves uses.[36]

The obstetric clinical care itself is no more complex for trans men than for a cisgender pregnancy, and the management of any obstetric complications that develop should be managed as standard clinical practice, irrespective of gender identity or previous testosterone use.[37] However, routine surveillance during pregnancy, such as ultrasound scans or pelvic examination, may be a source of distress.

In an online survey,[38] 41 self-identified trans men aged 28 years who used the pronouns *he* or *they* consented to share their experiences of fertility, pregnancy, and birth. Before conceiving, 25 of the men (61%) had used testosterone and 6 (24%) of these men had an unplanned pregnancy. Fertility is variously affected by testosterone, so that stopping hormone therapy often restores the ability to conceive. In this study, for those participants who stopped testosterone, 20 (80%) resumed menstruation within six months of cessation. Five trans men (20%) had already conceived before menstruation restarted. Most participants (88%) used their own eggs and their partner's sperm. Most of the men conceived within four months of trying, and only 7 percent used artificial fertility techniques. The participants thought of their pregnancy in a variety of ways, describing it as a *bridge to fatherhood*, and explaining themselves as the *carrier* or *gestational parent*.

Pregnancy and birth can be a psychologically difficult period for some trans men. During pregnancy there may be a conflict between gender identity and social norms that causes distress.[39] Birth may also be challenging. There is little data suggesting the optimal type of delivery, either by vaginal or caesarian section, for trans men, but special consideration should be given to ensure that health care staff are aware that the person's genitals may be a source of distress and may have changed in appearance due to testosterone exposure. After delivery, as for cis women, postpartum depression is common and for trans men may be further compounded by the lack of gender-appropriate resources.

Trans men who wish to transition surgically and carry a pregnancy in the future could consider keeping all their internal genitalia, or just having their ovaries removed by oophorectomy rather than having their womb removed by hysterectomy. Gestation can continue to birth without the need for ovaries as hormonal support with estrogen and progesterone can be administered. If a trans man does not wish to be the person that carries a pregnancy, then a partner or surrogate may provide alternative options.

It is important to note that although testosterone is likely to impair fertility, it is not a reliable form of contraception. Trans men should avoid unplanned pregnancy, as testosterone is harmful to the unborn child.

8.4.2 Trans Women

Pregnancy is currently not attainable for trans women, although it may be possible in the future. Uterus transplants have been performed in women with uterine factor infertility, leading to successful gestation and birth.[40] As for other transplants, immunosuppression is needed to prevent rejection; these medications may result in a higher-risk pregnancy due to the susceptibility to infection. Uterus transplantation is still an experimental procedure that needs further study of its potential opportunities for trans women.

The only record of a uterus transplant in a trans woman is the surgery performed for Lili Elbe in Germany in 1931. Sadly, she developed surgical complications and died three months after the operation. The potential for uterus transplant in modern times has only been recently reexplored.[41] These authors describe the potential of a combined uterus and vagina transplant, or a uterine transplant following prior vaginoplasty. The presence of a vagina is felt to be important to allow direct cervical visualization and biopsies, if needed, to assess for organ rejection. The surgical techniques required may be slightly different from those in cis women as the ligaments used for fixation of the uterus in cis women are not present. Hormonal therapy before and after uterus transplant would need to be changed for the trans women. Although progesterone is not generally given for hormone therapy in trans women, it would be essential after a uterus transplant, as taking estrogen without progesterone can lead to endometrial hyperplasia and potentially endometrial carcinoma. A hormone regimen in which estrogen is taken every day and progesterone for the last 14 days of the month, known as cyclical or sequential therapy, would produce a menstrual bleed, providing reassurance that the womb is healthy.

Hypothetically, achieving pregnancy after a uterus transplant would be possible using estrogen to stimulate growth of the lining of the womb or endometrium, followed by progesterone to maintain the lining for embryo implantation. However, there are some further considerations for trans women during pregnancy, as their pelvis may be narrower with a smaller opening if estrogen was not commenced early in life. Further research is needed to determine the feasibility of uterine transplant for trans women in practice, and whether it can lead to a healthy birth.

8.5 CHEST/BREASTFEEDING

8.5.1 Trans Men

It is important to consider the use of appropriate language to describe the trans male experience of feeding their child. If a parent is incorrectly described as *mother*, or terms such as *breasts* or *breastfeeding* are used, this could cause distress if such terms do not align with the person's gender identity. For example, all 22 participants in one Canadian survey referred to their upper front torso as their *chest* and avoided the term *breasts*. They variously referred to the process of feeding as *breastfeeding, nursing, chestfeeding, feeding,* and *mammal feeding*. For brevity, this section will refer to this procedure as *chestfeeding*.

The decision to chestfeed depends on the physical, emotional, logistical, and social factors familiar to all parents. People who have had chest surgery should be aware that their residual tissue may or may not enlarge during pregnancy. Although there are no data, it has been proposed that the type of chest surgery may influence a person's potential to chestfeed. Chestfeeding is more likely to be possible if there is sufficient glandular tissue and a place for the baby to latch onto, but the outcome for any individual is difficult to predict.

Some trans men who have given birth and who have had previous chest surgery may produce sufficient milk to feed their child, while others may experience swelling but without milk production. Some trans men will have had no changes to their chest. An American study of 41 trans men reported that those who used testosterone before pregnancy were less likely to chestfeed, but it is unclear if this was personal choice or a direct consequence of previous hormone treatment.[42] Another study[43] of 22 self-identified trans masculine individuals recruited through the Internet showed that 16 chose to chestfeed for at least some period of time, 4 did not attempt chestfeeding, and the remainder had not delivered. Nine of these participants had had chest reconstruction surgery before pregnancy. Irrespective of whether a man decides to chestfeed, they should be aware of the potential for mastitis, an inflammation of breast tissue that commonly occurs after delivery.

If the baby's nutritional needs are not met through exclusive chestfeeding, parents may need to use an additional form of feeding to provide sufficient milk. Supplemental feeding systems use thin tubes that rest next to the nipple and allow additional feed in conjunction with the parent's milk without the need for a bottle or teat. The pouch attached to the tube can be filled with donor milk or artificial formula. A parent that did not give birth may be able to induce lactation or restart lactation to feed babies or children to whom they did not give birth.

The decision to restart testosterone therapy in someone currently feeding their child with their own milk depends on weighing the various risks and benefits. There is some evidence that an elevated testosterone level may suppress lactation,[44] and there is the potential to pass a small amount of testosterone to the baby during feeding, although the available research shows no clear evidence of harm.[45] Conversely, testosterone therapy may be of significant benefit to the well-being of the parent. If the decision is made to restart testosterone, then it is sensible to monitor the baby for signs of testosterone exposure known as hyperandrogenism.

8.5.2 Trans Women

A recent report has described the first use of hormone therapy to start lactation in a trans woman planning to breastfeed her adopted infant. She had been on combination hormonal therapy that included estrogen, spironolactone, and progesterone for six to seven years and had mature Tanner stage 5 breasts. She had not had any gender-affirming surgery, including breast augmentation. The medical team used evidence from other contexts to design a hormonal protocol. It is known that to induce lactation, estrogen and progesterone should be increased to mimic the levels observed in pregnancy. In general, estrogen levels increase from the first trimester (188–2,497 pg/ml or 690–9,166 pmol/l) to the second (1278–7,192 pg/ml or 4,692–26,402 pmol/l) and third trimester (6,137–13,460 pg/ml or 22,539–49,412 pmol/l) of pregnancy; and progesterone rises from the start (4.73–50.74 ng/ml or 15.04–161.35 pmol/l) to the end (58.7–214.0 ng/ml or 186.67–680.52 nmol/l) of pregnancy.[46] The use of other medications such as the milk-producing galactagogues, in this case off-label use of the antisickness tablet domperidone, and a breast pump for five minutes three times daily can increase the levels of other hormones, such as oxytocin and prolactin, that are important for lactation. The trigger for the start of milk release is a sudden drop in estradiol and progesterone levels similar to what happens after birth.

The lactation induction protocol used for this woman and the hormone levels are shown in Table 8.1. Spironolactone was continued for androgen blockade throughout treatment and while breastfeeding; this was felt to be appropriate as available evidence suggests only 0.2 percent of the dose is passed into breast milk, an amount thought not to be harmful.[47] After three months of hormonal therapy the woman was making eight ounces of milk daily. A reduction in estrogen and progesterone was timed to occur two weeks before delivery of the baby. The woman was able to exclusively breastfeed her newborn for six weeks, and the child's pediatrician reported normal growth. The child then received supplementary formula in addition to the breast milk, and this combination feeding continued beyond six months.

Although this case had a positive outcome, the optimal regimen to enable breastfeeding remains unknown. It is interesting that in this case the measured estradiol and progesterone levels were not as high as their reported pregnancy reference ranges, yet lactation was still successful. Perhaps her prolactin level, which was four to five times the upper limit of the nonpregnant range (1.4 to 24.0 pg/ml), was important in milk production. Areas for future research include the optimal hormone doses and blood levels, the frequency and duration of mechanical stimulation with the pump, and the possible need for additional medications such as the galactagogues. Despite its limitations, this report is important as it demonstrates for the first time that functional lactation is achievable for trans women.

Table 8.1 Hormone Protocol Used to Induce Milk Expression in the Breasts of a Trans Woman

Timing	Estrogen	Progesterone	Galactagogue and Mechanical Breast Stimulation
Start	Estradiol 2 mg orally twice a day	Progesterone (micronized) 100 mg orally twice a day	
Starting blood levels	Estradiol 63 pg/ml	Progesterone 8 ng/ml	Prolactin 10 ng/nl
Initial treatment	Estradiol 2 mg orally twice a day	Progesterone (micronized) 100 mg orally twice a day	Domperidone 10 mg and breast pump 5 minutes per breast three times daily
Day 28 blood levels	Estradiol 129 pg/ml	Progesterone 6 ng/ml	Prolactin 148 ng/nl
Treatment at 1 month	Estradiol 8 mg orally daily	Progesterone (micronized) 200 mg orally twice a day	Domperidone 20 mg four times a day and breast pump 5 minutes per breast six times daily
Day 56	Estradiol 34 pg/ml	Progesterone 4 ng/ml	Prolactin 143 ng/nl
Treatment at 2 months	Estradiol 12 mg orally daily	Progesterone (micronized) 400 mg orally twice a day	Domperidone 20 mg four times a day and breast pump 5 minutes per breast six times daily
Day 70	Estradiol 33 pg/ml	Progesterone 5 ng/ml	Prolactin 115 ng/nl
Treatment at 3 months (2 weeks before birth)	Estradiol patch 25 mcg daily (low-dose)	Progesterone (micronized 100 mg daily)	Domperidone 20 mg four times a day and breast pump 5 minutes per breast six times daily

SUMMARY

Hormonal and surgical interventions have an unpredictable and potentially irreversible effect on fertility. For people who wish to have genetically related children, it may be helpful to store gametes, eggs or sperm, or an embryo to facilitate the possibility of a future pregnancy. Sometimes, the decision to preserve fertility or not is a difficult one, especially in the very young for whom avoiding puberty with GnRH blockers may be lifesaving. Pregnancy after fertility preservation is not guaranteed, and the artificial fertility techniques required to conceive might be difficult to access or be too costly. For people who have not yet reached a mature age, the techniques to produce a viable pregnancy are still in the early phase of development.

Conversely, for those people who did not preserve fertility before transition, there is still the opportunity to have biological children as long as sterilizing surgery has not been performed. Trans men are successfully completing pregnancy with increasing visibility post-transition, and they may be able to chest-feed their child if they so desire. For this reason, it is important not to assume trans men will wish to have their ovaries and uterus removed. Trans women on hormones may still have some sperm production after hormone therapy, allowing fertility. The ability to carry a pregnancy has not yet been achievable for trans women, but the first hormonal stimulation of breastfeeding has recently been reported.

Chapter 9

ANCILLARY PROCEDURES AND OTHER INTERVENTIONS

So that trans people can feel more comfortable in their new gender role, several additional medical treatments and support programs are available. These include speech therapy and facial hair electrolysis for trans women, as hormone therapy has no effect on voice pitch nor does it remove facial hair. Other surgical techniques for trans women include voice-box surgery and facial feminization surgery. Trans men can take advantage of voice training if testosterone treatment does not lower the voice pitch sufficiently.

9.1 SPEECH THERAPY

Speech therapy can be undertaken mainly by trans women to feminize their voice so that it more closely approximates that of a cisgender woman. To some extent, a convincing visual presentation can compensate for a less than acceptable female voice if passing is one of the trans woman's goals. Interpersonal communication, primarily by means of voice and mannerisms, is important for some trans women's acceptance into their feminine gender role.[1] The situation is rather complicated because a higher fundamental speech pitch does not guarantee that a trans woman will communicate without detection of her former gender identity. For example, in social situations, trans women may need to relinquish any previous tendency to lead in conversational speech when with a group of men. To effectively assimilate if that is their desire, trans women should wait their turn in the conversation just as many cisgender women feel obliged to do until their male acquaintances become more enlightened.[2]

The main difference between men's and women's voices is fundamental pitch. When compared with a typical woman's voice, the fundamental frequency and the resonant frequencies, or formants, are lower in men's voices. The fundamental frequency is the lowest frequency produced by the person's vocal apparatus. All other frequency components of the voice are multiples of this fundamental frequency. The various formants result from different types of resonances resulting from changes in the internal structure of the oral cavities. Whereas the fundamental frequency for men's voices lies between 107 Hz and 132 Hz, the female fundamental frequency lies between 196 Hz and 224 Hz.[3] So that trans women can more adequately mimic female speech, the fundamental frequency needs to be raised to about 160 Hz.

Other aspects of feminine speech are different from masculine speech. For example, women differ from men in their pronunciation of the *TH* in English words like *TH*is and *TH*in. Also, their speech shows a more dynamic intonation pattern during the pronunciation of a phrase. Most people have noted, for example, the tendency for women to raise the pitch of their voice at the end of a phrase or sentence, a characteristic that only tends to occur in male speech when a question is being asked.[4]

When trans women who had received estrogen therapy for at least 18 months say sentences, first in a female voice and then in a male voice, the average duration of isolated words is longer in the female version of the message. When speaking in a female voice, the fundamental frequency is higher, the pitch range is larger, but the loudness level is lower. The central frequency of the third formant, produced by a reduced mouth cavity length, tends to be higher in female speech than in male speech. This effect can be produced by retracting the corners of the mouth, a characteristic feature of female speaking, as well as by appropriate placement of the tongue.[5] Female-sounding trans female voices are correctly detected 99 percent of the time by naïve listeners, indicating that speech therapy for trans women is often quite successful.

To make their voices sound more feminine, trans women should pronounce consonants precisely and employ a softer voice tone. Trans women whose voices are most often perceived as female tend to be short in stature with height less than 170 cm, or 5'7". So, an effective combination for a trans woman being able to pass is a high fundamental frequency and a short stature.[6]

Even when trans women increase their voice pitch so that it lies within the female range, good female voice quality is often elusive. Since male vocal cords have a greater mass than female vocal cords, the air pressure in the voice box needed to start them vibrating is greater, leading to a generally lower pitch range. Also, as the male vocal tract is longer than that of a woman, the basic resonances are about 20 percent lower in pitch and have different resonance characteristics from those of the female voice. For these reasons, a successful imitation of the female voice requires painstaking training to realign the formant resonances. This is no easy task. Speakers with higher vowel formants, important for vowel identification, are more likely to be perceived as female even without too much of an increase in average pitch. However, training the voice to produce appropriate formants is difficult for birth-assigned males who have been exposed to higher levels of testosterone than females.

At a more global level, male speech indicates competitiveness whereas women speak in a more cooperative style. Female speech contains adjectives that do not add to the meaning of a sentence but make it sound more polite: words such as *lovely, divine,* and *cute.* Women also tend to add questions at the end of sentences such as *don't you;* for example, "I think this is a lovely outfit, *don't you?*" Women also tend to add suggestions of uncertainty to their speech, such as *perhaps* and *I wonder if.* Some commentators have suggested that the uncertainty associated with female speech reflects their perceived lower status in society. However, their use of uncertainty might reflect women's superior verbal communication skills when compared with those of men. Whereas women's conversation is collaborative and built upon shared understanding, men often avoid discussing personal issues and instead prefer factual topics such as sport, current events, and so on.[7]

Successful passing by trans women requires use of language that is more characteristic of women than men. They should be willing to listen to, rather than interrupt another person's conversation move their mouths more when speaking; and smile more frequently.[8] Of course, many women would be offended by gender stereotypes and suggest instead that these speech differences between women and men are not so obvious these days!

Social aspects of the communication skills of 47-year-old trans women when compared with those of a group of cisgender women of similar age indicated that trans women have more communication problems than do cisgender women. Such problems include the use of a convincing vocal tone to communicate a message, prolonged conversations due to excessive talkativeness, listening skill problems, losing track of conversations when there is a lot of surrounding noise, and understanding what is being said in group conversations. Adequate communication also depends on the trans woman's satisfaction with her voice as indicated by her confidence when talking to others.[9]

The most important strategy, at least initially, for using speech therapy to help trans women acquire female speech is to work on head resonance and voice volume while training the voice to have a lighter, more feminine character. Also important is intonation variability, with greater variation in voice pitch being required to approximate female speech. Delicate and light articulation, shortening of the vocal tract, and lowering of volume are also needed to produce a convincing female voice. Possible changes in speech rate as well as coughing and laughing in a feminine manner are also important aspects of speech training.

Useful strategies for improving female speech quality include having the trans woman categorize her own voice in terms of masculine and feminine voice standards and minimize chest resonance by employing auditory feed-back when listening to speech samples. The different effects of chest versus head resonance can be felt and heard by placing fingers of the same hand above and below the voice box and then producing resonance by humming consonants such as *m* and *n*. Another effective strategy is to raise and lower voice pitch in a glissando or sliding fashion, aiming always to increase the overall pitch of the voice. Vibrations are only felt above the voice box when there is adequate head resonance. The female voice should be based on head resonance but with no falsetto, the latter being a male strategy to produce a false high-pitched female-sounding voice.

Voice training should begin by using vowels formed by the front of the mouth, then progressing to words, followed by sentences, poetry, stories, and finally spontaneous speech. Practice with phrases regularly used by women in normal speech is important so that trans women can become more confident when speaking in real-life situations. Reciting poetry and children's stories in a highly modulated manner also helps produce a proper female voice tone. Learning appropriate feminine gestures to accompany the newly acquired speech is also important. Enunciating words by emphasizing initial conso-nants and learning to pronounce these words rather delicately is a worthwhile strategy. A slightly faster speech rate without sacrificing precise pronunciation also makes the speech sound more feminine.[10]

In social situations, any deficiency in voice credibility can be overcome to some extent by a convincing female presentation in other ways, such as in appear-ance, mannerisms, and so forth. Trans women are still more likely to be addressed as men over the telephone than in real life, indicating that physical appearance plays an important role in passing. One useful trick, of course, is to always intro-duce oneself with a female name when answering the telephone and prior to initiating a conversation. This strategy almost always works, provided the funda-mental voice pitch and other voice resonances are close to the female range.

The measured average fundamental frequency of 14 trans women's speech ranged from 130 to 207 Hz. There was no difference in average fundamental frequency between the five women who had experienced some voice training and those who had not, suggesting that voice training was inadequate for some of the trans women. The higher the fundamental frequency of the trans woman's voice, the higher was the femininity rating when only the voice was heard without seeing the person, as is the case over the telephone.[11]

9.1.1 Research Findings in Voice Therapy for Trans People

In this section we discuss some more research findings on voice therapy for trans women in greater detail. We will observe that the speech patterns reported in these studies differ over a range of fundamental frequencies and formant patterns, suggesting that there are large individual differences in how these women acquire a convincing female voice.

In one study, the success of speech therapy was evaluated using 10 trans women aged 45, seven of whom had undergone genital surgery. The women had received between 10 and 90 speech therapy sessions. Their current speech, evaluated on average four years since their last speech therapy lesson, indicated that the gains of 43 Hz on average following speech therapy were not maintained. Instead, there was a reduction in fundamental frequency from 168 Hz upon discontinuation of speech training to 147 Hz at follow-up, this latter value being higher the larger the number of speech therapy sessions. This fundamental frequency was still higher than the starting value of 126 Hz. Although the follow-up fundamental frequency was now slightly below the female range for seven of the women, most were still satisfied with their voice. Perhaps they found other ways to compensate for any gender ambiguity in their speech.[12]

We now explore male and female voice characteristics in greater detail. The male average fundamental frequency is 128 Hz with a range of 60Hz to 260 Hz and the female average fundamental frequency is 227 Hz with a range of 128 Hz to 520 Hz. A gender-ambiguous range has an average fundamental frequency of 160 Hz with a range of 128 Hz to 260 Hz. The female voice has about 20 percent higher resonance frequencies known as formants than does the male voice because of a shorter vocal tract in women, 17.5 cm for men and 14.7 cm for women. An increase in formant 1, F1, the lowest pitched frequency resonance, occurs when the mouth is opened wide and the tongue position lowered. A forward position of the tongue causes an increase in the second format, F2, a higher-pitched resonance frequency than F1. Retracting the corners of the mouth while smiling shortens the oral cavity, resulting in an increase in the third formant, F3, an even higher-pitched frequency resonance than either F1 and F2, and one that is so important for producing a convincing female voice. Lip rounding should be avoided as it lowers all formant frequencies. An overall headier sound is also important. Female speech has a more variable intonation pattern than male speech. The female voice has greater frequency changes, called jitter, and fewer changes in amplitude or shimmer than does a male voice. A breathier voice is also perceived as more feminine.[13]

In an appendix to the review article cited in note 13, some useful hints for enhancing one's female voice are provided. Pronunciation and other speech features characteristic of a female voice include:

1. Use of /-ing/ rather than /-in/ as a more accurate pronunciation of the present participle verb ending,

2. Greater precision when pronouncing the voiced *th* in *this*,

3. Using extra words to denote feelings or emotional states,

4. The use of nurturing phrases such as *I know how you feel*,

5. Discussion of personal relationships and the sharing of thoughts and feelings,

6. A minimal use of rude words and avoiding an assertive conversational style,

7. Using lots of adjectives such as *lovely*, *beautiful* as well as similarly pleasant adverbs,

8. Using repetitions like *very-very* and *teeny-weeny*,

9. Using intensifiers such as the word *so* in *It was so exciting*, and

10. Using tag questions such as *It's lovely, isn't it?*

Female communication includes more mimicking head movements, smooth body movements, greater use of hands with arms closer to the body, undulating hip movements, more expressive leg and foot movements, crossing the legs at the ankle rather than the knee, leaning toward the conversation partner, friendlier facial expressions, and making good eye contact. Other characteristic female behaviors include smiling, occasional touching, initiation of hugging, standing closer to other women, and more appropriate attire and etiquette.

Trans men have fewer speech problems than trans women as testosterone therapy causes a steady decrease in fundamental voice frequency. In a survey of 16 trans men, none of whom had received any voice therapy, 14 reported a lower and heavier voice since starting testosterone therapy. For most of these trans men, the change in voice quality occurred within three months of starting testosterone therapy.

Trans men are usually pleased with their new masculine voice, most indicating scarcely any difference between their voice and that of a cisgender male. Reassuringly, they are no longer addressed as a woman even on the telephone. Over a four-month period following the start of testosterone therapy, the maximum pitch that could be obtained decreased from 800 Hz to approximately 500 Hz for one man, and from 500 Hz to around 350 Hz for another. There were corresponding decreases in the fundamental voice frequency to around 125 Hz for both men. However, there was no increase in voice noisiness and voice frequency instability.[14]

Trans men pass more readily if they adopt male conversation strategies such as telling people what they want rather than asking for it. A trans person's ability to pass requires the attainment of verbal, grammar, and conversational skills in addition to having to master changes in fundamental pitch and fluctuations in speech dynamics. Trans men usually have an easier task in this respect than do trans women.

Older males in the age range 65 to 88 years speak with a fundamental frequency of about 127 Hz, whereas women of the same age group have a voice fundamental frequency of about 175 Hz. There is a positive relationship between the mean fundamental frequency measured by voicing a sustained *ah* sound and rated femininity that accounts for 60 percent of rated femininity with this sound. This femininity rating increases to almost 80 percent for sustained speech, with 26 percent of the relationship with rated femininity the fundamental frequency coming from fluctuations in voice frequency. It is interesting to note that self-rated femininity of voice and listener rating of femininity agree about 73 percent of the time, a value that is higher the longer the course of voice training.[15]

9.1.2 A Summary of Speech Therapy Findings

The goal of speech therapy in trans women is to increase the voice pitch and to acquire intonation and stylistic skills that mimic female speech as closely as possible. Although trans women's speech may not qualify as being distinctly feminine, when coupled with a convincing visual presentation few if any problems passing in a female gender role are experienced. By contrast, most trans men have a convincing male voice after just a few months of testosterone therapy.

The important aspects of voice that are reflected in gender recognition are fundamental frequency or pitch, variation in fundamental frequency as an indicator of intonation, and the first three vowel formant frequencies as indicators of resonance. Precise articulation is another gender marker in speech. Breathiness is often considered a feature of female speech even when its speech analog, the difference between the first and second formants, does not assist gender recognition. Entering vocal fry, a wobbly low pitch voice, is a sure sign of masculinity and needs to be avoided by trans women who are training their voice to become more feminine. A voice is best perceived as female if the fundamental frequency is above 180 Hz and the pitch range is from 140 Hz to 300 Hz, with predominantly upward intonation assisting female gender recognition and falling intonation reflecting a male voice. A more variable speech pattern in all possible ways is more characteristic of female voices. Lip rounding is characteristic of male speech, whereas lip spreading, as if smiling, is more characteristic of female speech.[16]

Altering oral resonance by retracting the corners of the mouth and spreading lips as if smiling, together with tongue placement toward the front of the mouth are supposed to allow the voice to be perceived as more feminine. A 2007 study used the vowel sounds *ah*, *ee*, *aw* that cause the tongue position to move from the back to the front of the mouth and the lips to move from an open to a closed pout position. Following training to improve resonance, there was an overall increase in each of the first three formants for all three vowels, and a corresponding increase in voice femininity ratings. However, this desired outcome did not happen for every one of the trans women who participated in the study.[17]

9.2 VOICE-BOX SURGERY FOR TRANS WOMEN

The voice is the most difficult aspect of adjusting to a new lifestyle for trans women; unconvincing voice and speech create problems of social identity and difficulty in assimilation. As voice training does not always produce a satisfactory outcome for all trans women, some of them resort to surgical techniques so that they can live more comfortably in their affirmed gender. Surgery to increase voice pitch has been claimed to improve gender identity, body image, self-esteem, and general well-being. A reduction of the laryngeal prominence, commonly referred to as the Adam's apple, using a surgical procedure known as thyroid chondroplasty or more simply, a tracheal shave, is also beneficial. This procedure can be performed either prior to the social transition or during genital surgery. Surgical techniques for raising voice pitch have generally involved reducing the vocal cord mass, shortening the vocal cords, or increasing vocal cord tension. Medical tests conducted preoperatively can be used to estimate the increase in voice fundamental pitch that might be reasonably expected from these surgical procedures.

9.2.1 Cricothyroid Approximation Surgery

Vocal cord length is determined by the relative positions of the cricoid, or lower cartilage, and the thyroid, or upper cartilage, which are both located in front of the larynx. The effect of surgery can be mimicked manually by pushing up the lower margin of the cricoid cartilage with the right index finger while simultaneously pressing down on the thyroid notch with the tip of the left index finger. If this manual procedure results in an increase in voice pitch, voice-box surgery may be effective. Such voice-box surgery is known as *cricothyroid approximation surgery*.

One type of voice-box surgical procedure involves increasing vocal cord tension by inserting two small metal plates to connect the cricoid and thyroid cartilages using wire sutures. This procedure does not interfere with the internal structure of the larynx. If the surgery is unsuccessful as indicated by no substantial increase in voice pitch, then the previous voice-box configuration can be restored by removing the mini-plates during follow-up surgery. The operation produces an approximation of the normal female thyroid and cricoid cartilage relationship, leading to greater tension between them and a subsequent increase in fundamental voice pitch.

Reports on the results of cricothyroid approximation surgery were obtained from 28 trans women aged 44. Twelve of the trans women had taken speech therapy prior to voice surgery. Over half the women indicated their concern about their voice in public life, especially when using the telephone. Prior to surgery they had employed various strategies to make their speaking voice more feminine, such as raising vocal pitch, speaking more melodiously and softly, and when their confidence was low, by speaking less often in social groups. Following surgery, some of these trans women reported that they felt less feminine if they did not adjust their voice as they had learned during voice training, whereas 62 percent reported that they were pleased with the voice surgery outcome. Satisfied clients were more likely to be accepted as a woman in public, including over the telephone. They felt more comfortable in social situations and did not relapse into a male-sounding voice except occasionally among their own family members. Even with successful voice surgery, follow-up speech therapy is worthwhile.

After voice-box surgery, the fundamental voice pitch increased by a small amount in some unsuccessful cases to almost double the previous fundamental frequency when the surgery had been successful. Whereas none of the women spoke in the female range before the operation, 28 percent could achieve this range immediately afterward, with another 38 percent achieving some greater success a year later. On the other hand, good cosmetic results with only inconspicuous scarring were achieved for 90 percent of clients following the much simpler technique of thyroid chondroplasty, or Adam's apple reduction surgery, a procedure that had been performed at the same time as voice-box surgery for these patients.[18]

When trans women's speech is compared before and after cricothyroid approximation surgery, the average most common, or modal, frequency increases from 142 Hz before surgery to 186 Hz after surgery. There is about a 50 percent chance of the voice being perceived as female when the modal frequency is 173 Hz, with 100 percent accurate identification occurring when the modal frequency reaches 238 Hz. Whereas prior to surgery the trans women's voice had two dominant frequencies, one below 150 Hz and the other over 200 Hz, surgery removed the lower frequency, leading to less voice strain, a desirable outcome for many trans women. Two of 14 trans women showed no change in voice pitch following surgery, indicating an 85 percent success rate overall.

For another 21 trans women who had undergone cricothyroid approximation surgery, the average increase in fundamental frequency was 71 Hz two weeks after the operation and a lower value of 57 Hz at the six-month follow-up. There was a 10 percent increase in voice irregularity two weeks after surgery that reduced to 3 percent at follow-up. Only 38 percent of these women had a speaking voice in the female range six months after surgery.[19]

Another version of cricothyroid approximation surgery raises the voice pitch by using nylon sutures that join the cricothyroid and thyroid bones at four sites to reinforce the contraction of the cricothyroid muscle that joins the thyroid bone to the voice-box cover. It is wise to decrease the cricothyroid distance more than would be required because after surgery the sutures tend to loosen a little.

Medical imaging is a reliable method for evaluating the effects of cricothyroid approximation surgery. When CAT scans were used to measure the cricothyroid interbone distance one week before and one week after surgery, the average cricothyroid distance was 10 mm prior to surgery and 4 mm after surgery, resulting in a decrease in cricothyroid distance of 6 mm. The average voice pitch increased from 118 Hz prior to surgery to 226 Hz after surgery, resulting in a substantially closer approximation to female voice pitch.[20]

The success of cricothyroid approximation surgery as well as thyroid chondroplasty was investigated for 42 trans women aged 39 who had undergone either or both surgical procedures within an eight-year period. Only four trans women had requested a repeat cricothyroid procedure to fix an unsatisfactory initial outcome. Overall, 81 percent of the women were satisfied with the incision scar on the neck following surgery, and 86 percent of those having thyroid chondroplasty were satisfied with the cosmetic appearance of the surgical incision on their neck and of course a reduction in their Adam's apple prominence, a sure male gender marker.

Following cricothyroid approximation surgery, 79 percent of the trans women reported an immediate improvement in female voice quality, whereas the remainder had a more prolonged recovery from surgery followed by a steady improvement in voice quality. Of those who undertook prior speech therapy without surgery, only 45 percent had experienced an improvement in their ability to achieve a female voice range. Cricothyroid approximation surgery had its maximum effect on the most prominent, rather than average, voice frequency. This effect might result from the large variability in pitch that occurs during normal female speech.

Voice-box surgery can reliably increase voice pitch from the male range to a fundamental pitch above 215 Hz, with large individual differences occurring within that range. Although intensive speech therapy also increases average vocal pitch toward the female range, the resulting speech still lacks the quality of the cisgender female voice. Acquiring the appropriate formant frequencies as well as inflecting the voice appropriately are skills that must be mastered to more closely approximate female speech.[21]

Unfortunately, cricothyroid approximation surgery is not without its problems. Surgical complications include difficulty in swallowing, a sore throat, frequent throat-clearing, and vocal fatigue. Some of these problems persist a year after surgery, but fortunately by then they are only about half as frequent as the number of problems that can occur immediately after the surgery. Some people report an adverse effect of surgery on their singing voice. However, these occasional problems resolve with time and most women are pleased with their voice quality following surgery. Ironically, successful surgery depends on the presurgical pitch range being within the masculine range with no evidence of voice strain resulting from long-term voice therapy. Since successful voice therapy relies on forcing the voice from its normal masculine range toward a more feminine one, the effort required to achieve this can sometimes produce severe voice strain.

In another study, the results from 20 cricothyroid approximation surgery clients aged 46 were reviewed on average 22 months after surgery. Whereas prior to surgery the fundamental pitch was between 134 Hz and 145 Hz for sustained vowel and reading tasks, respectively, the corresponding follow-up values were within the 185 Hz to 202 Hz female range. So average pitch increased about half an octave following normal postoperative relaxation of the stretched vocal cords, compared with an initial octave increase in fundamental pitch immediately after surgery. The fundamental pitch when reading aloud was close to the 189 Hz value for cisgender women when they performed a similar task. There was no change in hoarseness or in voice-pitch range following surgery. Both the lower and upper limits of the voice range increased by about four semitones in each case. Fifty-eight percent of participants were satisfied with their voice, 33 percent were dissatisfied, and the remaining 9 percent were indifferent with respect to the outcome. Vocal quality was rated as clear by 42 percent, rough or hoarse by 23 percent, and fair by 35 percent of participants. Forty-seven percent of participants still had their voice mistaken as masculine on the telephone occasionally; 31 percent reported that they were never mistaken for a man, whereas the remaining 22 percent reported that they were often mistaken for a man. About 60 percent found an improvement in the femininity ratings of their laugh, whereas scarcely more than 40 percent reported that their coughing and throat-clearing were considered feminine after voice-box surgery. So, the overall success rate of cricothyroid approximation surgery in trans women in this report was just over 50 percent.[22]

In another study, success rates from cricothyroid approximation surgery were about 79 percent and 72 percent as judged by the trans women and their speech therapists, respectively. The average postoperative gain in fundamental frequency was 11 Hz, a rather small improvement. This result suggested that surgery be reserved for those who cannot acquire a feminine voice using speech therapy. The average fundamental frequency increased from 119 Hz before the surgery, a value similar to the mean frequency of 115 Hz for cisgender males, to 169 Hz after the surgery. This is at the lower limit of the female range and just a little below 183 Hz, the average fundamental frequency for cisgender females. It was interesting to note that having a gender-appropriate fundamental frequency was more important when visual cues of the speaker's gender were not present.[23]

9.2.2 Vocal Fold Shortening

A new technique for voice feminization surgery has been developed that involves vocal fold shortening and the re-creation of the anterior commissure.

For 137 trans women the fundamental frequency increased from 130 Hz before the surgery to 207 Hz six months afterward. Following surgery there was a clear increase in voice femininity as well as a more natural and softer voice tone.[24]

Voice-box surgery is a procedure of last resort for those trans women whose voice pitch cannot be successfully feminized using speech therapy. Although the surgery is reversible if performed correctly, the success rate is somewhere between 50 and 80 percent, and the procedure is considered to be slightly risky by surgical standards as afterward the voice may be not much better than it was before the surgery with some possibly lingering undesirable side effects, especially for those who use their voice for singing. Even when voice-box surgery is successful, trans women still need to learn feminine ways of speaking, no easy task irrespective of any feminization that might occur in their fundamental voice pitch.

9.3 HAIR REDUCTION AND FACIAL ELECTROLYSIS

Human hair grows in a cyclic manner with an anagen, or growth, phase, followed by a quiescent, or telogen, phase. There is also a catagen phase during which the hair is at an intermediate stage of growth. During the anagen phase, cell activity occurs in both the hair bulb and dermal papilla, causing the old hair to be pushed out and replaced by a new one. Anagen phase hair is most sensitive to the various hair removal methods, but unfortunately multiple hair removal treatments are almost always required as only some hair is in this growth phase at any one time.[25]

Most hair follicles are present at birth with just a few that stop growing hair beyond 40 years of age. Rudimentary hair follicles start producing hair as early as weeks 16 to 20 in the womb. The main hair shaft, which contains keratin proteins, grows within the outer hair root sheath, a part of the skin's epidermis. Male body and facial hair consists of terminal hairs that are longer, pigmented, and coarser in texture than vellus hair, the soft, colorless hair typically found on women. The hair follicles form groups known as follicle units, each of which contains two to four follicles together with sebaceous or oil glands and their associated connective tissues. Men and women have the same number of follicle units, but men have more terminal hair than women. Terminal hair in women occurs mainly in the genital region but can occur elsewhere on the body. For scalp hair, the anagen phase may last from two to six years, whereas for body hair this phase may last only three to six months.

Androgens such as testosterone cause hair follicles with vellus hair to produce terminal hair. Androgens also prolong the anagen phase of body hair but shorten the anagen phase of scalp hair. This leads simultaneously to robust body hair in men as well as baldness in those men with a genetic predisposition for the condition. Androgens also increase the oiliness of both skin and hair. This means that people with androgen insensitivity syndrome, a rare difference in sexual development in otherwise male bodies, have mostly vellus body hair. Finasteride inhibits 5α-reductase activity in human genital and pubic skin, leading to a decreased production of dihydrotestosterone and a reduction of body hair in trans women. Hair growth over the forearm and lower leg is less sensitive to the effects of androgens than is hair growth in other body regions.[26]

Several medications can be used to reduce body hair. High doses of spirono-lactone are needed to suppress hair growth, so side effects such as excessive urination, especially at night, and low blood pressure with associated head-aches and fatigue are possible. Cyproterone acetate may be used as an alterna-tive anti-androgen and is effective in reducing terminal hair growth in trans women.

Even when medications are used to accelerate body hair loss in trans women, they have little effect on facial hair. Consequently, more conventional manual methods of hair removal are required. Although shaving is the most common method of hair removal, it has the disadvantage of only cutting the hair at the surface of the skin, leading to relatively rapid regrowth. Shaving has no effect on hair thickness or growth rate. Another popular hair removal method involves plucking or waxing. Waxing removes the hair at its roots and can be effective for up to six weeks following treatment. The only minor side effects are ingrown hairs that can occasionally lead to irritation when regrowth occurs. Depilation creams can also be effective, but as they only dissolve the hair shaft using a chemical reaction, regrowth occurs within about two weeks. Occasion-ally skin irritation can result from the chemicals used in these preparations.

Electrolysis is a tedious, painful, and time-consuming procedure used for removing facial and body hair in trans women. A fine needle is carefully inserted into each hair follicle. A combination of applied heat and electrical current leads to the destruction of the follicular isthmus as well as the lower follicle. Galvanic electrolysis passes a direct current to the hair follicle, destroy-ing it, whereas thermolysis relies on the heat generated by alternating current to achieve much the same result. As there are approximately 40,000 hairs in the male beard and about 200 hairs can be removed per hour, at least 200 hours of electrolysis are needed to remove most of the facial hair. The process is complicated further by the fact that only hairs in their growth, or anagen, phase can be removed permanently. Other hairs will eventually return but with much less resilience, making the final few hours of hair removal much easier. It is generally accepted that permanent hair removal is possible using electrolysis, but it takes several hundred hours to achieve this goal with regular treatment of stray hair growth being necessary. Skin irritation from electroly-sis clears up within a day or two after each session.

As testosterone is responsible for beard growth in the first place, any residual testosterone in trans women will maintain a luxurious growth. Once the combination of estrogen and anti-androgen therapy has reduced the effect of testosterone sufficiently, the removal of facial hair is easier and less painful because of a decrease in hair diameter but not its length. So, starting electrolysis before estrogen therapy will be less effective. If full-time living as a woman starts about the same time as estrogen therapy, several days of beard growth will be necessary prior to each electrolysis session. This means that adequate passing as a woman is not always possible until facial electrolysis is reasonably well advanced.

Facial electrolysis is one of the most expensive and time-consuming procedures in a trans woman's transition. Laser treatment is a viable alternative that destroys the hair bulb. Effective laser treatment depends on melanin in the hair shaft that can conduct light energy to the hair bulb. Laser treatment is not so effective with gray hair and can cause damage to skin with a high melanin content if care is not taken.

A typical treatment uses long-pulsed ruby laser applied monthly to the beard and chest hair.[27] People with black hair require at least seven one-hour sessions to clear the beard and chest hair. Although no guarantee of permanence can be given, no significant regrowth generally occurs up to six months following laser treatment. Unlike electrolysis, regular maintenance treatment is required. A 90 percent average hair clearance rate occurs after about nine treatments. Laser's hair removal effectiveness decreases with both age and with the amount of previously experienced electrolysis.[28]

Electrolysis remains the best option for permanent facial hair removal. However, for younger trans women who have no gray hair, laser hair removal is a viable option provided the repeat treatments can be tolerated.

9.4 FACIAL GENDER CONFIRMATION SURGERY

To improve their ability to pass as women, some trans women undergo facial gender confirmation surgery.[29] This is a complex and expensive procedure to recontour the face, including nose, jawbone, orbital ridges of the eyes, and forehead to more closely approximate the female facial form. The orbital ridges above the eyes are more prominent in males than in females, leading to a strong impression of masculinity. By contrast, the bone surrounding the eyes is much rounder and relatively larger in females. The cheekbones are heavier and flatter in men. However, these bones are more prominent in women, leading to a clear facial impression of femininity.

As the female face is less muscular but contains more subcutaneous fat than the male face, it appears softer, more rounded, and friendlier than does the average male face. The forehead height is less in females, being about 6 mm shorter than that of males. As the nose appears generally larger in males than females, some reduction and contouring of the nose is an important part of facial feminization.[30] The female nose has a smaller bone structure than the male nose, its central region or dorsum is narrower with a slight curve, and the nostrils and the base of the nose are smaller. The angle between the central part of the nose tip and the upper lip is about five degrees larger in women than in men, with a similar larger angle between the forehead and dorsum for women. In feminizing rhinoplasty, the dorsum and tip of the nose are made smaller and the tip is rotated upward. Overall the technique is effective in feminizing the face with only a few complications including a temporary loss of sensation in the tip of the nose, some bleeding from the nose, and temporary bruising below the eyes. These postoperational effects are completely resolved within a week or two of surgery.[31] In a study of 200 successive cases, feminizing rhinoplasty increased the angle between the forehead and nose to a value that better approximated that commonly observed in cisgender women. This had a dramatic feminizing effect on the middle third of the trans women's face. A small amount of tissue can also be removed from directly below the nose to raise the upper lip to display more vermillion and upper teeth, and produce quite a nice additional feminizing effect.[32]

SUMMARY

Ancillary medical procedures, such as speech therapy, voice-box surgery, and facial electrolysis, may be important for trans women. Although the successful attainment of feminine speech habits is often achieved using voice training, a few trans women undergo voice-box surgery to further feminize their voice. Trans women often endure 200 hours or more of painful electrolysis to remove facial hair, although an increasingly larger number of them, mostly younger trans women, prefer laser hair removal, which is much quicker even though not guaranteed to be permanent. Facial feminization surgery is an expensive supplementary procedure used by trans women to enhance their feminine appearance. It can have dramatic life-changing effects that enhance a trans woman's ability to pass seamlessly in public, gain employment if that has been denied them, and allow them to acquire other worthwhile social benefits.

Chapter 10

SOCIETAL ISSUES FOR GENDER-DIVERSE PEOPLE

One of the most difficult issues for trans people is the stigma and discrimination they may face from family, friends, educational institutions, the law, and even from some members of the medical profession. A recent review[1] proposed three levels where discrimination and stigma can occur: at the individual level, at the interpersonal level, and in the wider society. At the individual level the trans person is likely to conceal, avoid, and internalize the stigma, seeking counseling and support group help if it becomes unbearable. Interpersonal stigma sometimes results from interactions with family, friends, and others, which may escalate to physical violence. Such issues as economic and gender inequality represent threats from the wider society and the law and social institutions that are not easily fixed. No matter the source of stigma and discrimination, the effects on a trans person's mental health can be debilitating, leading to the high rates of anxiety and depression discussed in earlier chapters. Much of the research summarized below relates to the experiences of trans women rather than trans men, probably a result of the complex issues many trans women have to deal with during their transition.

10.1 FAMILY AND SOCIAL ISSUES

One of the greatest fears of trans people is whether their immediate family, friends, and work colleagues will offer them support in what is a long and difficult process toward self-fulfillment and happiness. In many cases, those closest to the transitioning person find it difficult to cope, at least in the initial stages. This situation may lead to shunning by family and friends so that the trans person has no further contact with their family and, most painfully, with their children. Being denied their parental right to be with their children is heartbreaking and can lead to severe psychological difficulties. Sadly, this situation appears to be common, although there has been insufficient research to inform counselors and the distraught trans person about appropriate remediation.

Some trans people delay their transition or slow its progress in consideration of their family and to minimize family conflict. Sometimes close family members, such as their spouse, request that they not be seen expressing their confirmed gender at family events. For example, this older trans woman did not dress *en femme* in consideration of the perceived wishes of her aging mother:

> I can weave a path very easily that is kind to her and at the worst inconveniences me . . . and that's only for her sake. Under other circumstances it would be different and will be in the future but for her mental health and well-being and reduced trauma because she's expressed not wanting to see this then I'll honour that. . . . To me it's a minor inconvenience. So I can very comfortably live with that and it's a tiny kindness that I'm embarking on towards her and the same would apply to my daughter and my wife.[2]

Clearly, proper family counseling support is needed in such circumstances for those transitioning and their loved ones.

Five emotional stages experienced by families of trans people after they have learned about their loved one's intention to transition are denial, anger, bargaining, depression, and acceptance. The partners of trans people often report feelings of shock, horror, disbelief, anger, betrayal, self-blame, loss of self-esteem, and depression. Clearly, adjusting to the news that a loved one is transitioning is a traumatic experience for many people. Family counseling is needed so that loved ones can adjust to their changed circumstances and assist their trans relative. Such interventions should occur before the trans person and their family lose contact with each other.[3]

Marriage breakup is common when a spouse is trans. It is difficult to predict how tolerant the significant other will be once they discover their spouse's cross-gendered behavior. For this reason, many trans people find the revelation of their cross-gendered identity to be an emotional experience.

10.1.1 The Effects of Transition on Family Members

Transition can have a substantial effect on the trans person's children. Often the concern of courts when adjudicating divorce settlements is to minimize the conflict and trauma suffered by the child, possibly by minimizing contact between the trans person and their children. Some trans people give up being a parent because they fear their transition might be harmful to the child. When their former spouse is adamantly opposed to any further contact, the trans person might be resigned to the fact that any legal fight is a lost cause. In more amicable circumstances, the trans parent continues to live with their family during the real-life experience or else maintains frequent family contact while living apart.

These interview vignettes illustrate the poignancy of children's thinking and their continuing love for a parent who is either transitioning or has already transitioned. In the following excerpts the interviewer's questions and the young person's responses are contained in quotations.[4]

Conversation with a seven-year-old boy and his parent who is transitioning from male to female:

> The boy says, "Linda wants to be a woman. Linda wants to start a fresh life. She likes living as a woman. I think that is happy for her. At first (when I was 4½) I didn't quite understand. As I got older, I realized she must be happy living as a woman, so I'll just accept that."
>
> The interviewer asks, "Does Linda have a penis?"
>
> The boy replies, "She is going to have it taken off."
>
> The interviewer asks, "What is your worry?"
>
> The boy replies, "The thing I worry about is if he gets injections that the wrong amount would be given and something would go wrong. . . . Is there a chance he could die in the operation?"

Conversation with a seven-year-old girl and her parent who is transitioning from male to female:

> The interviewer asks, "Why does your daddy dress as a lady?"
>
> The girl replies, "It's a better life."

Conversation with a 10-year-old boy and his 11-year-old sister and their parent who is transitioning from male to female:

> The interviewer asks, "How do you feel about it?"
>
> The boy replies, "It's all right."
>
> The interviewer asks, "Why is your daddy doing this?"
>
> The boy replies, "He does not like being a man."
>
> The boy's sister says, "My dad's having a sex change. He is turning into a woman."
>
> The interviewer asks, "Why?"
>
> The boy's sister replies, "He feels like a woman."

The interviewer asks, "How do you feel about it?"

The boy's sister replies, "I feel OK about it."

Comments by a 14-year-old teenager when asked about her parent who is transitioning from female to male:

> "My mother's not happy in the body she is in. My mom is a lot happier since starting to live as who she wants to be. When I was 13, my mother said, 'I want to be a man, do you care?' I said, no, as long as you are the same person inside and still love me. I don't care what you are on the outside. . . . It's like a chocolate bar, it's got a new wrapper but it's the same chocolate inside."

These vignettes demonstrate that trans people can remain effective and loving parents and that young children can understand and empathize with their trans parent's situation. These cases demonstrate that gender identity confusion in the child with respect to their parent does not always occur. Any subsequent teasing the children might suffer from peers is no more of a problem than the teasing children get for a myriad of other reasons. The children's best interests are not served by the bullying tactic of trading off the children as scapegoats when one parent's need for retaliation results in opposing any contact between the trans parent and their children. Although divorce is inevitable in many cases, just as it is in most other situations of marital disharmony, it should not affect future contact between parents and their children, nor should it be necessary that married trans people cannot change the sex on their birth certificate following genital surgery just because the marriage would then appear to be same-sex, as was the case in all Australian states and territories until recently.

Children with trans parents rarely display gender-atypical behavior themselves, but they are affected by the marital discord that arises between the trans person and their other parent.[5] In some countries, the law claims to protect the mental health of a married trans person's children by exacerbating the anguish and despair experienced when the trans person is denied access to their children, often against the children's wishes. A parent's adverse reaction to a trans spouse may even reflect deficiencies in their own ability to adjust to change.

A married person's transition can have a devastating effect on maintaining the family, even when the time between initial announcement of intent and the completion of the actual transition can be up to 10 years. However, a longer delay for the transition can be beneficial to the children. Those children who are most embarrassed by their parent's transition are also the most affected socially. These children are also more likely to suffer a decline in their academic performance. A third of children use their previous word, such as *Dad*, when addressing their transitioning parent in public and another third use a nickname. The older the child, the more they are affected by their parent's transition. There appears to be no greater incidence of mental health issues in children of a trans parent than in other children from more traditional family circumstances.[6]

As discussed in Chapter 8, trans men, who are still able to undergo pregnancy to full term, face social stigma and a lack of support, mostly the result of discrimination from the family. For these trans men, family support is crucial. Some of them suffer postpartum depression, a not uncommon complication for cisgender women. Trans people who do wish to have children tend to be younger than those who are not so inclined.[7]

A survey of 10 gender therapists indicated they considered it is better for trans people to disclose their transition to their children as soon as possible. Because adolescent children might react badly to such news, a trans parent needs to be prepared for whatever might happen. Risk factors for the children's welfare include an abrupt separation between their parents, a spouse who is unsupportive of the transition, parental conflict, and personal difficulties experienced by one or both parents. Children fare better when they have a close emotional relationship with the nontransitioning parent, there is extended family support of the transitioning parent, and contact is maintained with both parents. Children also manage best when they are younger or mature-age, as teenage children have the most difficulty accepting their transitioning parent.[8] It is interesting that parents who view transsexuality as a biological condition are more accepting of their child's situation, as was implied by the survey results described in Chapter 1.[9]

The conflict between living a secret cross-gendered life and coming out to family and friends can lead to clinically significant levels of depression and anxiety. When a married man lives full-time as a woman most of the time but transgresses to being male when the situation demands it, problems of self-identity can often arise. There have been no follow-up investigations to determine if temporary switching of gender roles is successful, or perhaps stressful, despite it being necessary sometimes to maintain marital harmony.

Most trans women reveal their gender difficulties to their spouses before approaching a support group, although many access Internet support chat lines during their exploratory phase to maintain confidentiality. Concerns during the public outing phase include anxiety about how others will react to the news. Although many trans women are concerned about how their family and friends will react to their unexpected revelation, less than 25 percent report negative reactions. So, some of their initial fears are probably unfounded. However, it is worthwhile providing close relatives with as much information as possible about the transition process at the outset so that an informed discussion can occur with respect to family circumstances.[10]

The main reason for telling family, friends, and work colleagues about one's intention to transition is the need to be responsible and inform people who might be affected by it. Sharing the news with a female friend may be ego-boosting as her reaction is usually less stigmatizing than that of male relatives and friends. For some trans women, outing themselves is based on a prior conviction that other people's love for them will be maintained and support will be forthcoming. It is preferable to come out face-to-face and provide significant others with time to absorb the news. A subsequent discussion might elucidate the likely consequences of the transition. To reduce the burden on the trans person, some relatives might offer to inform other family members and to encourage them to also offer their support.[11]

The conditions under which a trans woman's identity might be confirmed by her social interactions with family, friends, and others have been investigated. Whereas earlier reports had claimed that most trans people suffer mental health problems derived mostly from adverse social reactions, interviews of mainly African American trans women sex workers in New York City indicated that depression is less prevalent when there is good support from family and friends. The benefits arising from such support are enhanced by being upfront about one's trans identity to close associates, by being successful in one's cross-gendered role, and by minimizing any conflict between one's trans identity awareness and social performance of the cross-gendered role. A trans person's self-esteem is enhanced when existing sexual partners negotiate a new role for themselves and their trans partner as well as when support is offered by parents, siblings, and more distant family members. Continued employment is a challenge that is both ego-boosting and financially rewarding for trans people.[12]

A study of young trans people showed that parental acceptance is important for minimizing the psychological distress caused by gender nonconformity. Having a low level of father acceptance produces increased distress and anxiety, especially when the level of gender nonconformity is high. A high level of father support maintains lower levels of distress and anxiety at all levels of gender nonconformity.[13]

Young trans people believe that their family is most supportive when as a result of such support they endure fewer instances of self-harm and experience reduced depressive symptoms and anxiety. There is also the boost to self-esteem and resiliency that good family support can bring. However, these young people must still contend with the distress caused by having a body that does not conform to their gender identity, as well as having to endure bullying by peers and others at school and elsewhere.[14]

Gender-diverse children who disclose their gender diversity to their teacher are more likely to suffer rejection than other children in the class. This form of victimization at the highest level has an adverse effect on the young person's self-confidence and school achievement. These children feel unsafe at school. Gender stereotypes often mean that young trans people are not addressed by their preferred name and pronoun. However, trans students can feel safer at school if their welfare is recognized by changes in the school rules and especially when they are supported by their teacher.[15]

Any anxiety and depression felt by trans people can be reduced by strong general social support for trans men and trans women and a connectedness to other members of the trans community, especially for trans women.[16] Occasionally, the relationships between various members of the trans community can be fickle. For example, it is not unusual for trans people to avoid contact with crossdressers. In some situations, being able to pass becomes a status symbol, the more physically attractive members avoiding those who are not as able to pass or do not choose to do so. Eventually, trans people tend to leave support groups to live a life of their own, whereas crossdressers thrive on the privacy these support groups offer.

Resilience in a sample of 230 trans woman aged 19 to 59 was investigated by showing that the risk of major depression is reduced by their being involved with the trans community, but only when the experienced level of abuse from external sources was high. There was not so much need for community involvement when trans women experienced little or no abuse.[17]

The Internet provides an almost unlimited information resource for trans people with its informative webpages, videos, and entertainment. Particularly helpful are stories and advice offered by members of the trans communities and their supporters, as well as the many opportunities to share experiences with peers located anywhere in the world. To a large extent, the Internet allows otherwise lonely trans people to enjoy an online social life in a safe environment. The Internet has allowed political activism to prosper within trans communities for the betterment of all its members, some of whom use pseudonyms for privacy protection. Many trans people feel empowered by engaging with others in the online world, something they cannot easily achieve in the outside world.[18]

10.1.2 Relationship Issues for Trans People

The sexual preferences of trans people is an interesting issue. Frank Lewins,[19] who interviewed trans women and trans men using probably biased sampling, discovered that trans women in stable relationships tend to be sexually involved with women rather than men. After genital surgery these women indulge in what appears to be a gynephilic relationship.

In another study, older trans women aged 50 to 67 years were interviewed about their relationships with women. Eighty-two percent of the 17 woman were living as trans full-time and 43 percent had had genital surgery. These women's gender expression reflected the various phases of lifestyle exploration and experimentation. They had experienced a second adolescence and maturation as well as their re-gendering as a woman and achieving their own body-mind congruence, especially after genital surgery. This was something their female partners appreciated.[20]

A survey of 796 trans people 16 years and older in Sweden showed that 4 percent identified as nonbinary, with most of them saying they were either bisexual or queer. In terms of relationships, 38 percent had one sexual partner, 14 percent had more than one sexual partner, and 34 percent were not in a sexual relationship. Important for sexual health were satisfactory experiences with the physical (39%), emotional (23%), and relational (38%) aspects of sex. About half had been exposed to offensive treatment in the last three months, and 30 percent had been forced to have sex against their will. Most of the people surveyed were aware of safe sex practices.[21]

Another survey of 207 young people involved mostly trans feminine people and those who were assigned female at birth, many of whom identified as queer and pansexual. Slight aggressive behaviors directed toward these young people included the use of transphobic terminology, the assumption of a universal trans experience, disapproval of the trans experience, preference for a gender binary classification, assumption of sexual pathology, and questioning the legitimacy of the trans person's affirmed gender. Most of these so-called microaggressions were instigated by cisgender friends. Distress was caused when those people who initiated the microaggressions were close friends, especially those who identified as LGBT and who placed undue emphasis on the trans person's sexuality. The following quotation comes from a trans man who participated in this interview study:

> I lost some friends because they were disgusted by me being trans; it really hurt especially since a lot of them were gay- and lesbian-identified, and I could not understand how one marginalized community would be disgusted by me. It just really hurt me. I ended relationships with these people.[22]

Since 1997, representatives with a trans background have been elected to the board of the World Professional Association of Transgender Health. This marked a turning point as consumers as well as gender specialists now contribute to revisions of the Standards of Care, the procedures recommended for the treatment of trans people who wish to transition. A greater number of trans people have opted not to disappear into the cisgender world but to remain active in the various political movements that support gender-diverse people.[23]

To summarize, perhaps the most difficult challenge for trans people is maintaining their family relationships. For those who have children, the reaction to their new lifestyle is often acceptable to the children but devastating for their partner. Because of the stressful situations that can often arise, proper care of the trans person is essential.

10.1.3 Care of Trans and Gender-Diverse People

Caring for gender-diverse people is especially important. Like other minorities, trans people experience prejudice and other negative responses from caregivers. This is an unfortunate situation as trans people deserve the very best care on offer. In nursing situations, accommodating a trans person in a gender-segregated hospital ward can be a problem, especially when inappropriate and abusive language is used by the staff.[24]

Sixty percent of trans people experience some form of harassment or violence, and 37 percent experience economic discrimination. Drug and alcohol abuse by trans people often results from low self-esteem and a lack of educational and job opportunities. Because of harassment and family difficulties, some gender-diverse youth leave home and fend for themselves with inadequate resources. This leads to an increase in homelessness and substance abuse, especially alcohol, cocaine, and methamphetamines. Prejudice from health service providers can prevent these young people from obtaining urgent help. Also, black market hormone overdose is a further medical complication, especially when the client is too poor to afford hormone treatment or has not been approved for hormone use by a doctor.[25]

The care of older trans people is problematic because there is no guarantee that aged-care facilities will treat such people with dignity. Problems occur when religious aged-care agencies reject trans people, and other agencies offer less than adequate medical care. As discussed later in this chapter, this is an urgent issue for those concerned about an aging trans population.[26]

10.1.4 The Social Life of Trans People

The need for trans people to pass is relaxed in many progressive gender-diverse communities to provide space and acceptance of androgynous and gender-ambiguous people. Katrina Roen[27] refers to the binary gender status quo as *either/or* and compares this with a more flexible gender presentation as *both/neither*. *Either/or* trans people frequently aspire to a life of stealth, even isolating themselves from other trans people. This occurs despite people such as Kate Bornstein[28] proclaiming that such behavior is politically unwise, especially when the majority of trans people are stigmatized. Bornstein claims that passing represents shame, capitulation, invisibility, lies, and self-denial. Perhaps the gender diversity represented by *both/neither* is just as acceptable and as liberating as is racial and religious diversity.

Roen interviewed gender-diverse people to obtain information on the importance of passing. One of those interviewed, who presented as *both/neither*, could not obtain a position in a college course even though she had the necessary qualifications. Some trans women maintained a *both/neither* orientation in private and in thoughts about their situation, especially during transition, but felt some pressure to conform to an *either/or* presentation in public. Some of these people reported that their medical advisers would consider a *both/neither* presentation as politically radical, leading to problems in obtaining approval for gender-affirming surgeries. Most of them thought that a trans woman's "goal was to live as an ordinary woman . . . and ordinary women don't mix in trans-sexual circles."[29] By contrast, most of the trans men had no trouble passing as male so the *both/neither* category had little relevance for them.

It has been suggested that a trans woman who has not had any surgeries could still call herself a woman despite having residual male genitals. A trans woman's ability to pass successfully in everyday life is unrelated to the existence of male or surgically constructed genitals, these being generally hidden from public view. The critical event for such a person is the decision to live full-time as a woman with hormone assistance rather than feeling obliged to undergo genital surgery. Successfully living full-time as a woman is the primary qualification for being trans so that sex, as represented by external genitals, is irrelevant.

When trans women socially transition, many wish to be perceived as a woman rather than as someone in transition. Often initial outings in public are carefully planned, being limited to relatively safe places such as trans-friendly venues and driving there in their own car to avoid the perceived risk of exposure in public transport. Support groups are important at this stage despite the anxiety that sometimes results from intolerance from seasoned trans women. In addition to socialization at support groups, trans women enjoy receiving advice on makeup, hairstyles, and the other accoutrements to enhance their ability to pass as women.

The coming-out phase allows trans people to adjust so they can live as convincingly as possible as their true selves.[30] Many trans people agree that "passing . . . is the most important aspect of the whole thing. If you can't do that, I don't see the point of living this way."[31] Once passing is mastered to their satisfaction, many trans women no longer require trans community support and live as a woman, perhaps in stealth mode. For such people, being seen in public with an obviously trans person risks revealing their own background. An alternative view from a so-called gender radical is that "passing is more a fear that has to be overcome and when I overcame that fear to be nonchalant about it, I didn't care that I passed or not."[32] Nevertheless, people who maintain an androgynous appearance are often ridiculed and stigmatized. They run the risk of suffering emotional and physical abuse. Hence many trans women strive to be passable and live anonymously in society as women.

Many trans women value their feminine appearance as confirmation of their affirmed gender identity. This reflects the cultural importance of women looking like women; the more attractive they are, the more confident they feel in social situations. Many trans women appreciate that crossdressers can feel and look feminine occasionally, whereas for many full-time trans women the need to be seen as feminine is perpetual. Although there was pressure to conform to gender expectations when they were young, some trans women recall experiencing a childhood in which they were much more comfortable playing with girls and associating with a female group. When they were required to be with boys, many trans women report memories of anxiety, failure, and a loss of self-esteem. To tolerate this situation better, many of them were loners as young people.

Further into their transition, some trans women resort to drugs and alcohol to conceal the mismatch between their identity as female, and the role expected of them by family and peers. In desperation, a small number mutilate their genitals to reinforce their affirmed sexual identity. As has been frequently observed, 44 percent of a group of trans women had engaged in hypermasculine activities such as serving in the military to compensate for, and possibly obliterate, their gender-incongruent feelings.

As trans women become more immersed in their own culture and identify increasingly more often as female, they start to question their own sexual orientation. Although most react cautiously to advances by men, they may consider sex with men as a way to validate their womanhood. Many trans women consider this aspect of their transition to be rather problematical, probably because few middle-aged trans women report being androphilic prior to their transition.

Since Benjamin's[33] early work on transsexuality, adopting as complete a feminine lifestyle as possible during the social transition is thought to be important. In a study of experiences of passing involving four trans women and eight trans men who were undergoing medical treatment, five of them had begun their transition after an acute emotional crisis. One of these, a 56-year-old trans woman, decided to transition because she felt increasingly unattractive due to aging, undoubtedly a risky justification for transition. Most of the trans women had served in the armed forces, which provided an opportunity for them to prove their masculinity in the hope of curing their gender issues. Most had experienced physical or psychological abandonment by their same-sex parent during childhood, a few had crossdressed as children, and most of this very small clinical sample were chronically depressed and anxious.

A common misassumption made by clinicians is that trans people will want to have genital and other surgeries, pass as a man or woman, and thereafter live their lives by being as indistinguishable as possible from cisgender people of their affirmed gender. Trans people also need to acquire legal and social documentation appropriate to their new gender role. However, difficulties can arise irrespective of whether a trans person wishes to pass. Those who pass but live in stealth must hide their past life, often leading to confusion for others and stress for themselves. A trans man or trans women living in stealth is much less likely to serve as a role model for other trans people, especially those who are in transition and who cannot pass easily. On the other hand, those who do not pass may have difficulty in obtaining employment, their ambiguous appearance prejudicing both their own safety as well as their relations with family and friends. A division of the trans community based on ability to pass leads to distressing disagreements that prejudice any cohesive attempt to obtain justice for all trans people. Generally, trans people who pass without problems, especially those who are postoperative, aspire to, and acquire, a higher status than many others within the trans community.[34]

A study of the romantic lives of 569 trans men showed that 52 percent were living in a relationship that was associated with fewer symptoms of depression, especially if there was adequate social support.[35] For these men the need to pass as men is rarely a consideration in their social interactions.

In an online study involving 255 transgender Australians, 87 birth-assigned females and 168 birth-assigned males, the most common incidents of victimization involved direct personal abuse, being socially excluded, and the spreading of personal rumors. Verbal harassment, employment exclusion, and health care discrimination were other serious concerns. Overall, 69 percent of these trans people had been victimized at some time in their lives. Almost 60 percent of respondents had presented with depressive symptoms, about 44 percent had previously attempted suicide, 30 percent had a problem with alcohol, and 19 percent were having problems with other substances. Most of the trans people had limited social support, and there was a slight tendency for victimization to be associated with having less support from others. Beneficial for trans men were committed relationships, current employment, having had some form of gender confirmation surgery, and having no issue with alcohol use or any suicide attempt.[36]

Many trans people experience problems when outing themselves at work. For some, this leads to demotion, harassment, and eventually to either dismissal or voluntary resignation. For those requiring the most social support, the loss of professional identity and their previous level of income is further exacerbated by the loss of family and close friends. Most trans people are challenged by their initial attempts at living full-time as their true selves. The reactions of their employer as well as the attitude toward them from members of the wider community determine whether their public acceptance is tolerable. For some trans people, passing is paramount, whereas for others just being themselves is more important.

Of concern, the trans community itself can be a source of distress for some trans people, especially when postoperative trans people who can pass as socially acceptable men and women establish themselves at the peak of a *trans hierarchy*. Ways that trans people can cope with transphobia in the workplace include modification of their presentation and appearance, being emotionally remote at work, making and retaining good relations with coworkers, using outside assistance such as counseling when needed, being better than most of their coworkers at the job, and seeking leadership roles in the organization.[37]

A recent study showed that more trans women than trans men report discrimination at work. Coworker support helps, but there is no benefit from being open about one's trans status to management and coworkers.[38] However, because many trans people have been stigmatized by a mental illness diagnosis, it is difficult to avoid prejudice and transphobia in the workplace. Many members of the public want to distance themselves from people diagnosed with mental illness because of their fear and misunderstanding of mentally ill people. The situation for trans women is not helped by cisgender men perceiving them as a threat to male values, whereas symbolically joining the ranks of *masculine women* makes trans men's passage in the workplace somewhat easier.

In a study that used fictitious statements of employment experience, hiring decisions were affected by a perception that trans people's presumed mental illness diagnosis was a negative when it came to recommending they be hired for a job. In composing these recommendations, participants considered possible mental health problems for trans men. However, for trans women, any possible mental health reasons for not offering them a job were overshadowed by the applicant's transgender status. To that extent, presenting as male would have discounted any negative feelings that might have occurred regarding the applicant's transgender status.[39]

High rates of unemployment and underemployment among trans people can be the cause and result of mental health problems, no doubt affected by the consequent financial difficulties and possible homelessness. However, employment can have its drawbacks, especially when work colleagues produce higher levels of internalized stigma, and when the trans person's associated mental health problems are considered too difficult to disclose to an employer. Effective stress-reduction strategies include maintaining one's distance from threatening experiences in the workplace and employing emotion-regulating strategies and positive thinking to cope with transphobia, should it be experienced.[40]

10.2 RELIGIOUS AND ETHICAL ISSUES

Acceptance into society's institutions, such as organized religions, is important for trans people. Considerable harm can result from institutionalized prejudice by a majority directed against an already disenfranchised minority.

Ethical issues of concern to Christians in their dealings with trans people include questions of gender, the impact of gender status on an individual's participation in religious events, the acceptability of genital surgeries, and whether the church should solemnize marriages involving one or more trans person. Like the general community, many religious people were exposed to the idea of gender diversity when media reports of successful genital surgeries first appeared. Christians often oppose such surgery because it does not relate to procreation, and it does not appear to be medically necessary.[41] This is a common attitude among the religious that is inconsistent with the presumed biological basis of gender diversity, as we showed in a summary of results from an Internet survey in Chapter 1.

Some scriptures stipulate that crossdressing is as inappropriate a behavior as genital mutilation, the implicit assumption being that no one can interfere with one's preordained gender or sexual identity. This modern interpretation of scripture ignores the elevated position accorded castrated males, or eunuchs, in many ancient societies. For example, consider the following biblical edict from Matthew (19:12):

> For there are some eunuchs, which were so born from their *mother's* womb: and there are some eunuchs, which were made eunuchs of men: and there be eunuchs, which have made themselves eunuchs for the kingdom of heaven's sake. He that is able to receive *it*, let him receive *it*.

Based on this biblical excerpt, a Christian should welcome trans people into all religious activities including the sacrament of marriage. Of special significance is maintaining a legally valid marriage between a man and a woman when a person has transitioned from their birth-assigned sex by mutual consent of both parties. According to many religions, no outside agent can separate those who have been formally united by the acquiescence of God. This would imply that such an apparently same-sex marriage cannot be annulled!

Some religious people fail to understand why anyone would want surgery to alter a healthy body, especially when they believe wrongly that the long-term benefits of such a procedure have not been fully researched and documented. Their reservations are reinforced by the occasional incidents of postsurgical regret accompanied by what they might see as personal disabilities such as depression and prostitution. Our better understanding of the possibility of a positive impact of a parent's transition on their family life with its associated loving support from spouse and children cannot justify the bigotry toward trans people that emanates from some religious organizations.[42]

In most religions, a marriage involving at least one trans person remains valid provided it involves a union between a man and a woman. However, a problem arises when the legally accepted sexual designation of the trans people involved is based on biological criteria, rather than on social aspects of gender expression as recognized by the trans person's relatives and friends. For example, a preoperative trans woman might want to marry a cisgender man but for health reasons cannot endure genital surgery and thereby be able to change the sex designator on her birth certificate. Such a union might be considered same-sex, leading to the marriage not being recognized in some countries.

The theological status of a reconstructed sex organ, as opposed to a God-given one, is an interesting issue. It has been stated that "human sexuality is an artifact, and that artifactual sexuality is real sexuality."[43] So, is a surgically con-structed sexual organ an artifact? The extent to which the sexed nature of such an artifact can constitute the trans person's true sex is an interesting question. Maybe the resolution of such a dilemma might itself become a criterion for sex determination. However, when legislating sexual relationships within a marriage, society should really play no role in documenting a person's *real sex* since this is a private matter between the partners. As people generally infer a person's sex from their gender expression, everyone should have a right to express themselves in whatever way they feel most comfortable.

Many world religions are accepting of gender-diverse members of their communities, particularly the dharmic religions such as Buddhism and Hin-duism, as well as other spiritual entities such as Pagan, Celtic, and Wiccan groups. The Unitarian church is also accepting of gender-diverse Christian believers. The most common religious alliances of trans people are to Protes-tant groups (15%) and nonspecific spirituality (19%), whereas a slightly larger number of trans elders report being atheist, agnostic, or having no religion at all (19%).

10.3 LEGAL ISSUES

In many places, the law has made life difficult for trans people. Not only is the social stigma they suffer legitimized by law enforcement agencies, but institu-tions that most people take for granted have not made a trans person's life any easier. For example, a legal marriage is difficult to obtain for many trans peo-ple. Also, gaining appropriate employment and Social Security rights presents many challenges.

A person's legal sex in most countries is based on genital appearance as determined by medical staff at birth. This sex designation is recorded officially by the state on the person's birth certificate. For trans people, their birth certificate contains the wrong legal sex until it can be changed following genital surgeries. Recent exceptions to this archaic rule include the relaxed gender recognition policies of Argentina, Malta, Portugal, Ireland, and several others.

In some countries like Thailand, sexual orientation and gender identity are conflated so that a trans woman and an effeminate gay man would belong to a similar category. Despite its highly regarded medical services for trans people, Thailand only recognizes a person's sex, in any legal proceedings including the sex designation on a birth certificate and passport, as that person's birth-assigned sex, which cannot be changed following genital surgery.[44]

10.3.1 Marriage Law

Legal aspects of marriage recognition when there is at least one trans person involved present difficult problems for all concerned, especially when in former times a judge could insist that sex was determined by a person's chromosomes. Later, legal judgment recognized the increasing social acceptance of trans people, in particular the legal recognition of the new sexual identity of postoperative trans people. Since it is inappropriate for such people to live in a sexual limbo, recognition of a trans person's right to marry should occur under all circumstances.

One judge stated that "[i]f a society accepts that transsexualism is a serious and distressing medical problem, and allows those who suffer from it to undergo drastic treatment in order to adopt a new gender and thereby improve their quality of life, then reason and common humanity alike suggest that it should allow such persons to function as fully as possible in their new gender."[45] Also, Professor Gooren, a prominent researcher from the Netherlands, suggested that "[it] is reasonable to require from the law that it makes provision for those rare individuals in whom the formation of gender identity has not followed the course otherwise so reliably prognosticated by the external genitalia."[46] Human rights and natural justice require the law to be flexible enough to accommodate individual cases rather than adhering to biological misinterpretations deemed appropriate for all.

In some countries, sex is defined in two different ways, one emphasizing psychological and anatomical gender harmony, the other based on social and cultural gender consistency. Much of the law relating to sex is affected by a disguised form of homophobia as well as by strict adherence to the sex categories of male and female. Some legislators believe that trans people are homosexual, an attitude that is also shared by some members of the medical profession, some lawyers and doctors basing their professional judgments on the normativity of a heterosexual lifestyle.[47]

Legal judgments regarding marriage involving at least one trans person depend on whether sexual intercourse is necessary for the marriage to be legitimate. Otherwise there is no reason why marriages involving preoperative and nonoperative trans people cannot be legally validated. Reliance on fundamental biology such as the necessity of XX chromosomes for women and XY chromosomes for men pathologizes the trans person's body, which has been altered, at least by hormone therapy, at great personal cost.

In an Australian case, legal sex was defined more generally as

> the person's biological and physical characteristics at birth (including gonads, geni-
> tals and chromosomes); the person's life experiences, including the sex in which he
> or she is brought up and the person's attitude to it; the person's self-perception as a
> man or a woman; the extent to which the person has functioned in society as a man
> or a woman; any hormonal, surgical or other medical sex reassignment treatments
> the person has undergone, and the consequences of such treatment; and the person's
> biological, psychological and physical characteristics at the time of the marriage,
> including (if they can be identified) any biological features of the person's brain that
> are associated with a particular sex. . . . [P]ost-operative transsexuals will normally
> be members of their reassigned sex.[48]

This definition was based on current scientific knowledge in 2001 and extended the legal definition of sex to include both psychological and lifestyle aspects.

The same judge in this case noted, "failure to recognize the sex of post-operative [trans people] raises serious issues of human rights, such that the question arises whether the failure can be permitted on the basis of the margin of appreciation allowed to States under the [Australian] Constitution. It is clear that a decision in favor of the applicants would be more in accord with international thinking on human rights than a refusal of the application." Consequently, it was ruled that "post-operative transsexuals should be treated as members of the sex to which they have been assigned."[49]

10.3.2 Documentation Amendment and Employment Discrimination

Legal consideration of claims for employment discrimination by trans people requires the removal of prejudice. Generally, trans people are not protected by employment antidiscrimination legislation except in a few enlightened juris-dictions. Moreover, such people are not always included in the gay, lesbian, and bisexual campaigns for equality. Sometimes prejudicial judgments arise not from being affirmed surgically as male or female but merely from changing one's gender presentation. Some employers get away with such illegal dis-crimination by claiming that trans employees might adversely affect their cus-tomers' confidence, and of course their own bottom line! The situation is much worse in those jurisdictions that prosecute anyone who crossdresses in public.[50]

Sometimes it is difficult to determine a trans person's gender status, espe-cially if they pass well. This desirable situation from the passing trans person's perspective has produced difficulties in sexual harassment cases when defen-dants claim they were misled about a person's true sex. For example, if a court determines that harassment was based on a change in sex, rather than sex itself, then the protection afforded by sex antidiscrimination legislation may not apply. In some situations, such harassment may even be legally sanctioned.

Of course, the basic requirement in employment is competence on the job, and this should not be compromised by discrimination based on gender presentation or current sexual status.

Receiving medical benefits is often problematic as some courts refuse to recognize the medical diagnosis of gender dysphoria as either a disability or a medical condition. However, some enlightened jurisdictions recognize any DSM-diagnosed psychiatric condition as a disability, resulting in assistance being offered. This situation is one of the few ways in which trans people might benefit from the pathologization of their condition other than access to medical insurance for gender-affirmative medical interventions for which a medical diagnosis is required. How the newly defined gender incongruence condition in a sexual health section of the recently revised International Classification of Diseases, version 11 will influence the law and resolve the above issues will have to await its future implementation.

The relationship between discrimination based on sex and that based on gender diversity is interesting, especially when the trans person can avail themselves of sex discrimination legislation. This type of direct sex discrimination can occur when legal sex prevents a person from taking advantage of opportunities available to others, such as wearing the clothes, makeup, jewelry, and hairstyle of their affirmed gender and accessing gender-appropriate bathroom and changing room facilities. Such violation of individual rights might involve the allocation of childcare and other female jobs exclusively to cisgender women, as well as sexual harassment and discrimination directed against gender-diverse people and discrimination against those who violate sex-delineated dress codes.

The major forms of discrimination against trans people include sanctions toward those who are on hormone therapy and who are considering gender-affirming surgeries; restrictions on the use of single-sex locations and activities; and importantly, their inability to change their legal sex on official documents such as passports and birth certificates. The medical standards required for gender-affirming surgeries are more stringent than those applying to informed consent in irreversible, and potentially risky, elective procedures such as sterilization, organ donation, and cosmetic surgery. There is always the fear that the client will change their mind after proceeding with irreversible medical procedures, a situation that can deter a judge in some jurisdictions from authorizing even a name change as an initial step toward gender-affirming surgeries.

The medical and legal communities often serve as gatekeepers for society's disapproval of something as radical as what some call a sex change. In a poignant quote, Anna Kirkland suggested that "transsexuals wanted to have more and better information about their condition; to dispel ignorance about transsexualism among gender professionals and the public; to obtain better services; to lessen the financial burdens of surgery; and finally, to be treated with the same level of [*sic*] respect as patients with other conditions."[51] That such a situation has been more the exception than the rule represents a travesty of justice.

It is ironic that trans people have had to present themselves as ill or distressed to qualify for and obtain gender-affirming surgeries. Yet, following surgery, they must present as well-adjusted people to convince a court that they are a *real* man or a *real* woman. In many instances, being a postoperative trans person is equivalent to relegating one's parental responsibilities following separation and divorce, such is the disruption that is sometimes caused to their previous lifestyle and personal reputation. It is also clear that those trans people who wish to benefit from living appropriately as their affirmed sex should not violate society's binary gender norms but instead be perceived as "acceptable" in what is often a patriarchal society. Interestingly, the strategies required of trans women to be successful in legal matters are often those condemned by some radical feminists.[52]

The restriction society imposes on gender-diverse people of all persuasions has increased during the last couple of years as conservative forces impose more and more draconian measures to stymie the chances of these vulnerable people and their supporters. As we have seen, the medical and legal professions can impose sufficient constraints on gender-diverse people's lives to jeopardize their happiness and stifle their ambitions. When those seeking medical interventions do not have to be diagnosed as mentally ill, we will know that society wants trans people to enjoy the same privileges and rights as everybody else. As despotic regimes and fundamentalists of all persuasions impose more restrictions on trans people's freedoms, it is so important that all humane people act on these vulnerable people's behalf before it is too late.

10.3.3 Violence and the Violation of Human Rights

The rights of trans people are often compromised by institutionalized violence instigated by various countries and states. Transphobia is deeply entrenched in society's institutions, leading to prejudice based on a presumption that trans people are health hazards, a threat to public morality, and evidence of a decadent culture. Even greater hazards for trans people exist in societies where state-sponsored violence is rife. In many places, trans people are denied public-sector jobs, dismissed from employment once their lifestyle has been discovered, and frequently singled out for harassment. Much of this antagonism from social institutions has been eulogized in the interest of maintaining the nuclear family against possible disruption.

Semilegal police violence directed at trans people is difficult to eliminate due to vaguely worded regulations and arrest procedures during which the police can interpret the law in any way they like. Particularly distressing has been the targeting of trans people by police forces in countries that sanction torture and killings in holding cells. In these places, some more privileged trans people can avoid the ingrained state-instituted violence meted out to their less fortunate counterparts by using their better bargaining power with corrupt officials.[53]

Violence toward trans people risks damaging their physical and mental health, a situation that must be addressed by their medical advisers. Surprisingly, schools are hazardous places for gender-diverse students, those suffering harassment often leaving school voluntarily to minimize the adverse effects of bullying. Many societies believe that trans women threaten male privilege and the social order, and so deserve retribution.[54]

Violence against trans people, as has been documented worldwide by Amnesty International, violates the International Covenants on both Civil and Political Rights as well as that on Economic, Social, and Cultural Rights. For example, the United Nations Human Rights Convention and the European Convention on Human Rights forbid discrimination against trans people.

An international survey of some 300 trans people revealed that they were more likely to suffer violence and victimization than others in the community. Unfortunately, trans people are also less likely to receive supportive medical care and counseling. Despite legal protection, trans people receive insufficient medical and legal intervention following physical and sexual attacks. Trans women also suffer from misogynistic crimes perpetrated mostly by men, thus increasing their burden of stigma and fear.[55]

The Yogyakarta Principles are based upon international human rights law that applies to any gender-diverse person no matter where they live. These principles emphasize human dignity, self-determination, bodily integrity, and protection from medical abuse. They apply especially to those trans people who are subjected to psychological diagnoses so that they can obtain medical assistance to facilitate their transition. There may be a case for these diagnoses being needed, for example, so that some trans people in the United States who are lucky enough to have medical insurance can gain access to sponsored medical services to support their transition. However, this pathologization of the transition process to benefit a few should not impose a burden on healthy trans people elsewhere. What is needed instead is a proper informed consent process as is the case for most other medical procedures, an exception being when a trans person might have been diagnosed with a serious illness that precludes a medical transition. Furthermore, all recognition of gender by governments and others should not require the medicalization of a condition that is a normal state of the human experience.[56]

This branding of gender-diverse people as mentally ill is a serious violation of their human rights. It is one way that medical and other professionals have primed the general community to look down upon gender-diverse people as stereotypically inferior human beings. If they are not banished completely, some countries will still arrange for trans people to spend time in locked psychiatric facilities should they desire any medical intervention. There is little that professionals have done in these countries to encourage the full participation of trans people in education and work. As is the case in a few enlightened countries, gender-diverse people should be allowed to confirm their own legal identities, nonbinary gender identities should be appropriately recognized, and trans partners in a marriage should never be forced to divorce before being able to obtain official recognition of their affirmed gender. In mid-2018 those countries that have completely depathologized gender diversity include Argentina, Bolivia, Colombia, Denmark, Ireland, Malta, and Norway. Extra security precautions at airports and international borders are making it increasingly difficult for trans people to travel and to immigrate to foreign countries. Extra training on trans issues needs to be taken by law enforcement agencies and immigration officers.[57]

Violence against gender-diverse people has not been forestalled with 2,649 reported killings in 69 countries having occurred between 2008 and September 30, 2017, with many more murders going unreported. Gender-diverse people worldwide pay homage to all these unnecessary deaths on the Transgender Day of Remembrance held on November 20 every year. In addition to life-threatening violence, there are restrictions on the use of bathroom and changing room facilities as well as participation by gender-diverse people in sports designated for their affirmed gender.

10.4 AGING AND TRANS ELDERS

When people get older they are often more susceptible to health issues, and in their more senior years require special care. Older trans people face these same age-related challenges as well as other demands that confront a minority who have been subjected to the ravages of discrimination, job loss, loss of family and friends, and in some cases, homelessness. In this section we examine the challenges older trans people face as they transition from a life of individual responsibility to one where help from others, not always desired, is necessary for their continuing good health.

Significant issues for trans elders include the quality of their social support systems; their desire for close relationships and intimacy; safe, secure, and affordable living arrangements; the avoidance of violence and abuse; the availability of affordable and accepting health care; and the availability of friends and family to support them in end-of-life preparations. Not only do trans elders have to contend with ageism like other older people, but transphobia also raises its ugly head in many situations, even during health care consultations. Health care agencies and those involved in aged care need to have special training so that they can respectfully assist trans elders.[58]

Based on data from 2010, it is estimated that there are almost three million trans people in the United States aged 65 and older, about 0.4 percent of the population, and a worldwide population of up to 12 times that. These numbers are expected to increase rapidly over time as more trans people who transitioned in the last 40 years reach retirement and beyond. Like older people everywhere, trans elders can suffer from memory loss and dementia, as well as additional risks of depression and suicide. Many trans seniors live alone, so opportunities for socializing and communication with supportive others are vital. We are not certain what the long-term effects of hormone therapy are, so there may be health complications resulting from previous medical interventions that are unique to trans elders.[59] It could be that long-term estrogen therapy in trans women can induce a type of brain atrophy that is evident in some trans women over the age of 65 and that is a side effect of the replacement of testosterone by estrogen.[60]

Educators and providers of care to older trans people need to understand their own attitudes toward gender-diverse people and how these attitudes affect their ability to care for such people in the health care system, especially in aged-care facilities. These professionals need to understand that every person is different and comes to care with their own personal life history. Caregivers need to be up-to-date with the latest developments in appropriate care for minorities who may have been disadvantaged at various stages of their lives. Appropriate pronouns should be used in all discussions with trans elders, and proper outreach to families and other caregivers is required, including providing services that enhance trans elders' cognitive and emotional welfare.

One way to avoid embarrassment when speaking with trans elders is to not use gendered words until you first ask the person how they want to be addressed, for example, by saying *How may I help you?*, rather than *How may I help you, Sir?* Using the person's first or full name is also a polite thing to do. It is important that trans people agree to care rather than it be tacitly assumed that they need it. Trans elders should be accommodated in accordance with their affirmed gender, their health records being especially protected should they have been diagnosed with a mental illness in the past, such as gender identity disorder, that is only related to their gender variance and otherwise is no indicator of mental ill-health.[61]

Despite the onset of physical and other debilitating disorders in later life, many trans elders have been surprisingly resilient. Some trans elders have relatively large social networks, and they participate in spiritual and religious activities at a rate not dissimilar to cisgender people of the same age. Nevertheless, some older trans people maintain their earlier reluctance to access appropriate health care when needed.

Compared with their cisgender counterparts, trans elders tend to have a lower income, and they are less likely than their cisgender peers to have a power of attorney for health care and a will that they have shared with family and trusted others. Many trans elders suffer from a lack of exercise and have a higher obesity level than similarly aged people. In the past, many trans elders would have experienced victimization and consequently were likely to have had to conceal their trans identity. Trans elders often have poorer physical health, a greater level of disability, and are more likely to report depression and perceived stress than cisgender seniors. These findings suggest that the disadvantage trans people have endured during their more active years continues when they become seniors.[62]

More than half of those trans elders aged over 55 have lost close friends because of their transgender status. In the United States, 44 percent of trans elders live alone compared with 18 percent of the general population. Many of them have lost contact with their children and other members of their family. Because some trans elders have suffered violence and abuse in the past, it is important to provide safe living places for them as they get older. There is always the risk of the planned suicide that needs to be seriously addressed by aged-care workers and mental health professionals. The development of Alzheimer's disease and other forms of dementia are obvious risks with this disadvantaged population.[63]

A larger number of older trans women have been married than have older trans men. However, for those trans elders who are not in a relationship, finding someone to care for them in old age is difficult. Thirty percent of older trans people have no idea who will be caring for them in the future. This is a greater worry for the 34 percent of disabled trans elders who live alone. Their worries, in order of reported importance, are becoming unable to care for themselves, becoming sick, having to depend on others, and acquiring a dementing illness. Despite their concerns, 61 percent of older trans people, especially those over 60 years old, believe that they would be treated with dignity and respect by health care professionals.[64]

Older trans people are often interested in engaging in religious and spiritual experiences, possibly as a consequence of having suffered depression and social isolation due to the loss of friends and close relatives. Trans elders are unwilling to discuss their end-of-life requests with religious leaders but are more likely to do so with a spouse if they have one, a family member, or even professional caregivers, lawyers, and financial planners. Some trans elders have a will and slightly fewer have a power of attorney compared with the general population. Some trans elders indicated that they would attempt to get their affairs in order and discuss their death if it was imminent. Successful aging is associated with being or having been in the upper income bracket, and not being disabled. Less successful aging is associated with being alone and having few friends. However, religion plays no role in determining whether a trans person is likely to age successfully.[65]

SUMMARY

Trans people often suffer debilitating hardship and distress upon informing their family, friends, and workmates of their impending transition. Of special concern is the effect of a trans person's transition announcement on their partner and children, and how they will all cope following such a revelation. Unfortunately, this situation is often a precursor of marriage break-up, sometimes demanded by the trans person's professional advisers, with the real prospect of the trans person never being allowed to see their children again. This devastating situation, which occurs even when the children report few problems with their parent's transition, is the precursor of ill-health for the trans partner. Once the trans person has been able to deal with family and friends, they are then required to adjust to their new lifestyle by expressing their affirmed gender identity for all to see.

In some societies, trans people have to deal with religious and ethical challenges that often punish them for being their true selves. Such harassment, implicit or explicit, alienates some religious teaching from the realm of human rights and stretches the limits of ethical behavior toward another human being. An institutionalized and sanctioned form of such bigotry and prejudice occurs in societies that routinely demonize trans people to such an extent that trans people wonder whether they deserve to exist at all.

Legal constraints that prevent trans people from enjoying a lifestyle that is taken for granted by others are based on the inflexibility of the law when something as fundamental as gender (read *sexual*) identity is involved. Perhaps the most vexing problem affecting all trans people is the difficulty some of them experience in changing their designated sex on identity papers such as their birth certificate and passport. For those trans people who are already married, or who wish to marry after surgery, the legal system's reluctance to reassign legal sex so that such marriages can be officially recognized has resulted in several notable instances of court action. Despite some initial disappointments in such cases, recent legal judgments offer hope to trans people that their human rights are finally being recognized. However, in areas such as discrimination at work and elsewhere, trans people still suffer from legal inconsistencies that encourage violence toward, and harassment of, them.

Trans elders are almost an unstudied group among the gender-diverse communities. Their main worries are whether they will be able to live a comfortable, healthy, and stress-free life without having to deal with any of the traumas that many of them experienced previously. These include their loss of family, friends, employment, and safe living conditions. Some trans elders would have been living away from a supportive family earlier in their lives and must now contend with the possibility of discrimination and distress brought on by an intolerant health service and an ill-prepared aged-care system. End-of-life preparations will be difficult for some trans elders, especially those who have lost family and have no one close by to help them. Yet many trans elders have learned to be resilient, and they are now free to indulge in social and spiritual activities that offer them hope as they enjoy their senior years.

Chapter 11

CURRENT GUIDELINES AND FUTURE PROSPECTS

In this concluding chapter, we summarize the current state of play in transgender health, propose some promising improvements in the care of gender-diverse people, and offer some novel ideas about the important role that gender, in all its variations, plays in the lives of people everywhere. We mention some interesting directions for research in transgender health, hoping that others will take up some of these ideas and develop their own innovative research programs. We examine issues of social concern as they impact gender-diverse people, especially the increase in intolerance that seems to pervade the modern world. We conclude with some speculation about the origin of gender in humans and explore its implications for the welfare not only of gender-diverse people worldwide but their loved ones and supporters.

11.1 THE CURRENT STATE OF PLAY IN TRANSGENDER HEALTH

Transgender health care provision has changed radically since the previous version of this book published in 2006.[1] The models of care continue to become more centered on the person, rather than on their health care providers, as discussed in the next section. The understanding of medical therapy is also leaps ahead of what it was a decade ago. The hard work of clinical teams in Europe, the United States, and elsewhere has clarified the need for equitable and client-focused access to transition care, and the safety of the hormonal and surgical regimens available has been steadily improving.

We have seen GnRH analogs become well established as essential interventions for young people who are distressed by their looming puberty. The studies that have followed young people into adulthood have looked carefully at the benefits of hormonal and surgical intervention and weighed them against the potential adverse effects. There is now some evidence for the optimal types of estrogen and the transdermal route of administration to reduce the risk of thrombosis in trans feminine people as they reach middle age.

There is still much work to be done and many questions to be answered. When is the best time to start estrogen or testosterone in adolescence? Should surgery wait until adulthood? Exactly how should hormones be started and adjusted to achieve a person's goals? What are the effects on transition across a person's whole life? Are newer medical therapies, such as GnRH antagonists, going to be useful in the long run? Can we adjust hormone levels precisely enough to deliver evidence-based care to nonbinary people? How can we ensure that the opportunity for fertility preservation and starting a family are accessible for those who want to have biologically related children? Will artificial reproductive techniques become viable for people who have not gone through puberty? How can we ensure that gestational care and parenting are well supported? What surgical options can be developed for trans masculine and nonbinary people so that these procedures deliver what these special people need? Are the surgical outcomes going to be as good or better for young people who have already accessed GnRH analog treatment? Will surgical options, including facial surgery, be publicly funded? Will voice surgery be safe and effective for all trans feminine people who want it?

There has been an exponential increase in the publications related to transgender health. The series of important position papers in *The Lancet* from 2016[2] has brought the field into the medical mainstream. This bodes well for the future of research and the translation of that information into clinical care. The future is looking bright for transgender health care.

11.2 IMPROVEMENTS IN TRANSGENDER HEALTH CARE AND GUIDELINES FOR CARE

A complete paradigm shift has been occurring for the care of trans and gender-diverse people of all ages, but especially for young people. The pathologizing treatment protocols of the past in which mental health professionals searched for evidence of mental illness in normally developed gender-diverse people only to find none in most people are gradually being replaced with client-centered treatment programs. However, many clinicians working in transgender health cannot resist being the gatekeepers who control the future lives of their brave trans clients, and who in many cases make their client's angst even worse by doing so. Now we are on the threshold of a new era of informed consent, client-affirmed care. This means that the gender-diverse person, and their parent or guardian in the case of young people, can demand their treatments of choice provided it is medically safe to do so. The medical practitioner's job is merely to support the trans person's transition, nothing more and nothing less, because we all know that what was once a mental illness is now *a matter of diversity, not pathology!*

The mistaken belief that most adolescents get over their gender confusion and eventually accept a gendered expression consistent with their birth-assigned sex, designated *desistence* as if these young people were disguised criminals, was based on a perverse form of protective prejudice rather than good science. If during adolescence a trans person has doubts about their future, there are still quite a few options for a later-life transition as has occurred for all those older trans people who have affirmed their gender later in life and made a successful transition. Of course, it is possible that nonbinary young people correctly decide that a full or partial medical transition is not right for them. This, of course, is their right, and well-informed clinicians are now assisting such people to live happy and productive lives. As we saw in Chapter 7, the standardized protocols designed for the care of binary-gender identifying trans people can be somewhat modified to cater to this more diverse population.

What we do know from the groundbreaking research being performed by those conducting the TransYouth Project[3] at the University of Washington in the United States is that young people who can socially transition at their own pace, without constraints being imposed by others, can lead happy and successful lives with more or less the same mental health as their cisgender peers. So why do these young children need to be diagnosed with an illness by a mental health professional before they are provided medical care? It is the lack of support from parents, peers, schools, and others that causes these young people so much anguish that in some cases their mental health is seriously affected. This cruelty to brave young people can lead to self-harm and worst of all, suicide.

So it is recommended that carers listen to their child's own account of exactly who they are, respecting their choice of name and pronoun, and making sure that their children are valued and supported. It is also important to ensure that parents and significant others learn more about gender diversity in all its forms so that they can appreciate the needs and aspirations of trans people and ensure that they receive the best care possible. The family should realize that any attempt to make the lives of children and young gender-diverse people under their care any more difficult than they already might be is a type of child abuse that needs to be outlawed.

One of the goals of this book has been to provide the latest scientific knowledge in the field of transgender health and to outline the best ways trans people can be supported by their professional advisers. Family doctors and other members of the caring professions need to be sufficiently well informed to understand this new form of care and to make sure that the child's welfare is their number one priority.[4] It is important for everyone to learn more about the needs of the gender-diverse community and offer support without judgment and prejudice. Gender diversity has always been an important part of the human condition from ancient times to the present and in all peoples no matter where they reside.

A study has shown that adult trans people who underwent treatment by a psychiatrist and those who either did not use a psychiatrist or faked their stories to obtain treatment had similar outcomes. The trans women had better social and mental health outcomes but no change in employment outcomes following treatment, irrespective of whether a psychiatrist was involved. A similar result occurred for the trans men. Those who were noncompliant and did not bother with psychiatric help achieved their hormone treatment and legal name change about the same time as those who were compliant, but the noncompliant trans people were able to have surgery much sooner. These results suggest that involvement of a mental health professional in the transition process may not always be necessary, unless, of course, the person has been diagnosed with a mental illness that is unrelated to their gender diversity, or else they require support to assist with adjustment issues.[5]

As we saw in Chapters 6 and 7, the international standard for treating gender dysphoria as a medical condition is the World Professional Association for Transgender Health's (WPATH) Standards of Care for Gender Identity Disorders, Seventh Version, published in 2011. A new Eighth Version is scheduled for publication in 2019 when it is expected that the updated Standards of Care will include a diagnosis similar to gender incongruence, which is contained in the most recent International Classification of Diseases (ICD), Version 11 published in 2018. This diagnosis is now located in the Sexual Health section of the ICD and does not imply any accompanying mental ill-health.

Those caring for trans people should emphasize the flexibility of the Standards of Care guidelines and adapt their treatment strategies to suit each individual client. The guidelines offer minimum standards to ensure that overseas candidates for surgery, for example, have followed approximately the same preoperative evaluation as have locals. Departures from the Standards of Care guidelines used by individual gender services and professionals should be published in writing for the protection of all involved.

According to the current Standards of Care guidelines still being used by many professional services involved in the care of trans people in 2018, before starting medical treatment the trans person should have received at least some counseling, preferably performed by a mental health professional with specialist skills in gender issues. Sometimes this stipulation can be waived if the client has been living for some time in the desired gender role, and especially when self-administered hormones have been used without medical supervision. A trial hormone treatment can be useful because withdrawal of hormones, albeit unlikely, can occur within the first three months without lingering side effects. This trial period enables clients to decide if they want to continue with the treatment after having experienced both the beneficial and possibly undesirable side effects of hormone therapy. Evaluating the effects of a low-dose hormone trial is a diagnostic procedure that is far better and cheaper than multiple psychotherapy sessions and the administration of numerous useless psychological tests that some gender services employ. It is felt that such a low-dose hormone strategy can reduce the risk of self-harm and suicide that often accompanies the extended delays that some trans people face before being offered conventional treatment.

A trans person can request genital surgery when two independent professionals provide evidence that the client has successfully completed at least a year of real-life experience in the opposite-gender role. During this period, there should be an improvement in the client's adjustment without contraindications such as serious medical complications, substance abuse, and exacerbated mental illness. Most surgeons also request medical reports on hormone levels and the candidate's overall state of general health. This cautious approach is discriminatory simply because those requesting procedures involving cosmetic surgeries, for example breast enlargement, and other invasive and potentially more risky procedures never have to be assessed for their preoperational state of mind.

Many trans people have trouble changing their names and sex on legal documents, gaining access to their children after divorce, and acquiring medical insurance for genital surgery and other procedures. Although most trans people want their condition to be a normal variation of human experience, they simultaneously fear the consequences of being denied access to hormonal and surgical treatments if they do not have a recognized medical diagnosis.

On a positive note, some progressive gender services *accompany* clients through their attainment of a full medical transition rather than simply *working on* them. For example, the program at the University of Michigan in the United States is supportive, consultative, and caring, its aim being "the non-destructive self-actualization of the client."[6]

Information on the client's current physical health and medical history, developmental factors, socioeconomic situation, as well as a family history going back at least two generations, if possible, should be available. Since many middle-aged clients regret not having transitioned when they were younger, consultation with their family due to the social consequences of transition is desirable. Although such clients have experienced many years of suffering, they have often considered the comfort of others, especially their family and friends, rather than themselves, and so deserve special consideration.[7]

Some trans people seek only partial gender reassignment, for example, men who live full-time as women without hormones and surgery, and those requesting hormones to enhance their passability or to feel more comfortable living as women. The transition consultant should recognize that some trans people are not interested in passing and have no intention of actually becoming a woman. This situation complicates the evaluation process as many gender services still assume that, except for medical complications, all accepted clients will eventually progress to genital and other surgeries.[8] It is hoped that current and future services for trans people recognize these different requirements and allow their clients to pursue whatever procedures they feel most comfortable undertaking.

11.3 SUGGESTIONS FOR RESEARCH IN TRANSGENDER HEALTH

Future research in transgender health needs to concentrate on health delivery, theory and methodology, psychosocial issues, and individual differences. We need to understand and remove the barriers trans people experience when they try to obtain timely medical assistance. We need to learn more about how gender identity develops and changes over the lifespan, the ways trans people cope with stigma and stress, and the similarities and differences between various members of the gender-diverse community.[9] There has been little research on resilience among members of the trans community, and more longitudinal research on this topic and many others needs to be done.

Innovations in research methodology include the use of a two-stage gender/ sex question that first asks for a person's gender identity, including a way-out option for those who do not have any gender affiliation. The second part of the question asks for the person's sex assigned at birth, most likely corresponding to what was recorded on their birth certificate. It is important to reach out to the full diversity of the trans community when designing a research project and sending out an invitation for participants. Researchers cannot assume that gender-diverse people will make themselves available to researchers without them being told what will be involved if they decide to participate in the project and how the outcomes of the research will benefit the gender-diverse community. It is important to include checks to see if recruitment via mobile devices and Internet methods is representative of the wider trans communities. It is crucial to inform participants of the research findings, preferably by peer-reviewed open-access journal articles and summary documents distributed to all participants. Proper engagement with the trans community is required at all stages of the research.[10]

More sophisticated data analysis procedures need to be employed, especially in surveys that almost invariably just state the descriptive statistics. Based on popular accounts of the survey results, we can get the picture readily that self-harm and suicidal thoughts are common, especially among young gender-diverse people. Yet we cannot tell exactly who are at the greatest risk from such life-threatening situations. We have little knowledge about the basic psychological characteristics, the gender identities, and the social circumstances of those in greatest need of help. These surveys provide general findings for a relatively large sample of self-selected respondents, but no information is provided on individual cases. An individualized approach will surely require the use of mobile and wearable devices to maintain constant monitoring of those gender-diverse people who are at greatest risk—but only if they approve the use of such potentially invasive technology. Examples of the use of wearable technologies for continuous monitoring of depression and more serious mental health conditions, such as bipolar disorder, are now being developed.[11]

11.4 THE IMPACT OF EXTREME VIEWS ON THE WELFARE OF GENDER-DIVERSE PEOPLE

Recently there has been an increase in the power bestowed upon political leaders who hold extreme conservative views. Much of the resulting degradation of the rights of gender-diverse people has been encouraged by a new breed of populist politics. The policies adopted by some of these political leaders pander to the views of those people who have a narrow worldview. This situation can lead to the invention of dogma arising from preconceived notions about the absoluteness of gender as no more than birth-assigned sex, frequently embossed in the warm glow of religious righteousness. On another level, some otherwise highly educated feminist radicals have sought to demonize trans women with a similar brand of gender absoluteness that is enshrouded in the superiority of birth-assigned sex. These people have been cowardly enough to focus their vile platitudes upon young gender-diverse people and their supporters, often the mother. These besieged young people and their families cannot readily defend themselves against the constant diatribe they receive to their faces and in the compliant media.

This onslaught upon gender-diverse people is having an adverse effect on their physical and mental health. When the Trump administration in the United States threatened to define all trans people in terms of their birth-assigned sex rather than accepting their self-affirmed gender, there was a quadrupling of calls to emergency suicide prevention phone lines in that country. The offence generated by such an autocratic, unscientific imposition has created anxiety in the minds of even the most resilient of trans people. Hopefully, this book will provide sufficient scientific backing for anyone or any group that opposes these restrictions.

It is difficult to anticipate the consequences of this intolerance toward gender-diverse folk, except that the public exposure of an increasingly larger number of trans people has garnered support from many agencies, not least some of the most prominent employers in the United States. As we write this, the Transgender Day of Remembrance, November 20, 2018, has just passed. This is a day on which gender-diverse people worldwide light candles in memory of all those trans people who have been murdered, often quite violently, over the previous 12 months. Wouldn't it be lovely if there were no more of these terrible events to remember?

Although some would want all gender-diverse people banished, there are many other more insightful, humane, and caring people and organizations whose role has been to make life easier for trans people. The Mermaids in the United Kingdom and Transcend in Australia are just two of many charities that have been set up to assist young trans people, their families, and supporters. These organizations play an important role in providing meetup opportunities for young trans people and their families, and in lobbying government and other agencies to obtain a better deal for young trans people. Young trans people have also played crucial roles in fighting courageously to make their own lives and those of their friends more palatable. In Australia, a young trans woman was not only nominated for the Young Australian of the Year award, but she and her supporters convinced one of the highest courts in the land to change the law so that young trans people could gain access to hormone therapies without having to obtain prior court approval, a uniquely bizarre situation that arose in Australia from an unfortunate legal precedent. These groups and many others throughout the world have a strong presence on social media so that even the most isolated of trans people, young and old, can always remain connected to kindred folk from whom they can gain respect and support.

Over the last few years, not only have there been more books published on important trans issues from a clinical and research perspective, but authors of children's books have focused on stories that highlight the experiences of gender-diverse young people, a notable example being the Australian author Jo Hirst's *The Gender Fairy*.[12] There are trans people of all ages who have achieved great things on stage, in the movies, on the catwalk, in politics, and in the professions. These people serve as examples to young trans people who are unsure about how their futures might turn out. With proper support from family, peers, and community, these people can achieve at least as much as any of their cisgender peers. Their resilience, courage, and determination, often in adverse circumstances, allow these brave people to succeed where many of their cisgender peers might falter.

11.5 WHERE DOES GENDER COME FROM? A POSTSCRIPT SPECULATION

When people complete an intelligence or personality test, more often than not their only certain indication that their gender is being evaluated is when they tick a box to indicate whether they are male or female. This information is only used to classify them for an analysis of gender differences. However, as we have seen in this book, not everyone taking the test will identify as male or female. This situation makes us wonder whether there are any useful tests for assessing gender and its associated behaviors. In most situations this has simply meant that psychologists, for example, prefer to just identify differences in behavior between people they assume identify with a binary gender rather than assessing these differences over a wide range of gender identities, including none. This would be the case for the psychological test just mentioned.

As we saw in Chapter 2, although there are some gender differences observed in behavior, many of these are culturally determined and do not reflect any discoverable brain differences that can be used to identify gender by using as evidence any specific brain locations or functions. It is easier to accept the idea that gender is represented just about everywhere in the brain, perhaps as many complicated interacting processes, as implied by the diagram on the cover of this book, or similarly by a mosaic of different processes and associated structures. Like the beautiful fractal images that are used to speed up graphics in computer games, the closer you examine these patterns, the more complicated they appear.

Damian Kelty-Stephen and colleagues[13] have used the concept of intersectionality, the fact that a complicated phenomenon such as gender cannot be dissected into its constituent parts, to investigate gender as an inherently complex cognitive–social process that operates over a multitude of different levels, in this instance syllables, words, phrases, and sentences contained in a short written story. Consistent with this idea, people can express their individuality while interacting with their environment in all its forms, physical, mental, and social. In a sense, gender encompasses all that we wish to know about a person, their personality, their intelligence, their motivations, and their basic desires, as well as how they are impacted upon by the environment, both social and natural.

Kelty-Stephen asked people to read one of two concocted stories, one describing a typically male role and experience, and the other replacing the male experience by one that was typically female. When the main character's gender was revealed for the first time halfway through the story, those who saw an opposite gender identification to what they had expected based on the previous context were quite surprised. For example, this would occur soon after reading the name *Tom* when they had thought all along that they were reading about a woman. This surprise was indicated by a sudden increase in reading times for words more commonly associated with the unexpected gender revelation. By noting that readers normally process language at the various levels of syllable, word, phrase, and sentence, the researchers were able to predict quite accurately the reading times for each individual word in the sentence, provided the representation of gender was sufficiently complex to accommodate the way gender-relevant information is expressed in written prose. This is certainly not represented by something simple such as ticking Male or Female or even drawing a cross on a line with Male at one end and Female at the other.

Perhaps this finding might simply indicate how people anticipate the meaning of words and sentences in a short story and might have nothing special to say about gender. However, what the results show is that people might have a basic need to know what a person's gender is, whether or not that preconceived gender is the correct one. A similar situation might occur if instead of describing a person's gender-stereotypical behavior in words, it is done using images. This situation more closely approximates trans people's early experiences in public, when for some of them there is a strong need to be perceived by others as a member of their affirmed gender. Their safety may depend on their passing seamlessly in public.

Clearly, most people's understanding of gender is a simplistic one. Rather, gender must encompass all that is characteristic of a person's expression in words, in their appearance, and in their social interactions. It makes you wonder, therefore, whether any sensible meaning can be attributed to terms such as *gender dysphoria* or *gender incongruence*, diagnostic labels for those who seek medical help prior to transition. As gender is such a complex phenomenon, just like personality and intelligence, how would people feel if they had to endure the labels *intelligence dysphoria* or *intelligence incongruence*, or even *personality dysphoria* or *personality incongruence* should they deviate somewhat from the intelligence and personality that people expect of them? With disbelief or disgust, most probably!

11.6 GENERAL CONCLUSIONS

We have provided readers of varying backgrounds with a reasonably comprehensive account of gender diversity, its long human history, its widespread expression in all modern human societies, and the scientific evidence for its existence in behavior, as well as part of brain structure and function. We have highlighted the challenges many gender-diverse people face when they try to live normal productive lives in societies that frequently frustrate and impede their ability to do so. With our emphasis on transgender health for those gender-diverse people who wish to avail themselves of medical and psychological interventions, we have provided the most up-to-date information available on clinical practice, and we have offered suggestions for a more humane, client-centered approach to care. We hope that this book will be read widely by trans people, their families and friends, and especially by those professionals who treat trans people, including the family doctor.

Still, many questions remain unanswered. What exactly is gender? Why do a lot of people ignore its rich variety of forms and instead remain fixated on birth-assigned sex as its preferred proxy? How can we convince more government agencies to fund the medical needs of trans people in the same way they fund the more expensive medical requirements of cisgender people? When will gender-diverse people have the same human rights as other community members, especially in societies that impose unbearable constraints on their lives? Perhaps definitive answers and resolutions of these matters will take some time, but we hope that time will come before long because our gender-diverse friends deserve better than they have now.

APPENDIX: RESOURCES

This appendix contains a list of resources for trans people, their supporters, and professional advisers. More detailed information and links to Internet resources are contained in the webpage for this book at http://AGuideTo TransgenderHealth2019.online

RESOURCES FOR TRANS PEOPLE AND PROFESSIONALS

The main professional body for transgender health is the World Professional Association for Transgender Health (WPATH). The WPATH webpage (http:// www.wpath.org) has resources such as the latest version of the Standards of Care and information about professional activities, including its biennial conference. WPATH publishes *The International Journal of Transgenderism*.

There are local branches of WPATH in a number of countries and regions, such as the Australia and New Zealand Professional Association for Transgender Health (ANZPATH, https://www.anzpath.org/), the Canadian Professional Association for Transgender Health (CPATH, http://www.cpath.ca /home/), the European Professional Association for Transgender Health (EPATH, https://epath.eu/), and the United States Professional Association for Transgender Health (USPATH, https://www.wpath.org/uspath).

The U.K. Gender Identity Research & Education Society (GIRES) also has free training in transgender health for professionals, including general practitioners. https://www.gires.org.uk/e-learning/caring-for-gender-noncon forming-young-people/

Fenway Health, part of the National LGBT Education Center in Boston, MA, United States, has free courses on transgender health for professionals. https://www.lgbthealtheducation.org/

Global Action on Trans Equality (GATE) is an international agency that works for the benefit of trans* people everywhere. GATE publishes reports of international significance. http://transactivists.org/

Transgender Europe (TGEU) fights for the rights of trans* people through-out Europe. https://tgeu.org/

The Gender Trust in the United Kingdom distributes information of interest to trans* and gender-diverse people and their supporters. http://www.gender trust.org.uk/

GLAAD (GLBTQ Legal Advocates & Defenders) is a wide-ranging U.S. organization founded in 1985 that supports the LGBTIQ communities with special groups for trans* and gender-diverse people of all ages. https://www .glaad.org/

The National Center for Transgender Equality, founded in 2003 by Mara Keisling, fights for the rights of transgender people throughout the United States. https://transequality.org/

The Transgender Law Center is the largest organization that fights for the civil rights of transgender and gender-diverse people in the United States. https://transgenderlawcenter.org/

Gender Spectrum is a U.S. organization that assists trans* children and teen-agers, their families, and supporters. https://www.genderspectrum.org/

Gender Diversity is a U.S. organization for trans* people and their supporters that conducts educational programs and runs the annual Gender Odyssey conference in Seattle, WA. http://www.genderdiversity.org/

Transgender Victoria represents the needs of transgender and gender-diverse people in the Australian state of Victoria. https://transgendervictoria.com/

RESEARCH ON TRANSGENDER HEALTH

Organizations that perform research on transgender health include:

The Gender Identity Research & Education Society (GIRES) in the United Kingdom promotes and collates research on transgender health performed in the United Kingdom and elsewhere. https://www.gires.org.uk/

The Center of Excellence for Transgender Health at the University of California, San Francisco, United States, performs research and has a professional training program. http://transhealth.ucsf.edu/

The TransYouth Project at the University of Washington, Seattle, United States, is conducting research on young trans people. https://depts.washington.edu /scdlab/research/transyouth-project-gender-development/

The National LGBT Health Education Center, Boston, United States, produces educational and research materials on transgender health. https://www .lgbthealtheducation.org/

The Transgender Research Group at the University of Waikato in New Zealand has recently produced culturally sensitive guidelines for supporting trans and gender-diverse people in that country. https://researchcommons.waikato .ac.nz/bitstream/handle/10289/12160/Guidelines%20for%20Gender%20 Affirming%20Health%20low%20res.pdf?sequence=2&isAllowed=y

Transgender Studies Quarterly is a U.S. journal that publishes peer-reviewed articles on mostly trans* culture and articles that challenge the pathologization and victimization of the trans* experience. https://read.dukeupress.edu /tsq

Transgender Health is an open-access U.S. journal that publishes peer-reviewed research focusing on all aspects of transgender health. https://www.liebertpub .com/loi/trgh

TransParent, for parents of trans youth seeking support. http://transparentusa .org/

The Philadelphia Trans Wellness Conference, held annually in Philadelphia, PA, United States, covers a wide range of health issues for professionals and trans* community members. https://www.mazzonicenter.org/trans-wellness

SUPPORT FOR FAMILY AND FRIENDS

A number of government- and community-funded organizations exist to support trans people, young and not-so-young. These include:

Mermaids is a U.K. organization that supports transgender and gender-diverse children. https://www.mermaidsuk.org.uk/

The Gender Centre in Sydney, Australia, supports gender-diverse people and their supporters. https://gendercentre.org.au/

Hunter New England Health in Newcastle, Australia, has some useful information for young people, their family, and supporters. http://www.hnekidshealth.nsw.gov.au/gender

In Australia there are support lines for gender-diverse people of all ages at https://qlife.org.au/ and for young trans* people at http://www.genderhelpforparents.com.au/

OTHER USEFUL INFORMATION

A lot of information for trans and gender-diverse people is available on Facebook and other social media platforms. Facebook has many groups, both open and closed, that can be used by trans* and gender-diverse people to share experiences, gain information, and indulge in discreet communication with other people. Many of these groups have a parallel presence on Twitter, Instagram, and other commonly used social media platforms.

There are many series of videos on YouTube about trans* issues including the continuing video diaries of trans* people of all ages. Of special interest are various people's experiences of transition as well as their progress through living full-time in their affirmed gender and undergoing various surgeries and such ancillary procedures as speech training and hair removal.

Worthwhile YouTube subscriptions include *The Story of Jazz. A Transgender Child*, *Her Story Show*, and *GoCharlie*.

NOTES

PREFACE

1. Shakin, M., Shakin, D., and Hall, S. (1985). Infant clothing: Sex labeling for strangers. *Sex Roles* 12:955–964.

2. Bornstein, K. (1994). *Gender outlaw.* New York: Routledge, p. 63.

3. See http://sandystone.com/hale.rules.html. Downloaded on August 17, 2018.

4. The term *gynephilia* was reportedly first used by Kurt Freund, a noted sexologist. The terms *gynephilic* and *androphilic* were recommended in: Diamond, M. (2002). Sex and gender are different: Sexual identity and gender identity are different. *Clinical Child Psychology and Psychiatry* 7:320–334.

CHAPTER 1

1. Sweileh, W.M. (2018). Bibliometric analysis of peer-reviewed literature in transgender health (1900–2017). *BMC International Health and Human Rights*, 18, 16, https://doi.org/10.1186/s12914-018-0155-5. Marshall, Z., Welch, V., Minichiello, A., Swab, M., Brunger, F. and Kaposy, C. (2019). Documenting research with transgender, non-binary, and other gender diverse (trans) individuals and communities: Introducing the global trans research evidence map. *Transgender Health* 4:68–80.

2. Vedeler, H.T. (2008). Reconstructing meaning in Deuteronomy 22:5: Gender, society, and transvestitism in Israel and the Ancient Near East. *Journal of Biblical Literature* 127:459–476.

3. Cited in Benjamin, H. (1966). *The transsexual phenomenon.* New York: The Julian Press.

4. Liveley, G. (2003). Tiresias/Teresa: A man-made-woman in Ovid's Metamorphoses 3.318–38. *Helios* 30:147–162.

5. Endres, N. (2015). Galli: Ancient Roman priests. *GMBLQ Encyclopedia*. Downloaded from http://www.glbtqarchive.com/ssh/galli_S.pdf on August 17, 2018.

6. Vedeler, H.T. (2008). op. cit., p. 476.

7. Bullough, V.L. (1974). Transvestites in the Middle Ages. *American Journal of Sociology* 79:1381–1394.

8. Feinsod, M. (2013–2014). A distant reflection: The physician in the eye of the Jewish medieval satirist Kalonymus ben Kalonymus (1287–1337?). *Korot* 22: 243.

9. Warren, C.A.B. (2014). Gender reassignment surgery in the 18th century: A case study. *Sexualities* 17:872–884.

10. *The Hull Packet and Original Weekly Commercial, Literary and General Advertiser*, May 29, 1810.

11. Ellis, H. (1928). *Studies in the psychology of sex, Vol. 7, Eonism and other supplementary studies*. Philadelphia: H.A. Davis.

12. In Spanish, *mujerado* means *having been transformed into a woman*.

13. Brooks, R. (2012). Transforming sexuality: The medical sources of Karl Heinrich Ulrichs (1825–95) and the origins of the theory of bisexuality. *Journal of the History of Medicine and Allied Sciences* 67:177–216.

14. Ekins, R. and King, D. (2001). Pioneers of transgendering: The popular sexology of David O. Cauldwell. *International Journal of Transgenderism* 5. Downloaded from https://www.atria.nl/ezines/web/IJT/97-03/numbers/symposion/cauldwell_01.htm on August 18, 2018.

15. Pfäfflin, F. (1997). Sex reassignment, Harry Benjamin, and some European roots. *International Journal of Transgenderism* 1. Downloaded from https://www.atria.nl/ezines/web/IJT/97-03/numbers/symposion/ijtc0202.htm on August 18, 2018.

16. Haire, N. (1930). *Encyclopaedia of sexual knowledge*. London: Encyclopaedic Press. Summary compiled by S. Johnson.

17. A difference in sexual development, previously known as an *intersex* condition, often involves malformation of the genitals so that it is difficult to determine a child's birth sex by simple inspection. Some of these differences in sexual development arise from genetic variations that produce the wrong body chemistry. This can lead to masculinization of female bodies and feminization of male bodies. Klinefelter syndrome, which occurs in about 1 in 750 male births, is characterized by a lack of body and pubic hair, underdeveloped testicles, infertility, as well as some loss in cognitive function. Some breast development can occur at puberty, but generally most people with the syndrome live their lives unaffected. Nieschlag, E. (2013). Klinefelter syndrome: The commonest form of hypogonadism, but often overlooked or untreated. *Deutsches Ärzteblatt International* 10: 347–353.

18. Elbe, L. and Hoyer, N. (2004). *Man into woman. The first sex change, a portrait of Lili Elbe: The true and remarkable transformation of the painter Einar Wegener*. London: Blue Boat Books.

19. Gilpin, D.C., Raza, S. and Gilpin, D. (1979) Transsexual symptoms in a male child treated by a female therapist. *American Journal of Psychotherapy* 33:453–463.

20. Ettner, R. (1999). *Gender loving care: A guide to counseling gender-variant clients*. New York: Norton & Company.

21. Michel, A., Mormont, C. and Legros, J.J. (2001) A psycho-endocrinological overview of transsexualism. *European Journal of Endocrinology* 145:365–376.

22. Schaefer, L.C. and Wheeler, C.C. (1995) Harry Benjamin's first ten cases (1938–1953): A critical historical note. *Archives of Sexual Behavior* 24:73–93.

23. Hill, D.B. (2008). Dear Doctor Benjamin: Letters from transsexual youth (1963–1976). *International Journal of Transgenderism*, 10, 149–170.

24. Gay and Lesbian Historical Society of Northern California. (1998). MTF transgender activism in the Tenderloin and beyond, 1966–1975: Commentary and interview with Elliot Blackstone. *Gay & Lesbian Quarterly* 4:349–372.

25. A movie about the Compton Cafeteria riot can be viewed on https://www.youtube.com/watch?v=WmR3KQ9K-Zk downloaded on August 18, 2018.

26. A detailed account of transgender history is contained in the book by Meyerowitz, J. (2002) *How sex changed: A history of transsexuality in the United States*. Cambridge, MA: Harvard University Press.

27. Cohen-Kettenis, P.T., and Gooren, L.J.G. (1999). Transsexualism: A review of etiology, diagnosis and treatment. *Journal of Psychosomatic Research* 46:315–333.

28. Fisk, N. (1973) Gender dysphoria syndrome (The how, what, and why of a disease). In D. Laub & P. Gandy (Eds.), *Proceedings of the Second Interdisciplinary Symposium on Gender Dysphoria Syndrome*. Palo Alto, CA: Stanford University Press, pp. 7–14.

29. Winter, S. (2017). Gender trouble: The World Health Organization, the International Statistical Classification of Diseases and Related Health Problems (ICD)-11 and the trans kids. *Sexual Health*, 14:423–430. Winter, S., Diamond, M., Green, J., Karasic, D., Reed, T., Whittle, S., et al. (2016). Transgender people: Health at the margins of society. *The Lancet*, http://dx.doi.org/10.1016/S0140-6736(16)00683-8.

30. Bullough, V.L. (2003) The contributions of John Money: A personal view. *Journal of Sex Research* 40:230–236.

31. Damodaran, S.S. and Kennedy, T. (2000). The Monash Gender Dysphoria Clinic: Opportunities and challenges. *Australasian Psychiatry* 8:355–357. Erasmus, J., Bagga, H., and Harte, F. (2015). Assessing patient satisfaction with a multidisciplinary gender dysphoria clinic in Melbourne. *Australasian Psychiatry*, 23, 158–162.

32. Murjan, S., Shepherd, M. and Ferguson, B.G. (2002). What services are available for the treatment of transsexuals in Great Britain? *Psychiatric Bulletin* 26:210–212.

33. Weitze, C. and Osburg, S. (1996). Transsexualism in Germany: Empirical data on epidemiology and application of the German Transsexuals' Act during its first ten years. *Archives of Sexual Behavior* 25:409–425.

34. Ruan, F.-F. and Bullough, V.L. (1988). The first case of transsexual surgery in mainland China. *Journal of Sex Research* 25:546–547.

35. Stryker, S. (1998). The transgender issue: An introduction. *Gay & Lesbian Quarterly* 4:152.

36. Broad, K.L. (2002). GLB + T?: Gender/sexuality movements and transgender collective identity (de)constructions. *International Journal of Sexuality and Gender Studies* 7:241–264.

37. This is difficult to quantify, but Titman 2014 from www.practicalandrogyny.com has reported that 0.4 percent of the U.K. population define as nonbinary when given a three-way choice that includes this as an option. In younger transgender people, 13 percent of 6,000 respondents to the National Transgender Discrimination Survey conducted at the University of California chose to describe their gender identity in their own terms, such as *genderqueer, gender rebel*, etc. https://transequality.org/issues/resources/national-transgender-discrimination-survey-full-report accessed on August 19, 2018.

38. Like all statistics related to the trans experience, regret rates for those who have undergone genital surgeries are difficult to determine. However, regret rates as low as 2 percent have been reported, these being comparable with, or perhaps less than, those associated with other surgeries such as those intended for aesthetic or other elective purposes.

39. Morris, R.C. (1995). All made up: Performance theory and the new anthropology of sex and gender. *Annual Review of Anthropology* 24:567–592.

40. Ibid., p. 579.

41. Ibid., p. 580.

42. Towle, E.B. and Morgan, L.M. (2002). Romancing the transgender native: Rethinking the use of the "Third Gender" concept. *Gay & Lesbian Quarterly* 8:469–497.

43. Brown, K. (2004). "Sistergirls"—Stories from indigenous Australian transgendered people. *Aboriginal and Islander Health Worker Journal* 28:25–26.

44. Kerry, S. (2018). Payback: The custom of assault and rape of sistergirls and brotherboys; Australia's trans and sex/gender diverse first peoples. *Violence and Gender* 5:37–41.

45. Bockting, W.O. and Cesaretti, C. (2001). Spirituality, transgender identity, and coming out. *Journal of Sex Education and Therapy* 26:291–300.

46. Sinnott, M. (2000). The semiotics of transgendered sexual identity in the Thai print media: Imagery and discourse of the sexual other. *Culture, Health & Sexuality* 2:425–440.

47. Littlewood, R. (2002). Three into two: The third sex in Northern Albania. *Anthropology & Medicine* 9:37–50.

48. McLelland, M. (2002). The newhalf net: Japan's "intermediate sex" on-line. *International Journal of Sexuality and Gender Studies* 7:163–175.

49. Ramaswami, M. (2003). Essentialism, culture, and beliefs about gender among the Aravanis of Tamil Nadu, India. *Sex Roles* 49:489–496.

50. http://www.dailymail.co.uk/news/article-3384847/Dame-Edna-creator-Barry-Humphries-provokes-outrage-transgender-campaigners-says-sex-change-surgery-self-mutilation-attacks-Caitlyn-Jenner-latest-outburst.html accessed on August 19, 2018.

51. Some earlier examples include Boylan, J.F. (2003). *She's not there. A life in two genders.* New York: Broadway Books; Clark, S. (2004). *Running to normal.* Available from http://www.iUniverse.com, accessed August 19, 2018; Cummings, K. (1993). *Katherine's diary.* Melbourne: Mandarin; McCloskey, D.N. (1999). *Crossing. A memoir.* Chicago: University of Chicago Press; Morris, J. (1974). *Conundrum.* London: Faber & Faber.

52. This book by Anne Reid is an especially candid and informative story written by the wife of a trans woman: Reid, A.M. (2018). *She said, she said: Love, loss, & living my new normal.* Sydney: A Sense of Place Publishing.

53. Landén, M. and Innala, S. (2000). Attitudes toward transsexualism in a Swedish national survey. *Archives of Sexual Behavior* 29:375–388.

54. Ibid., pp. 376–377.

55. https://www.researchgate.net/publication/271131673_Attitudes_Towards_Transsexual_and_Intersexed_People_An_International_Internet_Survey, downloaded on August 19, 2018.

56. Rogers, L. (1999). *Sexing the brain.* London: Weidenfeld & Nicolson.

57. Fine, C. (2010). *Delusions of gender: How our minds, society, and neurosexism create difference.* New York: W.H. Norton.

58. Raj, R. (2002). Towards a transpositive therapeutic model: Developing clinical sensitivity and cultural competence in the effective support of transsexual and transgendered clients. *International Journal of Transgenderism* 6. Downloaded from https://cdn.atria.nl/ezines/web/IJT/97-03/numbers/symposion/ijtvo06no02_04.htm on August 19, 2018.

59. van Kesteren, P.J., Gooren, L.J. and Megens, J.A. (1996). An epidemiological and demographic study of transsexuals in the Netherlands. *Archives of Sexual Behavior* 25:589–600.

60. Jarolím, L. (2000). Surgical conversion of genitalia in transsexual patients. *BJU International* 85:851–856.

61. Green, R. (2000). Family co-occurrence of "Gender Dysphoria": Ten sibling or parent–child pairs. *Archives of Sexual Behavior* 29:499–507.

62. Canner, J.K., Harfouch, O., Kodadek, L.M., Pelaez, D., Coon, D., Offodile, A.C., et al. (2018). Temporal trends in gender-affirming surgery among transgender patients in the United States. *JAMA Surgery* 153:609–616.

63. Olyslager, F. and Conway, L. (2007). On the calculation of the prevalence of trans-sexualism. Paper presented at the World Professional Association for Transgender Health Symposium, Chicago, Illinois. Downloaded from http://ai.eecs.umich.edu/people/conway /TS/Prevalence/Reports/Prevalence%20of%20Transsexualism.pdf on August 19, 2018.

64. Redfern, J.S. and Sinclair, B. (2014). Improving health care encounters and communication with transgender patients. *Journal of Communication in Healthcare* 7:25–40.

65. The most recent figures on prevalence and their sources are as follows: *1.3% transgender* in Shields, J.P., Cohen, R., Glassman, J.R., Whitaker, K., Franks, H. and Bertolini, I. (2013). Estimating population size and demographic characteristics of lesbian, gay, bisexual and transgender youth in middle school. *Journal of Adolescent Health* 52:248–250; *1.2% transgender* in Clark, T.C., Lucassen, M.F., Bullen, P., Denny, S.J., Fleming, T.M., Robinson, E.M., et al. (2014). The health and well-being of transgender high school students: Results from the New Zealand adolescent health survey (Youth'12). *Journal of Adolescent Health* 55:93–99; and *0.4% transgender* in Meerwijk, E.L. and Sevelius, J.M. (2017). Transgender population size in the United States: A meta-regression of population-based probability samples. *American Journal of Public Health* 107:e1–e8.

CHAPTER 2

1. Diamond, M. (2000). Sex and gender: Same or different? *Feminism & Psychology* 10:46–54.

2. *Gender dysphoria*, as a diagnosis, is described in the latest version of the *Diagnostic and Statistical Manual*, DSM-5, published by the American Psychiatric Association. Although this diagnosis is not intended to pathologize atypical gender expression, it is retained in a book of mental illnesses, possibly because some trans people require a diagnosis for their further medical treatments, including surgeries.

3. Deaux, K. (1985). Sex and gender. *Annual Review of Psychology* 36:51.

4. Collaer, M.L. and Hines, M. (1995). Human behavioral sex differences: A role for gonadal hormones during early development? *Psychological Bulletin* 118:55–107.

5. See Figure 1 in Redfern, J.S. and Sinclair, B. (2014). Improving health care encounters and communication with transgender patients. *Journal of Communication in Healthcare* 7:25–40.

6. Gustafson, M.L. and Donahoe, P.K. (1994). Male sex determination: Current concepts of male sexual differentiation. *Annual Review of Medicine* 45:505–524.

7. Ibid., Figure 2.1 on p. 507.

8. Dewing, P., Shi, T., Horvath, S. and Vilain, E. (2003). Sexually dimorphic gene expression in mouse brain precedes gonadal differentiation. *Molecular Brain Research* 118:82–90.

9. Hengstschläger, M., van Trotsenburg, M., Repa, C., Marton, E., Huber, J.C. and Bernaschek, G. (2003). Sex chromosome aberrations and transsexualism. *Fertility and Sterility* 79:639–640.

10. Henningsson, S., Westberg, L., Nilsson, S., Lundström, B., Ekselius, L., Bodlund, O., et al. (2005). Sex steroid-related genes and male-to-female transsexualism. *Psychoneuroendocrinology* 30:657–664.

11. Veale, J.F., Clarke, D.E. and Lomax, T.C. (2010). Biological and psychosocial correlates of adult gender-variant identities: A review. *Personality and Individual Differences*, 48:357–366.

12. McEwen, B.S. (1999). Permanence of brain sex differences and structural plasticity of the adult brain. *Proceedings of the National Academy of Sciences, USA* 96:7128–7130.

13. Swaab, D.F., Chung, W.C.J., Kruijver, F.P.M, Hofman, M.A. and Hestiantoro, A. (2003). Sex differences in the hypothalamus in the different stages of human life. *Neurobiology of Aging* 24:S1–S16.

14. Bishop, K.M. and Wahlsten, D. (1997). Sex differences in the human corpus callosum: Myth or reality? *Neuroscience and Biobehavioral Reviews* 21:581–601. Wahlsten, D. and Bishop, K.M. (1998). Effect sizes and meta-analysis indicate no sex dimorphism in the human or rodent corpus callosum. *Behavioral and Brain Sciences* 21:338–339.

15. See Figure 1 in Zhou, J.-N., Hofman, M.A., Gooren, L.L. and Swaab, D.F. (1995). A sex difference in the human brain and its relation to transsexuality. *Nature* 378:68–70.

16. Swaab, D.F., Chung, W.C.J., Kruijver, F.P.M, Hofman, M.A. and Ishunina, T.A. (2001). Structural and functional sex differences in the human hypothalamus. *Hormones and Behavior* 40:93–98.

17. Dournaud, P., Boudin, H., Schonbrunn, A., Tannenbaum, G.S. and Beaudet, A. (1998). Interrelationships between somatostatin sst2A receptors and somatostatin-containing axons in rat brain: Evidence for regulation of cell surface receptors by endogenous somatostatin. *Journal of Neuroscience* 18:1056–1071.

18. Savic, I. and Arver, S. (2011). Sex dimorphism of the brain in male-to-female transsexuals. *Cerebral Cortex* 21:2525–2533.

19. Goldstein, J.M., Seidman, L.J., Horton, N.J., Makris, N., Kennedy, D.N., Caviness, V.S., et al. (2001). Normal sexual dimorphism of the adult human brain assessed by *in vivo* magnetic resonance imaging. *Cerebral Cortex* 11:490–497.

20. Adinoff, B., Devous, Sr., M.D., Best, S.E., Chandler, P., Alexander, D., Payne, K., et al. (2003). Gender differences in limbic responsiveness, by SPECT, following a pharmacologic challenge in healthy subjects. *NeuroImage* 18:697–706.

21. Durston, S., Hulshoff, H.E., Casey, B.J., Giedd, J.N., Buitelaar, J.K. and van Engeland, H. (2001). Anatomical MRI of the developing brain: What have we learned? *Journal of the American Academy of Child and Adolescent Psychiatry* 40:1012–1020.

22. Rametti, G., Carrillo, B., Gómez-Gil, E., Junque, C., Zubiarre-Elorza, L., Segovia, S., et al. (2011). The microstructure of white matter in male and female transsexuals before cross-sex hormone treatment: A DTI study. *Journal of Psychiatric Research* 45:949–954.

23. Rametti, G., Carrillo, B., Gómez-Gil, E., Junque, C., Zubiarre-Elorza, L., Segovia, S., et al. (2012). Effects of androgenization on the white matter microstructure of female-to-male transsexuals: A diffusion tensor imaging study. *Psychoneuroendocrinology* 37:1261–1269.

24. See Figures 2 and 3 in Zhou, J.-N., Hofman, M.A., Gooren, L.L. and Swaab, D.F. (1995). A sex difference in the human brain and its relation to transsexuality. *Nature* 378:68–70.

25. Kruijver, F.P.M., Zhou, J.-N., Pool, C.W., Hofman, M.A., Gooren, L.J.G. and Swaab, D.F. (2000). Male-to-female transsexuals have female neuron numbers in a limbic nucleus. *Journal of Clinical Endocrinology and Metabolism* 85:2034–2041.

26. Chung, W.C.J., de Vries, G.J. and Swaab, D.F. (2002). Sexual differentiation of the bed nucleus of the stria terminalis in humans may extend into adulthood. *Journal of Neuroscience* 22:1027–1033.

27. The locations of these hypothalamic nuclei are described in both the text and figures of Kruijver, F.P.M., Balesar, R., Espila, A.M., Unmehopa, U.A. and Swaab, D.F. (2002). Estrogen receptor-α distribution in the human hypothalamus in relation to sex and endocrine status. *Journal of Comparative Neurology* 454:115–139.

28. Berglund, H., Lindström, P., Dhejne-Helmy, C. and Savic, I. (2008). Male-to-female transsexuals show sex-atypical hypothalamus activation when smelling odorous steroids. *Cerebral Cortex* 18:1900–1908.

29. Papageorgiou, C., Papageorgaki, P., Tolis, G., Rabavilas, A. and Christodoulou, G. (2003). Psychophysiological correlates in male to female transsexuals studied with a P300 investigation. *Psychological Medicine* 33: 555–561.

30. Govier, E., Diamond, M., Wolowiec, T. and Slade, C. (2010). Dichotic listening, handedness, brain organization, and transsexuality. *International Journal of Transgenderism* 12:144–154.

31. Zubiaurre-Elorza, L., Junque, C., Gómez-Gil, E., Segovia, S., Carrillo, B., Rametti, G., et al. (2012). Cortical thickness in untreated transsexuals. *Cerebral Cortex*, 23:2855–2862.

32. Zubiaurre-Elorza, L., Junque, C., Esther Gómez-Gil, E. and Guillamon, A. (2014). Effects of cross-sex hormone treatment on cortical thickness in transsexual individuals. *Journal of Sexual Medicine* 11:1248–1261.

33. Manzouri, A., Kosidou, K. and Savic, I. (2017). Anatomical and functional findings in female-male transsexuals: Testing a new hypothesis. *Cerebral Cortex* 27:998–1010.

34. See Figure 5 of Guillamon, A., Junque, C. and Gómez-Gil, E. (2016). A review of the status of brain structure research in transsexualism. *Archives of Sexual Behavior* 45:1615–1648.

35. Spizzirri, G., Duran, F.L., Chaim-Avancini, T.M., Serpa, M.H., Cavallet, M., Pereira, C.M.A., et al. (2018). Grey and white matter volumes either in treatment-naïve or hormone-treated transgender women: A voxel-based morphometry study. *Scientific Reports* 8:736. Downloaded from https://www.nature.com/articles/s41598-017-17563-z on August 21, 2018.

36. Manzouri, A., Kosidou, K. and Savic, I. (2017). Anatomical and functional findings in female-to-male transsexuals: Testing a new hypothesis. *Cerebral Cortex* 27:998–1010.

37. Frable, D.E.S. (1997). Gender, racial, ethnic, sexual, and class identities. *Annual Review of Psychology* 48:139–162, p. 144.

38. Kohlberg, L.A. (1966). A cognitive-developmental analysis of children's sex role concepts and attitudes, in E.E. Maccoby (Ed.), *The development of sex differences*. Stanford, CA: Stanford University Press, pp. 82–173.

39. Warin, J. (2000). The attainment of self-consistency through gender in young children. *Sex Roles* 42:209–231.

40. Martin, C.L., Ruble, D.N. and Szkrybalo, J. (2002). Cognitive theories of early gender development. *Psychological Bulletin* 128:903–933.

41. Campbell, A., Shirley, L. and Caygill, L. (2002). Sex-typed preferences in three domains: Do two-year-olds need cognitive variables? *British Journal of Psychology* 93:203–217.

42. Cohen-Kettenis, P.T. and Pfäfflin, F. (2003). *Transgenderism and intersexuality in childhood and adolescence: Making choices.* Thousand Oaks, CA: Sage Publications.

43. Brutsaert, H. (1999). Coeducation and gender identity formation: A comparative analysis of secondary schools in Belgium. *British Journal of Sociology of Education* 20:343–353.

44. Golombok, S. and Rust, G. (1993). The Pre-School Activities Inventory: A standardized assessment of gender roles in children. *Psychological Assessment* 5:131–136.

45. Albert, A.A. and Porter, J.R. (1988). Children's gender-role stereotypes: A sociological investigation of psychological models. *Sociological Forum* 3:184–210.

46. Martin, C.L., Ruble, D.N. and Szkrybalo, J. (2002). Cognitive theories of early gender development. *Psychological Bulletin* 128:911.

47. Barberá, E. (2003). Gender schemas: Configuration and activation processes. *Canadian Journal of Behavioural Science* 35:176–184.

48. Tenenbaum, H.R. and Leaper, C. (2002). Are parents' gender schemas related to their children's gender-related cognitions? A meta-analysis. *Developmental Psychology* 38:615–630.

49. Olson, K.R. (2017). When sex and gender collide. *Scientific American* 317:44–49.

CHAPTER 3

1. A quote from Ekins, R. and King, D. (2001). Transgendering, migrating and love of oneself as a woman: A contribution to a sociology of autogynephilia. *International Journal of Transgenderism* 5. Downloaded from https://cdn.atria.nl/ezines/web/IJT/97-03/numbers/symposion/ijtvo05no03_01.htm on August 22, 2018.

2. Ibid.

3. Mason-Schrock, D. (1996). Transsexuals' narrative construction of the "true self." *Social Psychology Quarterly* 59:176–192.

4. Gooren, L.J.G. (1993). Transsexualism, medicine and law. Closing speech at *The Council of Europe, 23rd Colloquy on European Law: Transsexualism, medicine and law*. Downloaded from http://library.transgenderzone.com/?page_id=1066 on August 22, 2018.

5. Kimura, D. (1996). Sex, sexual orientation and sex hormones influence human cognitive function. *Current Opinion in Neurobiology* 6:259–263.

6. Maccoby, E.E. and Jacklin, C.N. (1974). *The psychology of sex differences*. Stanford, CA: Stanford University Press.

7. Deaux, K. (1985). Sex and gender. *Annual Review of Psychology* 36:51.

8. Haraldsen, I.R., Opjordsmoen, S., Egeland, T. and Finset, A. (2003). Sex-sensitive cognitive performance in untreated patients with early onset gender identity disorder. *Psychoneuroendocrinology* 28:906–915.

9. van Goozen, S.H.M., Cohen-Kettenis, P.T., Gooren, L.J.G., Frijda, N.H. and van der Poll, N.E. (1994). Activating effects of androgens on cognitive performance: Causal evidence in a group of female-to-male transsexuals. *Neuropsychologia* 32:1153–1157.

10. Slabbekoorn, D., van Goozen, S.H.M., Megens, J., Gooren, L.J.G. and Cohen-Kettenis, P.T. (1999). Activating effects of cross-sex hormones on cognitive functioning: A study of short-term and long-term hormone effects in transsexuals. *Psychoneuroendocrinology* 24:423–447.

11. Alexander, G.M. (2003). An evolutionary perspective of sex-typed toy preferences: Pink, blue, and the brain. *Archives of Sexual Behavior* 32:7–14.

12. Thornhill, R. and Gangestad, S.W. (1999). Facial attractiveness. *Trends in Cognitive Sciences* 3:452–460.

13. See Figure 1 in Fellous, J.-M. (1997). Gender discrimination and prediction on the basis of facial metric information. *Vision Research* 37:1961–1973. The distances estimated from the face shown in Figure 1 of the above article are E3 = 6.4 cm, W4 = 8.5 cm, N2 = 1.5 cm, B2 = 1.1 cm, and L1 = 4.2 cm. Substituting these values into the Facial Masculinity Index equation produced a value of –2.9, suggesting that the face shown in Figure 1 of this article has feminine characteristics.

14. The preferred term is now *facial gender confirmation surgery*. Capitán, L., Simon, S., Berli, J.U., Bailón, C., Bellinga, R.J., Santamaría, J.G., et al. (2017). Facial gender confirmation surgery: A new nomenclature. *Plastic and Reconstructive Surgery*, 240:766e–767e.

15. Obleser, J., Eulitz, C., Lahiri, A. and Elbert, T. (2001). Gender differences in functional hemispheric asymmetry during processing of vowels as reflected by the human brain magnetic response. *Neuroscience Letters* 314:131–134.

16. Geschwind, N. and Galaburda, A.M. (1987). *Cerebral lateralization: Biological mechanisms, associations, and pathology.* Cambridge, MA: MIT Press.

17. Philips, S.U. (1980). Sex differences and language. *Annual Review of Anthropology* 9:523–544.

18. Argamon, S., Koppel, M., Fine, J. and Shimoni, A.R. (2003). Gender, genre, and writing style in formal written texts. *Text* 24:321–346. Koppel, M., Argamon, S. and Shimoni, A.R. (2002). Automatically categorizing written texts by author gender. *Literary and Linguistic Computing* 17:401–412.

19. Ho, S.M.Y. and Lee, T.M.C. (2001). Computer usage and its relationship with adolescent lifestyle in Hong Kong. *Journal of Adolescent Health* 29:258–266. Goswami, A. and Dutta, S. (2016). Gender differences in technology usage—a literature review. *Open Journal of Business and Management* 4:51–59.

20. Thomson, R. and Murachver, T. (2001). Predicting gender from electronic discourse. *British Journal of Social Psychology* 40:193–208.

21. Palanza, P. (2001). Animal models of anxiety and depression: How are females different? *Neuroscience and Biobehavioral Reviews* 25:219–233.

22. Woodhill, B.M. and Samuels, C.A. (2003). Positive and negative androgyny and their relationship with psychological health and well-being. *Sex Roles* 48:555–565.

23. Costa, Jr., P.T., Terracciano, A. and McCrea, R.R. (2001). Gender differences in personality traits across cultures: Robust and surprising findings. *Journal of Personality and Social Psychology* 81:322–331.

24. Lippa, R.A. (2001). On deconstructing and reconstructing Masculinity-Femininity. *Journal of Research in Personality* 35:168–207.

25. Visser, I. (2002). Prototypes of gender: Conceptions of feminine and masculine. *Women's Studies International Forum* 25:529–539.

26. Vingerhoets, A.J.J.M., Cornelius, R.R., van Heck, G.L. and Becht, M.C. (2000). Adult crying: A model and review of the literature. *Review of General Psychology* 4:354–377.

27. Sandnabba, N.K., Santtila, P., Wannäs, M. and Krook, K. (2003). Age and gender specific sexual behaviors in children. *Child Abuse & Neglect* 27:579–605.

28. Roberts, C.W., Goodman, M., Green, R. and Williams, K. (1987). Boyhood gender identity development: A statistical contrast of two family groups. *Developmental Psychology* 23:544–557.

29. Manning, K.E., Holmes, C., Sansfaçon, A.P., Newhook, J.T. and Travers, A. (2015). Fighting for trans* kids: Academic parent activism in the 21st century. *Studies in Social Justice* 9:118–135.

CHAPTER 4

1. Katz-Wise, S.L. & Budge, S.L. (2015). Cognitive and interpersonal identity processes related to mid-life gender transitioning in transgender women. *Counselling Psychology Quarterly* 28:162.

2. Katz-Wise, S.L., Budge, S.L., Fugate, E., Flanagan, K., Touloumtzis, C., Rood, B., et al. (2017). Transactional pathways of gender identity development in transgender and gender-nonconforming youth and caregiver perspectives from the Trans Youth Family Study. *International Journal of Transgenderism* 18:243–263.

3. Riggs, D.W. and Bartholomaeus, C. (2015). The role of school counsellors and psychologists in supporting transgender people. *The Australian Educational and Developmental Psychologist* 32:158–170.

4. Ibid., p. 164.

5. Ibid., p. 165.

6. Case, K.A. and Meier, S.C. (2014). Developing allies to transgender and gender-nonconforming youth: Training for counsellors and educators. *Journal of LGBT Youth* 11:62–82.

7. Riley, E.A., Sitharthan, G., Clemson, L. and Diamond, M. (2011). The needs of gender-variant children and their parents according to health professionals. *International Journal of Transgenderism* 13:54–63.

8. Once trans people have completed their transition, or even before then, most consider their sexual orientation relative to their affirmed sex and not their born sex. For example, a homosexual trans woman would have a female partner. However, to be more specific we will use the term *gynephilic* to indicate that this woman is in a relationship with a woman. If a woman is in a relationship with a man, we will say that she is *androphilic*.

9. Elliot, P. and Roen, K. (1998). Transgenderism and the question of embodiment. Promising queer politics? *Gay & Lesbian Quarterly* 4:259.

10. Lutz, D.J., Roback, H.B. and Hart, M. (1984). Feminine gender identity and psychological adjustment of male transsexuals and male homosexuals. *Journal of Sex Research* 20:350–362.

11. Devor, H. (1997). *FTM: Female-to-male transsexuals in society*. Bloomington: Indiana University Press.

12. Lee, T. (2001). Trans(re)lations: Lesbian and female to male transsexual accounts of identity. *Women's Studies International Forum* 24:347–357.

13. McCauley, E.A. and Ehrhardt, A.A. (1980). Sexual behavior in female transsexuals and lesbians. *Journal of Sex Research* 16:202–211.

14. Devor, H. (1993). Sexual orientation identities, attractions, and practices of female-to-male transsexuals. *Journal of Sex Research* 30:303–315.

15. Bullough, V., Bullough, B. and Smith, R. (1983). A comparative study of male transvestites, male to female transsexuals, and male homosexuals. *Journal of Sex Research* 19:238–257.

16. Veale, J.F., Clarke, D.E. and Lomax, T.C. (2008). Sexuality of male-to-female transsexuals. *Archives of Sexual Behavior* 37:586–597.

17. Simon, P.A., Reback, C.J. and Bemis, C.C. (2000). HIV prevalence and incidence among male-to-female transsexuals receiving HIV prevention services in Los Angeles County. *AIDS* 14:2953–2955.

18. Oggins, J. and Eichenbaum, J. (2002). Engaging transgender substance users in substance use treatment. *International Journal of Transgenderism* 6. Downloaded from https://cdn.atria.nl/ezines/web/IJT/97-03/numbers/symposion/ijtvo06no02_03.htm on August 23, 2018.

19. Hughes, T.L. and Eliason, M. (2002). Substance use and abuse in lesbian, gay, bisexual and transgender populations. *Journal of Primary Prevention* 22:263–298.

20. Schilder, A.J., Laframboise, S., Hogg, R.S., Trussler, T., Goldstone, I., Schechter, M.T., et al. (1998). "They don't see our feelings." The health care experiences of HIV-positive transgendered persons. *Journal of the Gay and Lesbian Medical Association* 2:103–111.

21. Kenagy, G.P. and Hsieh, C.-M. (2005). The risk less known: Female-to-male transgender persons' vulnerability to HIV infection. *AIDS Care* 17:195–207.

22. Dean, L., Meyer, I.H., Robinson, K., Sell, R.L., et al. (2000). Lesbian, gay, bisexual, and transgender health: Findings and concerns. *Journal of the Gay and Lesbian Medical Association* 4:102–151.

23. Murphy, T.E. (2001). Lesbian, gay, bisexual, and transgender medical students and their ethical conflicts. *Journal of the Gay and Lesbian Medical Association* 5:31–35.

24. Davis, S.A. and Meier, S.C. (2014). Effects of testosterone treatment and chest reconstruction surgery on mental health and sexuality in female-to-male transgender people. *International Journal of Sexual Health* 26:113–128.

25. Keo-Meier, C.L., Herman, L.I., Reisner, S.L., Pardo, S.T., Sharp, C. and Babcock, J.C. (2015). Testosterone treatment and MMPI-2 improvement in transgender men: A prospective controlled study. *Journal of Consulting and Clinical Psychology* 83:143–156.

26. Yalom, I. (2005). *Theory and practice of group psychotherapy* (5th ed.). New York, NY: Basic Books, pp. 92–93.

27. van Goozen, S.H.M., Cohen-Kettenis, P.T., Gooren, L.J.G., Frijda, N.H. and van de Poll, N.E. (1995). Gender differences in behaviour: Activating effects of cross-sex hormones. *Psychoendocrinology* 20:343–363.

28. Nuttbrock, L., Bockting, W., Rosenbaum, A., Mason, M., Macri, M. and Becker, J. (2012). Gender identity conflict/affirmation and major depression across the life course of transgender women. *International Journal of Transgenderism* 13:91–103.

29. Bailey, M.J., Dunne, M.P. and Martin, N.G. (2000). Genetic and environmental influences on sexual orientation and its correlates in an Australian twin sample. *Personality and Social Psychology* 78:524–536.

30. van Beijsterveldt, C.E.M, Hudziak, J.J. and Boomsma, D.I. (2006). Genetic and environmental influences on cross-gender behavior and relation to behavior problems: A study of Dutch twins at ages 7 and 10 years. *Archives of Sexual Behavior* 35:647–658.

31. Veale, J.F., Clarke, D.E. and Lomax, T.C. (2010). Biological and psychosocial correlates of adult gender-variant identities: A review. *Personality and Individual Differences* 48:357–366.

32. McManus, C. (2002). *Right hand, left hand: The origins of asymmetry in brains, bodies, atoms and cultures.* London: Phoenix.

33. Lippa, R.A. (2003). Handedness, sexual orientation, and gender-related personality traits in men and women. *Archives of Sexual Behavior* 32:103–114.

34. Green, R. and Young, R. (2001). Hand preference, sexual preference, and transsexualism. *Archives of Sexual Behavior* 30:565–574. Orlebeke, J.F., Gooren, L.J.G., Verschoor, A.M. and van den Bree, M.J.M. (1992). Elevated sinistrality in transsexuals. *Neuropsychology* 6:351–355.

35. Green, R. and Young, R. (2000). Fingerprint asymmetry in male and female transsexuals. *Personality and Individual Differences* 29:933–942. Slabbekoorn, D., van Goozen, S.H.M., Sanders, G., Gooren, L.J.G. and Cohen-Kettenis, P.T. (2000). The dermatoglyphic characteristics of transsexuals: Is there evidence for an organizing effect of sex hormones? *Psychoneuroendocrinology* 25:365–375.

36. Manning, J.T. (2002). *Digit ratio: A pointer to fertility, behavior, and health.* New Brunswick, NJ: Rutgers University Press.

37. Austin, E.J., Manning, J.T., McInroy, K. and Mathews, E. (2002). A preliminary investigation of the associations between personality, cognitive ability and digit ratio. *Personality and Individual Differences* 33:1115–1124.

38. Schneider, H.J., Pickel, J. and Stalla, G.K. (2006). Typical female 2nd-4th finger length (2D:4D) ratios in male-to-female transsexuals—possible implications for prenatal androgen exposure. *Psychoneuroendocrinology* 31:265–269.

CHAPTER 5

1. Herman-Jeglinska, A., Grabowska, A. and Dulko, S. (2002). Masculinity, femininity, and transsexualism. *Archives of Sexual Behavior* 31:527–534.

2. Scheim, A.I. and Bauer, G.R. (2015). Sex and gender diversity among transgender persons in Ontario, Canada: Results from a respondent-driven sampling survey. *Journal of Sex Research* 52:1–14.

3. Rider, G.N., McMorris, B.J., Gower, A.L., et al. (2018). Health and care utilization of transgender and gender nonconforming youth: A population-based study. *Pediatrics* 14:e20171683.

4. Ringo, C.P. (2002). Media roles in female-to-male transsexual and transgender identity formation. *International Journal of Transgenderism* 6. Downloaded from https://cdn.atria .nl/ezines/web/IJT/97-03/numbers/symposion/ijtvo06no03_01.htm on August 23, 2018.

5. Marone, P., Iacoella, S., Cecchini, M.G., Ravenna, A.R. and Ruggieri, V. (1998). An experimental study of body image and perception in gender identity disorders. *International Journal of Transgenderism* 2. Downloaded from https://www.atria.nl/ezines/web/IJT/97 -03/numbers/symposion/ijtc0501.htm on August 23, 2018.

6. Viglione, D.J. (1999). A review of recent research addressing the utility of the Rorschach. *Psychological Assessment* 11:251–265.

7. Tsushima, W.T. and Wedding, D. (1979). MMPI results of male candidates for transsexual surgery. *Journal of Personality Assessment* 43:385–387. Michel, A., Ansseau, M., Legros, J.J., Pitchot, W., Cornet, J.P. and Mormont, C. (2002). Comparisons of two groups of sex-change applicants based on the MMPI. *Psychological Reports* 91:233–240. Hartmann, U., Becker, H. and Rueffer-Hesse, C. (1997). Self and gender: Narcissistic pathology and personality factors in gender dysphoric patients. Preliminary results of a prospective study. *International Journal of Transgenderism* 1. Downloaded from https://cdn.atria.nl/ezines /web/IJT/97-03/numbers/symposion/ijtc0103.htm on November 8, 2018.

8. These statements are those that discriminate best for *Gd* obtained from Table 1 in Althof, S.E., Lothstein, L.M., Jones, P. and Shen, J. (1983). An MMPI Subscale (*Gd*): To identify males with gender identity conflicts. *Journal of Personality Assessment* 47:42–49.

9. These sample items are contained in Table 2 (trans females) and Table 3 (trans males) of Steensma, T.D., Kreukels, B.P.C., Jürgensen, M., Thyen, U., de Vries, A.L.C. and Cohen-Kettenis, P.T. (2013). The Utrecht Gender Dysphoria Scale: Validation Study. Downloaded from http://dare.ubvu.vu.nl/bitstream/handle/1871/40250/?sequence=8 on June 20, 2018. See also Schneider, C., Cerwenka, S., Nieder, T.O., Briken, P., Cohen-Kettenis, P.T., De Cuypere, G., et al. (2016). Measuring gender dysphoria: A multicenter examination and comparison of the Utrecht Gender Dysphoria Scale and the Gender Identity/Gender Dysphoria Questionnaire for Adolescents and Adults. *Archives of Sexual Behavior* 45:551–558.

10. Brems, C., Adams, R.L. and Skillman, G.D. (1993). Person drawings by transsexual clients, psychiatric clients, and nonclients compared: Indicators of sex-typing and pathology. *Archives of Sexual Behavior* 22:253–264.

11. Costa, Jr., P.T. and McCrae, R.R. (1992). The five-factor model of personality and its relevance to personality disorders. *Journal of Personality Disorders* 6:343–359.

12. Wolfradt, U. and Neumann, K. (2001). Depersonalization, self-esteem and body image in male-to-female transsexuals compared to male and female controls. *Archives of Sexual Behavior* 30:301–310.

13. Lippa, R.A. (2001). On deconstructing and reconstructing masculinity-femininity. *Journal of Research in Personality* 35:168–207.

14. See, for example, the conceptualization of two types of transsexual clients, primary and secondary, originally proposed in Harry Benjamin's 1966 book *The Transsexual Phenomenon*.

15. Cole, C.M., O'Boyle, M., Emory, L.E. and Meyer, W.J. (1997). Comorbidity of gender dysphoria and other major psychiatric diagnoses. *Archives of Sexual Behavior* 26:13–26.

16. National Institute of Mental Health. (2001). Borderline personality disorder. Bethesda, MD: National Institute of Mental Health, National Institutes of Health, U.S. Department of Health and Human Services (NIH Publication Number: 01-4928). Downloaded from https://www.nimh.nih.gov/health/publications/borderline-personality -disorder/bor derlinepersonalitydis-508-qf-17-4928_156499.pdf on August 23, 2018.

17. Miach, P.P., Berah, E.F., Butcher, J.N. and Rouse, S. (2000). Utility of the MMPI-2 in assessing gender dysphoric patients. *Journal of Personality Assessment* 75:268–279.

18. Rotondi, N.K. (2012). Depression in trans people: A review of the risk factors. *International Journal of Transgenderism* 13:104–116.

19. Hughto, J.M.W. and Reisner, S.L. (2016). A systematic review of the effects of hormone therapy on psychological functioning and quality of life in transgender individuals. *Transgender Health* 1:21–31.

20. This is a sample vignette of a feminine boy reported on p. 536 of Hill, D.B. and Willoughby, B.L.B. (2005). The development and validation of the Genderism and Transphobia Scale. *Sex Roles* 53:531–544.

21. Redfern, J.S. and Sinclair, B. (2014). Improving health care encounters and communication with transgender patients. *Journal of Communication in Healthcare* 7:25–40.

22. Shiffman, M., VanderLaan, D.P., Wood, H., Hughes, S.K, Owen-Anderson, A., Lumley, M.M., et al. (2016). Behavioural and emotional problems as a function of peer relationships in adolescents with gender dysphoria: A comparison with clinical and nonclinical controls. *Psychology of Sexual Orientation and Gender Diversity* 3:27–36.

23. Meyer, I.H., Brown, T.N.T., Herman, J.L., Reisner, S.L. and Bockting, W.O. (2017). Demographic characteristics and health status of transgender adults in select US regions: Behavior Risk Factor Surveillance System, 2014. *American Journal of Public Health* 107:582–589.

24. McCann, E. and Sharek, D. (2016). Mental health needs of people who identify as transgender: A review of the literature. *Archives of Psychiatric Nursing* 30:280–285.

25. Bockting, W.O., Miner, M.H., Swinburne Romine, R.E., Hamilton, A. and Coleman, E. (2013). Stigma, mental health, and resilience in an online sample of the US transgender population. *American Journal of Public Health* 103:943–951.

26. The citation is from p. 20 of Singh, A.A., Hays, D.G. and Watson, L.S. (2011). Strength in the face of adversity: Resilience strategies of transgender individuals. *Journal of Counselling & Development* 89:20–27.

27. Hepp, U. and Milos, G. (2002). Gender identity disorder and eating disorders. *International Journal of Eating Disorders* 32:473–478.

28. Hepp, U., Milos, G. and Braun-Scharm, H. (2004). Gender identity disorder and anorexia nervosa in male monozygotic twins. *International Journal of Eating Disorders* 35:239–243.

29. Fernández-Arana, F., Peri, J.M., Navarro, V., Badía-Casanovas, A., Turón-Gil, V. and Vallejo-Ruiloba, J. (2000). Transsexualism and anorexia nervosa: A case report. *Eating Disorders* 8:63–66.

30. Surgenor, L.J. and Fear, J.L. (1998). Eating disorder in a transgendered patient: A case report. *International Journal of Eating Disorders* 24:449–452.

31. Pregnancy as an example of a normal condition is a useful analogy to being trans, which without accompanying medical and psychological complications is itself a normal human condition. This example is contained in Roughgarden, J. (2004). *Evolution's rainbow: Diversity, gender, and sexuality in nature and people.* Berkeley, CA: University of California Press.

32. Richards, C. (2016). Trans and non-binary genders: Implications for applied clinical psychology. *Clinical Psychology Forum* 285:28–32.

33. Besser, M., Carr, S., Cohen-Kettenis, P., Connolly, P., de Sutter, P., Diamond, M., et al. (2006). Atypical gender development: A review. GIRES, King's Fund, April 2004. *International Journal of Transgenderism* 9:29–44.

34. Israel, G.E. and Tarver, D.E. (1997). *Transgender care: Recommended guidelines, practical information & personal accounts.* Philadelphia, PA: Temple University Press.

35. Dean, L., Meyer, I.H., Robinson, K., Sell, R.L., Sember, R., Silenzio, V.M.B., et al. (2000). Lesbian, gay, bisexual, and transgender health: Findings and concerns. *Journal of the Gay and Lesbian Medical Association* 4:102–151.

36. Michel, A., Mormont, C. and Legros, J.J. (2001). A psycho-endocrinological overview of transsexualism. *European Journal of Endocrinology* 145:365–376.

37. Perez-Brumer, A., Hatzenbueler, M.L., Oldenberg, C.E. and Bockting, W. (2015). Individual- and structural-level risk factors for suicide attempts among transgender adults. *Behavioral Medicine* 41:164–171.

38. Reisner, S.L., Vetters, R., Leclerc, M., Zaslow, S., Wolfrum, S., Shumer, D., et al. (2015). Mental health of transgender youth in care at an adolescent community health center: A matched retrospective cohort study. *Journal of Adolescent Health* 56:274–279.

39. Smith, E., Jones, T., Ward, R., Dixon, J., Mitchell, A. and Hillier, L. (2014). *From blues to rainbows: The mental health and well-being of gender diverse and transgender young people in Australia.* Downloaded from https://www.beyondblue.org.au/docs/default-source/research -project-files/bw0268-from-blues-to-rainbows-report-final-report.pdf on August 24, 2018.

40. Strauss, P., Cook, A., Winter, S., Watson, V., Wright Toussaint, D. and Lin, A. (2017). *Trans pathways: The mental health experiences and care pathways of trans young people. Summary of results.* Telethon Kids Institute, Perth, Australia.

41. Veale, J.F., Watson, R.J., Peter, T. and Saewyc, E.M. (2017) Mental health disparities among Canadian transgender youth. *Journal of Adolescent Health* 60:44–49.

42. Clark, B.A., Veale, J.F., Townsend, M., Frohard-Dourlent, H. and Saewyc, E. (2018). Non-binary youth: Access to gender-affirming primary health care. *International Journal of Transgenderism.* https://doi.org/10.1080/15532739.2017.1394954

43. McNeil, J., Bailey, L., Ellis, S., Morton, J. and Regan, M. (2012). *Trans mental health and emotional wellbeing study.* Edinburgh, UK: Scottish Transgender Alliance.

44. Veale, J., Saewye, E., Frohard-Dourlent, H., Dobson, S., Clark, B., et al. (2015). *Being safe, being me: Results of the Canadian trans youth health survey.* Vancouver, BC: Stigma and Resilience Among Vulnerable Youth Centre, School of Nursing, University of British Columbia.

45. Robinson, K.H., Bansel, P., Denson, N., Ovenden, G. and Davies, C. (2014). *Growing up queer: Issues facing young Australians who are gender variant and sexuality diverse.* Young and Well Cooperative Research Centre, Melbourne, Australia.

46. Glidden, D., Bouman, W.P., Jones, B.A. and Arculus, J. (2016). Gender dysphoria and Autism Spectrum Disorder: A systematic review of the literature. *Sexual Medicine Reviews* 4:3–14.

47. Statistical significance is shown when these two confidence intervals do not overlap, as occurs in this study.

48. Kristensen, Z.E. and Broome, M.R. (2015). Autistic traits in an Internet sample of gender variant UK adults. *International Journal of Transgenderism* 16:234–245.

CHAPTER 6

1. Cohen-Kettenis, P.T., Steensma, T.D. and de Vries, A.L. (2011). Treatment of adolescents with gender dysphoria in the Netherlands. *Child and Adolescent Psychiatric Clinics of North America* 20:689–700.

2. Newhook, J.T., Pyne, J., Winters, K., Feder, S., Holmes, C., Tosh, J., et al. (2018). A critical commentary on follow-up studies and "desistance" theories about transgender and gender-nonconforming children. *International Journal of Transgenderism* 19:212–224.

3. Winters, K., Newhook, J.T., Pyne, J., Feder, S., Jamieson, A., Holmes, C., et al. (2018). Learning to listen to trans and gender diverse children: A response to Zucker (2018) and Steensma and Cohen-Kettenis (2018). *International Journal of Transgenderism* 19:246–250.

4. Drummond, K.D., Bradley, S.J., Peterson-Badali, M. and Zucker, K.J. (2008). A follow-up study of girls with Gender Identity Disorder. *Developmental Psychology* 44:34–35.

5. Steensma, T.D., Biemond, R., de Boer, F. and Cohen-Ketternis, P.T. (2011). Desisting and persisting gender dysphoria after childhood: A qualitative follow-up study. *Clinical Child Psychology and Psychiatry* 16:499–516. Steensma, T.D., McGuire, J.K., Kreukels, B.P., Beekman, A.J. and Cohen-Kettenis, P.T. (2013). Factors associated with desistence and persistence of childhood gender dysphoria: A quantitative follow-up study. *Journal of the American Academy of Child and Adolescent Psychiatry* 52:582–590. Wallien, M.S. and Cohen-Kettenis, P.T. (2008). Psychosexual outcome of gender-dysphoric children. *Journal of the American Academy of Child and Adolescent Psychiatry* 47:1413–1423.

6. Olsen, J., Schrager, S.M., Belzer, M., Simons, L.K. and Clark, L.F. (2015). Baseline physiologic and psychosocial characteristics of transgender youth seeking care for gender dysphoria. *Journal of Adolescent Health* 57:374–380. Chen, M., Fuqua, J. and Eugster, E.A. (2016). Characteristics of referrals for gender dysphoria over a 13-year period. *Journal of Adolescent Health* 58:369–371. Holt, V., Skagerberg, E. and Dunsford, M. (2016). Young people with features of gender dysphoria: Demographics and associated difficulties. *Clinical Child Psychology and Psychiatry* 21:108–118.

7. Reed, B., Rhodes, S., Schofield, P. and Wylie, K. (2009). *Gender variance in the UK: Prevalence, incidence, growth and geographic distribution.* Ashstead, Surrey: Gender Identity Research and Education Society.

8. Hidalgo, M.A., Ehrensaft, D., Tishelman, A.C., Clark, L.F., Garofalo, R., Rosenthal, S.M., et al. (2013). The gender affirmative model: What we know and what we aim to learn. *Human Development* 56:285–290.

9. Hill, D.B., Menvielle, E., Sica, K.M. and Johnson, A. (2010). An affirmative intervention for families with gender variant children: Parental ratings of child mental health and gender. *Journal of Sex & Marital Therapy* 36:6–23.

10. Drescher, J., Cohen-Kettenis, P. and Winter, S. (2012). Minding the body: Situating gender identity diagnoses in the ICD-11. *International Review of Psychiatry* 24:568–577.

11. de Vries, A.L. and Cohen-Kettenis, P.T. (2012). Clinical management of gender dysphoria in children and adolescents: The Dutch approach. *Journal of Homosexuality* 59:301–320.

12. Ristori, J. and Steensma, T.D. (2016). Gender dysphoria in childhood. *International Review of Psychiatry* 28:13–20.

13. Ehrensaft, D. (2012). From gender identity disorder to gender identity creativity: True gender self child therapy. *Journal of Homosexuality* 59:337–356.

14. Winters, K., Newhook, J.T., Pyne, J. Feder, S., Jamieson, A., Holmes, C., et al. (2018). Learning to listen to trans and gender diverse children: A response to Zucker (2018) and Steensma and Cohen-Kettenis (2018). *International Journal of Transgenderism* 19:246–250.

15. Olson, K.R., Durwood, L. and McLaughlin, K.A. (2016). Mental health of transgender children who are supported in their identities. *Pediatrics* 137:e20153223. Durwood, L., McLaughlin, K.A. and Olson, K.R. (2017). Mental health and self-worth in socially transitioned transgender youth. *Journal of the American Academy of Child and Adolescent Psychiatry* 56:116–123.

16. Olson, K.R., Durwood, L. and McLaughlin, K.A. (2016). Mental health of transgender children who are supported in their identities. *Pediatrics* 137:e20153223.

17. Coleman, E., Bockting, W., Botzer, M., Cohen-Kettinis, P., DeCuypere, G., Feldman, J., et al. (2011). Standards of care for the health of transsexual, transgender, and gender-nonconforming people, version 7. *International Journal of Transgenderism* 13:165–232. Murchison, G. on behalf of the Human Rights Campaign Foundation, American Academy of Pediatrics and American College of Osteopathic Pediatricians (2016). Supporting & caring for transgender children. Downloaded from http://hrc.im/supportingtranschildren on July 1, 2018. Adelson, S.L., Stroeh, O.M. and Ng, Y.K. (2016). Development and mental health of lesbian, gay, bisexual, or transgender youth in pediatric practice. *Pediatric Clinics of North America* 63:971–983.

18. Winter, S., De Cuypere, G., Green, J., Kane, R. and Knudson, G. (2016). The proposed ICD-10 Gender Incongruence of Childhood diagnosis: A World Professional Association for Transgender Health membership survey. *Archives of Sexual Behavior* 45:1605–1614.

19. Drescher, J., Cohen-Kettenis, P.T. and Reed, G.M. (2016). Gender incongruence of childhood in the ICD-11: Controversies, proposal, and rationale. *Lancet Psychiatry* 3:297–304.

20. Hembree, W.C., Cohen-Kettenis, P.T., Gooren, L., Hannema, S.E., Meyer, W.J., Murad, M.H., et al. (2017). Endocrine treatment of gender-dysphoric/gender-incongruent persons: An Endocrine Society clinical practice guideline. *Journal of Clinical Endocrinology and Metabolism* 102:3869–3903.

21. Wood, H., Sasaki, S., Bradley, S.J., Singh, D., Fantus, S., Owen-Anderson, A., et al. (2013). Patterns of referral to a gender identity service for children and adolescents (1976–2011): Age, sex ratio, and sexual orientation. *Journal of Sex & Marital Therapy* 39:1–6. Aitken, M., Steensma, T.D., Blanchard, R., VanderLaan, D.P., Wood, H., Fuentes, A., et al. (2015). Evidence for an altered sex ratio in clinic-referred adolescents with gender dysphoria. *Journal of Sexual Medicine* 12:756–763.

22. Steensma, T.D., Wensing-Kruger, S.A. and Klink, D.T. (2017). How should physicians help gender-transitioning adolescents consider potential iatrogenic harms of hormone therapy? *AMA Journal of Ethics* 19:762–770.

23. Cohen-Kettenis, P.T. and van Goozen, S.H. (1997). Sex reassignment of adolescent transsexuals: A follow-up study. *Journal of the American Academy of Child and Adolescent Psychiatry* 36:263–271. Smith, Y.L., van Goozen, S.H., Kuiper, A.J. and Cohen Kettenis, P.T. (2005). Sex reassignment: Outcomes and predictors of treatment for adolescent and adult transsexuals. *Psychological Medicine* 35:89–99. de Vries, A.L., McGuire, J.K., Steensma, T.D., Wagenaar, E.C., Doreleijers, T.A. and Cohen-Kettenis, P.T. (2014). Young adult psychological outcome after puberty suppression and gender reassignment. *Pediatrics* 134:696–704.

24. Gridley. S.J., Crouch, J.M., Evans, Y., Eng, Y., Antoon, E., Lyapustina, M., et al. (2016). Youth and caregivers' perspectives on barriers to gender-affirming health care for transgender youth. *Journal of Adolescent Health* 59:254–261.

25. Lawlis, S.M., Donkin, H.R., Bates, J.R., Britto, M.T. and Conard, L.A.E. (2017). Health concerns of transgender and gender nonconforming youth and their parents upon presentation to a transgender clinic. *Journal of Adolescent Health* 61:642–648.

26. Telfer, M.M., Tolit, M.A., Pace, C.C. and Pang, K.C. (2017). *Australian Standards of Care and treatment guidelines for trans and gender diverse children and adolescents*. Melbourne: The Royal Children's Hospital.

27. Simons, L., Schrager, S.M., Clark, L.F., Belzer, M. and Olson, J. (2013). Parental support and mental health among transgender adolescents. *Journal of Adolescent Health* 5:791–793.

28. Steensma, T.D., Zucker, K.J., Kreukels, B.P., Vanderlaan, D.P., Wood, H., Fuentes, A., et al. (2014). Behavioural and emotional problems on the Teacher's Report Form: A cross-national, cross-clinic comparative analysis of gender dysphoric children and adolescents. *Journal of Abnormal Child Psychology* 42:635–647. de Vries, A.L., Steensma, T.D., Cohen-Kettenis, P.T., VanderLaan, D.P. and Zucker, K.J. (2016). Poor peer relations predict parent- and self-reported behavioral and emotional problems of adolescents with gender dysphoria: A cross-national, cross-clinic comparative analysis. *European Child & Adolescent Psychiatry* 25:579–588. Shiffman, M., VanderLaan, D.P., Wood, H., Hughes, S.K., Owen-Anderson, A., Lumley, M.M., et al. (2016). Behavioral and emotional problems as a function of peer relationships in adolescents with gender dysphoria: A comparison with clinical and nonclinical controls. *Psychology of Sexual Orientation and Gender Diversity* 3:27–36.

29. Olson, J., Forbes, C. and Belzer, M. (2011). Management of the transgender adolescent. *Archives of Pediatrics & Adolescent Medicine* 165:171–176.

30. de Vries, A.L., Doreleijers, T.A., Steensma, T.D. and Cohen-Kettenis, P.T. (2011). Psychiatric comorbidity in gender dysphoric adolescents. *Journal of Child Psychology and Psychiatry* 52:1195–1202.

31. Edwards-Leeper, L. and Spack, N.P. (2012). Psychological evaluation and medical treatment of transgender youth in an interdisciplinary "Gender Management Service" (GeMS) in a major pediatric center. *Journal of Homosexuality* 59:321–336.

32. de Vries, A. L., Noens, I. L., Cohen-Kettenis, P.T., van Berckelaer-Onnes, I.A. and Doreleijers, T.A. (2010). Autism spectrum disorders in gender dysphoric children and adolescents. *Journal of Autism and Developmental Disorders* 40:930–936.

33. Vocks, S., Stahn, C., Loenser, K. and Legenbauer, T. (2009). Eating and body image disturbances in male-to-female and female-to-male transsexuals. *Archives of Sexual Behavior* 38:364–377. Witcomb, G.L., Bouman, W.P., Brewin, N., Richards, C., Fernandez-Aranda, F. and Arcelus, J. (2015). Body image dissatisfaction and eating-related psychopathology in trans individuals: A matched control study. *European Eating Disorders Review* 23:287–293.

34. Strang, J.F., Meagher, H., Kenworthy, L., de Vries, A.L.C., Menvielle, E., Leibowitz, S., et al. (2018). Initial clinical guidelines for co-occurring Autism Spectrum Disorder and Gender Dysphoria or Incongruence in adolescents. *Journal of Clinical Child and Adolescent Psychology* 47:105–115.

35. de Vries, A.L., Kreukels, B.P., Steensma, T.D., Doreleijers, T.A. and Cohen-Ketternis, P.T. (2011). Comparing adult and adolescent transsexuals: An MMPI-2 and MMPI-A study. *Psychiatry Research* 186:414–418.

36. Durwood, L., McLaughlin, K.A. and Olson, K.R. (2017). Mental health and self-worth in socially transitioned transgender youth. *Journal of the American Academy of Child and Adolescent Psychiatry* 56:116–123.

37. Delemarre-van de Waal, H.A. and Cohen-Kettenis, P.T. (2006). Clinical management of gender identity disorder in adolescents: A protocol on psychological and paediatric endocrinology aspects. *European Journal of Endocrinology* 155:S131–S137.

38. Cohen-Kettenis, P.T. and van Goozen, S.H. (1998). Pubertal delay as an aid in diagnosis and treatment of a transsexual adolescent. *European Child & Adolescent Psychiatry* 7:246–248.

39. Mahfouda, S., Moore, J.K., Siafarikas, A., Zepf, F.D. and Lin, A. (2017). Puberty suppression in transgender children and adolescents. *The Lancet Diabetes and Endocrinology* 5:816–826.

40. Hembree, W.C. (2013). Management of juvenile gender dysphoria. *Current Opinion in Endocrinology, Diabetes and Obesity* 20:559–564.

41. de Vries, A.L., Steensma, T.D., Doreleijers, T.A. and Cohen-Kettenis, P.T. (2011). Puberty suppression in adolescents with gender identity disorder: A prospective follow-up study. *Journal of Sexual Medicine* 8:2276–2283. de Vries, A.L., McGuire, J.K., Steensma, T.D., Wagenaar, E.C., Doreleijers, T.A. and Cohen-Kettenis, P.T. (2014). Young adult psychological outcome after puberty suppression and gender reassignment. *Pediatrics* 134:696–704.

42. Costa, R., Dunsford, M., Skagerberg, E., Holt, V., Carmichael, P. and Colizzi, M. (2015). Psychological support, puberty suppression, and psychosocial functioning in adolescents with Gender Dysphoria. *Journal of Sexual Medicine* 12:2206–2214.

43. Khatchadourian, K., Amed, S. and Metzger, D.L. (2014). Clinical management of youth with gender dysphoria in Vancouver. *Journal of Pediatrics* 164:906–911.

44. Klink, D., Bokenkamp, A., Dekker, C. and Rotteveel, J. (2015). Arterial hypertension as a complication of triptorelin treatment in adolescents with gender dysphoria. *International Journal of Endocrinology and Metabolism* 2:00008.

45. Vlot, M.C., Klink, D.T., den Heijer, M., Blankenstein, M.A., Rotteveel, J. and Heijboer, A.C. (2017). Effect of pubertal suppression and cross-sex hormone therapy on bone turnover markers and bone mineral apparent density (BMAD) in transgender adolescents. *Bone* 95:11–19.

46. Cohen-Kettenis, P.T., Schagen, S.E., Steensma, T.D., de Vries, A.L. and Delemarre-van de Waal, H.A. (2011). Puberty suppression in a gender-dysphoric adolescent: A 22-year follow-up. *Archives of Sexual Behavior* 40:843–847.

47. Staphorsius, A.S., Kreukels, B.P., Cohen-Ketternis, P.T., Veltmann, D.J., Burke, S.M., Schagen, S.E., et al. (2015). Puberty suppression and executive functioning: An fMRI-study in adolescents with gender dysphoria. *Psychoneuroendocrinology* 56:190–199.

48. Leibowitz, S. and de Vries, A.L.C. (2016). Gender dysphoria in adolescence. *International Review of Psychiatry* 28:21–35.

49. Klotz, L., Boccon-Gibod, L., Shore, N.D., Andreou, C., Persson, B., Cantor, P., et al. (2008). The efficacy and safety of degarelix: A 12-month, comparative, randomized, open-label, parallel-group phase III study in patients with prostate cancer. *BJU International* 102:1531–1538.

50. Taylor, H.S., Giudice, L.C., Lessey, B.A., Abrao, M.S., Kotarski, J., Archer, D.F., et al. (2017). Treatment of endometriosis-associated pain with elagolix, an oral GnRH antagonist. *New England Journal of Medicine* 377:28–40.

51. Tack, L.J., Craen, M., Dhondt, K., van den Bossche, H., Laridaen, J. and Cools, M. (2016). Consecutive lynestrenol and cross-sex hormone treatment in biological female adolescents with gender dysphoria: A retrospective analysis. *Biology of Sex Difference* 7:14.

52. Tack, L.J.W., Heyse, R., Craen, M., Dhondt, K., Bossche, H.V., Laridaen, J., et al. (2017). Consecutive cyproterone acetate and estradiol treatment in late-pubertal transgender female adolescents. *Journal of Sexual Medicine* 14:747–757.

53. Peitzmeier, S., Gardner, I., Weinand, J., Corbet, A. and Acevedo, K. (2017). Health impact of chest binding among transgender adults: A community-engaged, cross-sectional study. *Culture, Health & Sexuality* 19:64–75.

54. Vrouenraets, L.J., Fredriks, A.M., Hannema, S.E., Cohen-Kettenis, P.T. and de Vries, M.C. (2015). Early medical treatment of children and adolescents with Gender Dysphoria: An empirical ethics study. *Journal of Adolescent Health* 57:367–373. Rosenthal, S.M. (2014). Approach to the patient: Transgender youth: Endocrine considerations. *Journal of Clinical Endocrinology and Metabolism* 99:4379–4389.

55. Leibowitz, S. and de Vries, A.L.C. (2016). Gender dysphoria in adolescence. *International Review of Psychiatry* 28:21–35.

56. Milrod, C. and Karasic, D.H. (2017). Age is just a number: WPATH-affiliated surgeons' experiences and attitudes toward vaginoplasty in transgender females under 18 years of age in the United States. *Journal of Sexual Medicine* 14:624–634. Khatchadourian, K., Amed, S. and Metzger, D.L. (2014). Clinical management of youth with gender dysphoria in Vancouver. *Journal of Pediatrics* 164:906–911.

57. Marinkovic, M. and Newfield, R.S. (2017). Chest reconstructive surgeries in transmasculine youth: Experience from one pediatric center. *International Journal of Transgenderism* 18:376–381.

58. van der Sluis, W.B., Bouman, M.B., de Boer, N.K., Buncamper, M.E., van Bodegraven, A.A., Neefjes-Borst, E.A., et al. (2016). Long-term follow-up of transgender women after secondary intestinal vaginoplasty. *Journal of Sexual Medicine* 13:702–710. Bouman, M.B., van der Sluis, W.B., van Woudenberg-Hamstra, L.E., Buncamper, M.E., Kreukels, B.P.C., Meijerink, W.J.H.J., et al. (2016). Patient-reported esthetic and functional outcomes of primary total laparoscopic intestinal vaginoplasty in transgender women with penoscrotal hypoplasia. *Journal of Sexual Medicine* 13:1438–1444.

59. Smith, Y.L., van Goozen, S.H. and Cohen-Kettenis, P.T. (2001). Adolescents with gender identity disorder who were accepted or rejected for sex reassignment surgery: A prospective follow-up study. *Journal of the American Academy of Child and Adolescent Psychiatry* 40:472–81.

60. de Vries, A.L., McGuire, J.K., Steensma, T.D., Wagenaar, E.C., Doreleijers, T.A. and Cohen-Kettenis, P.T. (2014). Young adult psychological outcome after puberty suppression and gender reassignment. *Pediatrics* 134:696–704.

CHAPTER 7

1. Coleman, E., Bockting, W., Botzer, M., Cohen-Kettinis, P., DeCuypere, G., Feldman, J., et al. (2011). Standards of Care for the health of transsexual, transgender, and gender-nonconforming people, Version 7. *International Journal of Transgenderism* 13:165–232. Hembree, W.C., Cohen-Kettenis, P.T., Gooren, L., Hannema, S.E., Meyer, W.J., Murad, M.H., et al. (2017). Endocrine treatment of gender-dysphoric/gender-incongruent persons: An Endocrine Society clinical practice guideline. *Journal of Clinical Endocrinology and Metabolism* 102:3869–3903.

2. Smith, E., Jones, T., Ward, R., Dixon, J., Mitchell, A. and Hillier, L. (2014). *From blues to rainbows: Mental health and wellbeing of gender diverse and transgender young people in Australia*. Melbourne: The Australian Research Centre in Sex, Health, and Society. ISBN 978121915628. Hyde, Z., Doherty, M., Tilley, P.J.M., McCaul, K.A., Rooney, R. and Jancey, J. (2014). *The first Australian national trans mental health study: Summary of results*. Perth, Australia: School of Public Health, Curtin University. Riggs, D.W., Coleman, K. and Due, C. (2014). Healthcare experiences of gender diverse Australians: A mixed-methods, self-report survey. *BMC Public Health* 14:230.

3. Cavanaugh, T., Hopwood, R. and Lambert, C. (2016). Informed consent in the medical care of transgender and gender-nonconforming patients. *AMA Journal of Ethics* 18:1147–1155.

4. Mamoojee, Y., Seal, L.J. and Quinton, R. (2017). Transgender hormone therapy: Understanding international variation in practice. *The Lancet Diabetes and Endocrinology* 5:243–246.

5. Colizzi, M., Costa, R. and Todarello, O. (2014). Transsexual patients' psychiatric comorbidity and positive effect of cross-sex hormonal treatment on mental health: Results from a longitudinal study. *Psychoneuroendocrinology* 39:65–73.

6. White Hughto, J.M. and Reisner, S.L. (2016). A systematic review of the effects of hormone therapy on psychological functioning and quality of life in transgender individuals. *Transgender Health* 1:21–31.

7. Colizzi, M., Costa, R. and Todarello, O. (2014). Transsexual patients' psychiatric comorbidity and positive effect of cross-sex hormonal treatment on mental health: Results from a longitudinal study. *Psychoneuroendocrinology* 39:65–73. Heylens, G., Verroken, C., De Cock, S., T'Sjoen, G. and De Cuypere, G. (2014). Effects of different steps in gender reassignment therapy on psychopathology: A prospective study of persons with a gender identity disorder. *Journal of Sexual Medicine* 11:119–126.

8. Manieri, C., Castellano, E., Crespi, C., Di Bisceglie, C., Dell'Aquila, C., Gualerzi, A., et al. (2014). Medical treatment of subjects with Gender Identity Disorder: The experience in an Italian public health center. *International Journal of Transgenderism* 15:53–65.

9. Smith, Y.L., van Goozen, S.H., Kuiper, A.J. and Cohen Kettenis, P.T. (2005). Sex reassignment: Outcomes and predictors of treatment for adolescent and adult transsexuals. *Psychological Medicine* 35:89–99.

10. den Heijer, M., Bakker, A. and Gooren, L. (2017). Long-term hormonal treatment for transgender people. *BMJ* 359:j5027.

11. Meyer, W.J. 3rd, Finkelstein, J.W., Stuart, C.A., Webb, A., Smith, E.R., Payer, A.F., et al. (1981). Physical and hormonal evaluation of transsexual patients during hormonal therapy. *Archives of Sexual Behavior* 10:347–356. Meyer, W.J. 3rd, Webb, A., Stuart, C.A., Finkelstein, J.W., Lawrence, B. and Walker, P.A. (1986). Physical and hormonal evaluation of transsexual patients: A longitudinal study. *Archives of Sexual Behavior* 15:121–138.

12. Giltay, E.J. and Gooren, L.J.G. (2000). Effects of sex steroid deprivation/administration on hair growth and skin sebum production in transsexual males and females. *Journal of Clinical Endocrinology and Metabolism* 85:2913–2921.

13. Irwig, M.S. (2017). Testosterone therapy for transgender men. *The Lancet Diabetes and Endocrinology* 5:301–311.

14. Wierckx, K., van de Peer, F., Verhaeghe, E., Dedecker, D., van Caenegem, E., Toye, K., et al. (2014). Short- and long-term clinical skin effects of testosterone treatment in trans men. *Journal of Sexual Medicine* 11:222–229.

15. Wierckx, K., van Caenegem, E., Schreiner, T., Haraldsen, I., Fisher, A.D., Toye, K., et al. (2014). Cross-sex hormone therapy in trans persons is safe and effective at short-time follow-up: Results from the European network for the investigation of gender incongruence. *Journal of Sexual Medicine* 11:1999–2011.

16. Ahmad, S. and Leinung, M. (2017). The response of the menstrual cycle to initiation of hormonal therapy in transgender men. *Transgender Health* 2:176–179.

17. Slabbekoom, D., van Goozen, S.H., Megens, J., Gooren, L.J. and Cohen-Kettenis, P.T. (1999). Activating effects of cross-sex hormones on cognitive functioning: A study of short-term and long-term hormone effects in transsexuals. *Psychoneuroendocrinology* 24:423–447.

18. Wierckx, K., Elaut, E., van Caenegem, E., van De Peer, F., Dedecker, D., van Houdenhove, E., et al. (2011). Sexual desire in female-to-male transsexual persons: Exploration of the role of testosterone administration. *European Journal of Endocrinology* 165:331–337.

19. Costantino, A., Cerpolini, S., Alvisi, S., Morselli, P.G., Venturoli, S. and Meriggiola, M.C. (2013). A prospective study on sexual function and mood in female-to-male transsexuals during testosterone administration and after sex reassignment surgery. *Journal of Sex & Marital Therapy* 39:321–335.

20. Cosyns, M., van Borsel, J., Wierckx, K., Dedecker, D., van de Peer F., Daelman, T., et al. (2014). Voice in female-to-male transsexual persons after long-term androgen therapy. *Laryngoscope* 124:1409–1414.

21. Rosenthal, S.M. (2014). Approach to the patient: Transgender youth: Endocrine considerations. *Journal of Clinical Endocrinology & Metabolism* 99:4379–4389.

22. Spratt, D.I., Stewart, I.I., Savage, C., Craig, W., Spack, N.P., Chandler, D.W., et al. (2017). Subcutaneous injection of testosterone is an effective and preferred alternative to intramuscular injection: Demonstration in female–to-male transgender patients. *Journal of Clinical Endocrinology and Metabolism* 102:2349–2355.

23. van Kesteren, P.J., Asscheman, H., Megens, J.A. and Gooren, L.J. (1997). Mortality and morbidity in transsexual subjects treated with cross-sex hormones. *Clinical Endocrinology (Oxford)* 47:337–342.

24. Bondy, C.A. and the Turner Syndrome Study Group. (2007). Care of girls and women with Turner syndrome: A guideline of the Turner Syndrome Study Group. *Journal of Clinical Endocrinology and Metabolism* 92:10–25.

25. de Blok, C.J.M., Klaver, M., Wiepjes, C.M., Nota, N.M., Heijboer, A.C., Fisher, A.D., et al. (2018). Breast development in transwomen after 1 year of cross-sex hormone therapy: Results of a prospective multicenter study. *Journal of Clinical Endocrinology and Metabolism* 103:532–538.

26. Fisher, A.D., Castellini, G., Ristori, J., Casale, H., Cassioli, E., Sensi, C., et al. (2016). Cross-sex hormone treatment and psychobiological changes in transsexual persons: Two-year follow-up data. *Journal of Clinical Endocrinology and Metabolism* 101:4260–4269.

27. Seal, L.J., Franklin, S., Richards, C., Shishkareva, A., Sinclaire, C. and Barrett, J. (2012). Predictive markers for mammoplasty and a comparison of side effect profiles in transwomen taking various hormonal regimens. *Journal of Clinical Endocrinology and Metabolism* 97:4422–4428.

28. Gooren, L.J., van Trotsenburg, M.A., Giltay, E.J. and van Diest, P.J. (2013). Breast cancer development in transsexual subjects receiving cross-sex hormone treatment. *Journal of Sexual Medicine* 10:3129–3134.

29. Saenger, P., Wikland, K.A., Conway, G.S., Davenport, M., Gavholt, C.H., Hintz, R., et al. (2001). The Fifth International Symposium on Turner Syndrome. Recommendations for the diagnosis and management of Turner syndrome. *Journal of Clinical Endocrinology and Metabolism* 86:3061–3069.

30. Rossouw, J.E., Anderson, G.L., Prentice, R.L., LaCroix, A.Z., Kooperberg, C., Stefanick, M.L., et al. Writing Group for the Women's Health Initiative Investigators. (2002). Risks and benefits of estrogen plus progestin in healthy postmenopausal women: Principal results from the Women's Health Initiative randomized controlled trial. *JAMA* 288:321–333. Cushman, M., Kuller, L.H., Prentice, R., Rodabough, R.J., Psaty, B.M., Stafford, R.S., et al. and Women's Health Initiative Investigators. (2004). Estrogen plus progestin and risk of venous thromboembolism. *JAMA* 292:1573–1580. Gurney, E.P., Nachtigall, M.J., Nachtigall, L.E. and Naftolin, F. (2014). The Women's Health Initiative trial and related studies: 10 years later, a clinician's view. *Journal of Steroid Biochemistry and Molecular Biology* 142:4–11.

31. Eden, J. (2017). The endometrial and breast safety of menopausal hormone therapy containing micronized progesterone: A short review. *Australian and New Zealand Journal of Obstetrics and Gynaecology* 57:12–15.

32. Elbers, J.M., Giltay, E.J., Teerlink, T., Scheffer, P.G., Asscheman, H., Seidell, J.C., et al (2003). Effects of sex steroids on components of the insulin resistance syndrome in transsexual subjects. *Clinical Endocrinology (Oxford)* 58:562–571.

33. Giltay, E.J. and Gooren, L.J.G. (2000). Effects of sex steroid deprivation/administration on hair growth and skin sebum production in transsexual males and females. *Journal of Clinical Endocrinology and Metabolism* 85:2913–2921.

34. Seal, L.J. (2016). A review of the physical and metabolic effects of cross-sex hormonal therapy in the treatment of gender dysphoria. *Annals of Clinical Biochemistry* 53:10–20.

35. Gómez-Gil, E., Zubiaurre-Elorza, L., Esteva, I, Guillamon, A., Godás, T., Cruz Almaraz, M., et al. (2012). Hormone-treated transsexuals report less social distress, anxiety and depression. *Psychoneuroendocrinology* 37:662–670.

36. Elaut, E., de Cuypere, G., de Sutter, P., Gijs, L., van Trotsenburg, M., Heylens, G., et al. (2008). Hypoactive sexual desire in transsexual women: Prevalence and association with testosterone levels. *European Journal of Endocrinology* 158:393–399.

37. Leinung, M.C., Feustal, P.J. and Joseph, J. (2018). Hormonal treatment of transgender women with oral estradiol. *Transgender Health* 3:74–81.

38. Casper, R.F. and Yen, S.S. (1981). Rapid absorption of micronized estradiol-17 beta following sublingual administration. *Obstetrics & Gynecology* 57:62–64. Price, T.M., Blauer, K.L., Hansen, M., Stanczyk, F., Lobo, R. and Bates, G.W. (1997). Single-dose pharmacokinetics of sublingual versus oral administration of micronized 17 beta-estradiol. *Obstetrics & Gynecology* 89:340–345.

39. Asscheman, H., Giltay, E.J., Megens, J.A., de Ronde, W.P., van Trosenburg, M.A. and Gooren, L.J. (2011). A long-term follow-up study of mortality in transsexuals receiving treatment with cross-sex hormones. *European Journal of Endocrinology* 164:635–642.

40. Meriggiola, M.C. and Gava, G. (2015). Endocrine care of transpeople part II. A review of cross-sex hormonal treatments, outcomes and adverse effects in transwomen. *Clinical Endocrinology (Oxford)* 83:607–615. Asscheman, H., Gooren, L.J. and Eklund, P.L. (1989). Mortality and morbidity in transsexual patients with cross-gender hormone treatment. *Metabolism* 38:869–873.

41. Gooren, L.J., Giltay, E.J. and Bunck, M.C. (2008). Long-term treatment of transsexuals with cross-sex hormones: Extensive personal experience. *Journal of Clinical Endocrinology and Metabolism* 93:19–25.

42. Toorians, A.W., Thomassen, M.C., Zweegman, S., Magdeleyns, E.J., Tans, G., Gooren L.J., et al. (2003). Venous thrombosis and changes of hemostatic variables during cross-sex hormone treatment in transsexual people. *Journal of Clinical Endocrinology and Metabolism* 88:5723–5729.

43. Ahmad, S., Barrett, J., Beaini, A.Y., Bouman, W.P., Davies, A., Greener, H.M., et al. (2013). Gender dysphoria services: A guide for general practitioners and other healthcare staff. *Sexual and Relationship Therapy* 28:172–185.

44. Dittrich, R., Binder, H., Cupisti, S., Hoffmann, I., Beckman, M.W. and Mueller, A. (2005). Endocrine treatment of male-to-female transsexuals using gonadotropin-releasing hormone agonist. *Experimental and Clinical Endocrinology & Diabetes* 113:586–592.

45. Gulmez, S.E., Lassen, A.T., Aalykke, C., Dall, M., Andries, A., Andersen, B.S., et al. (2008). Spironolactone use and the risk of upper gastrointestinal bleeding: A population-based case-control study. *British Journal of Clinical Pharmacology* 66:294–299.

46. Seal, L.J., Franklin, S., Richards, C., Shishkareva, A., Sinclaire, C. and Barrett, J. (2012). Predictive markers for mammoplasty and a comparison of side effect profiles in transwomen taking various hormonal regimens. *Journal of Clinical Endocrinology and Metabolism* 97:4422–4428.

47. Honer, C., Nam, K., Fink, C., Marshall, P., Ksander, G., Chatelain, R.E., et al. (2003). Glucacorticoid receptor antagonism by cyproterone acetate and RU486. *Molecular Pharmacology* 63:1012–1020.

48. Cremoncini, C., Vignati, E. and Libroia, A. (1976). Treatment of hirsuitism and acne in women with two combinations of cyproterone acetate and ethinylestradiol. *Acta Europaea Fertilitatis* 7:299–314. Frey, H. and Aakvaag, A. (1981). The treatment of essential

hirsuitism in women with cyproterone acetate and ethinyl estradiol. Clinical and endocrine effects in 10 cases. *Acta Obstetricia et Gynecologica Scandinavica* 60:295–300. Ylöstalo, P., Laakso, L., Viinikka, L., Ylikorkala, O. and Vihko, R. (1981). Cyproterone acetate in the treatment of hirsuitism. *Acta Obstetricia et Gynecologica Scandinavica* 60:399–401.

49. Gil, M., Oliva, B., Timoner, J., Maciá, M.A., Bryant, V. and de Abajo, F. J. (2011). Risk of meningioma among users of high doses of cyproterone acetate as compared with the general population: Evidence from a population-based cohort study. *British Journal of Clinical Pharmacology* 72:965–968.

50. Richards, C., Bouman, W.P., Seal, L., Barker, M.J., Nieder, T.O. and T'Sjoen, G. (2016). Non-binary or genderqueer genders. *International Review of Psychiatry* 28:95–102.

51. Koehler, A., Eyssel, J. and Nieder, T.O. (2018). Genders and individual treatment progress in (non-)binary trans individuals. *Journal of Sexual Medicine* 15:102–113.

52. Gooren, L.J. and Behre, H.M. (2008). Testosterone treatment of hypogonadal men participating in competitive sports. *Andrologia* 40:195–199.

53. Zitzmann, M., Faber, S. and Nieschlag, E. (2006). Association of specific symptoms and metabolic risks with serum testosterone in older men. *Journal of Clinical Endocrinology and Metabolism* 91:4335–4343.

54. Lackner, J.E., Rücklinger, E., Schatzi, G., Lunglmayr, G. and Kratzik, C.W. (2011). Are there symptom-specific testosterone thresholds in aging men? *BJU International* 108:1310–1315.

55. Gooren, L.J. (1987). Androgen levels and sex functions in testosterone-treated hypogonadal men. *Archives of Sexual Behavior* 16:463–473.

56. Shores, M.M., Matsumoto, A.M., Sloan, K.L. and Kivlahan, D.R. (2006). Low serum testosterone and mortality in male veterans. *Archives of Internal Medicine* 166:1660–1665.

57. Atsma, F., Bartelink, M.L., Grobbee, D.E. and van der Schouw, Y.T. (2006). Post-menopausal status and early menopause as independent risk factors for cardiovascular disease: A meta-analysis. *Menopause* 13:265–279.

58. Shahinian, V.B., Kuo, Y.F., Freeman, J.L. and Goodwin, J.S. (2005). Risk of fracture after androgen deprivation for prostate cancer. *New England Journal of Medicine* 352:154–164.

59. Klink, D., Caris, M., Heijboer, A., van Trotsenburg, M. and Rotteveel, J. (2015). Bone mass in young adulthood following gonadotropin-releasing hormone analog treatment in adolescents with gender dysphoria. *Journal of Clinical Endocrinology and Metabolism* 100:E270–E275.

60. Finkelstein, J.S., Lee, H., Leder, B.Z., Burnett-Bowie, S.A., Goldstein, D.W., Hahn, C.W., et al. (2016). Gonadal steroid-dependent effects on bone turnover and bone mineral density in men. *Journal of Clinical Investigation* 126:1114–1125.

61. Gambacciani, M., Cappagli, B., Ciaponi, M., Pepe, A., Vacca, F. and Genazzani, A. R. (2008). Ultra low-dose hormone replacement therapy and bone protection in postmenopausal women. *Maturitas* 59:2–6.

62. Popat, V.B., Calis, K.A., Kalantaridou, S.N., Vanderhoof, V.H., Koziol, D., Troendle, J.F., et al. (2014). Bone mineral density in young women with primary ovarian insufficiency: Results of a three-year randomized controlled trial of physiological transdermal estradiol and testosterone replacement. *Journal of Clinical Endocrinology and Metabolism* 99:3418–3426.

63. Weinand, J.D. and Safer, J.D. (2015). Hormone therapy in transgender adults is safe with provider supervision: A review of hormone therapy sequelae for transgender individuals. *Journal of Clinical & Translational Endocrinology* 2:55–60.

64. Dekker, M.J., Wierckx, K., van Caenegem, E., Klaver, M., Kreukels, B.P., Elaut, E., et al. (2016). A European Network for the Investigation of Gender Incongruence: Endocrine Part. *Journal of Sexual Medicine* 13:994–999.

65. Quinn, V.P., Nash, R., Hunkeler, E., Contreras, R., Cromwell, L., Becerra-Culqui, T.A., et al. (2017). Cohort profile: Study of Transition, Outcomes and Gender (STRONG) to assess health status of transgender people. *BMJ Open* 7:e018121.

66. Brown, G.R. and Jones, K.T. (2016). Mental health and medical health disparities in 5135 transgender veterans receiving healthcare in the Veterans Health Administration: A case-control study. *LGBT Health* 3:122–131.

67. Asscheman, H., Giltay, E.J., Megens, J.A., de Ronde, W.P., van Trosenburg, M.A. and Gooren, L.J. (2011). A long-term follow-up study of mortality in transsexuals receiving treatment with cross-sex hormones. *European Journal of Endocrinology* 164:635–642.

68. Dhejne, C., Lichtenstein, P., Boman, M., Johansson, A.L., Långström, N. and Lan-dén, M. (2011). Long-term follow-up of transsexual persons undergoing sex reassignment surgery: Cohort study in Sweden. *PLoS One* 6:e16885.

69. Wylie, W., Knudson, G., Khan, S.I., Bonierbale, M., Watanyusakul, S. and Baral, S. (2016). Serving transgender people: Clinical care considerations and service delivery models in transgender health. *Lancet* 388:401–411.

70. Irwig, M. S. (2017). Clinical dilemmas in the management of transgender men. *Current Opinion in Endocrinology, Diabetes and Obesity* 24:233–239.

71. Wierckx, K., Muller, S., Weyers, S., van Caenegem, E., Roef, G., Heylens, G. et al. (2012). Long-term evaluation of cross-sex hormone treatment in transsexual persons. *Journal of Sexual Medicine* 9:2641–2651.

72. Mueller, A., Haeberle, L., Zollver, H., Claassen, T., Kronawitter, D., Oppelt, P.G., et al. (2010). Effects of intramuscular testosterone undecanoate on body composition and bone mineral density in female-to-male transsexuals. *Journal of Sexual Medicine* 7:3190–3198. Pelusi, C., Costantino, A., Martelli, V., Lambertini, M., Bazzocchi, A., Ponti, F., et al. (2014). Effects of three different testosterone formulations in female-to-male transsexual persons. *Journal of Sexual Medicine* 11:3002–3011.

73. Shatzel, J.J., Connelly, K.J. and DeLoughery, T.G. (2017). Thrombotic issues in transgender medicine: A review. *American Journal of Hematology* 92:204–208.

74. Giltay, E.J. and Gooren, L.J.G. (2000). Effects of sex steroid deprivation/administration on hair growth and skin sebum production in transsexual males and females. *Journal of Clinical Endocrinology and Metabolism* 85:2913–2921.

75. Thiboutot, D.M. on behalf of the Global Alliance (2018). Practical management of acne for clinicians: An international consensus from the Global Alliance to Improve Outcomes in Acne. *Journal of the American Academy of Dermatology* 78:S1–S23.

76. Elamin, M.B., Garcia, M.Z., Murad, M.H., Erwin, P.J. and Montori, V.M. (2010). Effect of sex steroid use on cardiovascular risk in transsexual individuals: A systematic review and meta-analyses. *Clinical Endocrinology (Oxford)* 72:1–10.

77. Maraka, S., Sing Ospina, N., Rodriguez-Gutierrez, R., Davidge-Pitts, C.J., Nippoldt, T.B., Prokop, L.J., et al. (2017). Sex steroids and cardiovascular outcomes in transgender individuals: A systematic review and meta-analysis. *Journal of Clinical Endocrinology and Metabolism* 102:3914–3923.

78. Wierckx, K., Elaut, E., Declercq, E., Heylens, G., De Cuypere, G., Taes, Y., et al. (2013). Prevalence of cardiovascular disease and cancer during cross-sex hormone therapy in a large cohort of trans persons: A case-control study. *European Journal of Endocrinology* 169:471–478.

79. Ruetsche, A.G., Kneubuehl, R., Birkhaeuser, M.H. and Lippuner, K. (2005). Cortical and trabecular bone mineral density in transsexuals after long-term cross-sex hormonal treatment: A cross-sectional study. *Osteoporosis International* 16:791–798.

80. van Caenegem, E., Wierckx, K., Taes, Y., Dedecker, D., van de Peer, F., Toye, K., et al. (2012). Bone mass, bone geometry, and body composition in female-to-male

transsexual persons after long-term cross-sex hormonal therapy. *Journal of Clinical Endocrinology and Metabolism* 97:2503–2511.

81. Singh-Ospina, N., Maraka, S., Rodriguez-Gutierrez, R., Davidge-Pitts, C., Nippoldt, T.B., Prokop, L.J., et al. (2017). Effect of sex steroids on the bone health of transgender individuals: A systematic review and meta-analysis. *Journal of Clinical Endocrinology and Metabolism* 102:3904–3913.

82. van Kesteren, P., Lips, P., Gooren, L.J., Asscheman, H. and Megens, J. (1998). Long-term follow-up of bone mineral density and bone metabolism in transsexuals treated with cross-sex hormones. *Clinical Endocrinology (Oxford)* 48:347–354.

83. Beral, V., Banks, E. and Reeves G. (2002). Evidence from randomized trials on the long-term effects of hormone replacement therapy. *Lancet* 360:942–944.

84. Brown, G.R. and Jones, K.T. (2015). Incidence of breast cancer in a cohort of 5,135 transgender veterans. *Breast Cancer Research and Treatment* 149:191–198.

85. Grynberg, M., Fanchin, R., Dubost, G., Colau, J.C., Brémont-Weil, C., Frydman, R., et al. (2010). Histology of genital tract and breast tissue after long-term testosterone administration in a female-to-male transsexual population. *Reproductive BioMedicine Online* 20:553–538.

86. Ikeda, K., Baba, T., Noguchi, H., Nagasawa, K., Endo, T., Kiya, T., et al. (2013). Excessive androgen exposure in female-to-male transsexual persons of reproductive age induces hyperplasia of the ovarian cortex and stroma but not polycystic ovary morphology. *Human Reproduction* 28:453–461.

87. Urban, R.R., Teng, N.N. and Knapp, D.S. (2011). Gynecologic malignancies in female-to-male transgender patients: The need of original gender surveillance. *American Journal of Obstetrics and Gynecology* 204:e9–e12.

88. Futterweit, W. (1998). Endocrine therapy of transsexualism and potential complications of long-term treatment. *Archives of Sexual Behavior* 27:209–226.

89. Grynberg, M., Fanchin, R., Dubost, G., Colau, J.C., Brémont-Weil, C., Frydman, R., et al. (2010). Histology of genital tract and breast tissue after long-term testosterone administration in a female-to-male transsexual population. *Reproductive BioMedicine Online* 20:553–538.

90. Wylie, K.R., Barrett, J., Besser, M., Bouman, W.P., Bridgman, M., Clayton, A., et al. (2014). Good practice guidelines for the assessment and treatment of adults with gender dysphoria. *Sexual and Relationship Therapy* 29:154–214.

91. Silverberg, M.J., Nash, R., Becerra-Culqui, T.A., Cromwell, L., Getahun, D., Hunkeler, E., et al. (2017). Cohort study of cancer risk among insured transgender people. *Annals of Epidemiology* 27:499–501.

92. Peitzmeier, S.M., Khullar, K., Reisner, S.L. and Potter, J. (2014). Pap test use is lower among female-to-male patients than non-transgender women. *American Journal of Preventive Medicine* 47:808–812.

93. Reisner, S.L., Deutsch, M.B., Peitzmeier, S.M., White Hughto, J.M., Cavanaugh, T.P., Pardee, D.J., et al. (2018). Test performance and acceptability of self- versus provider-collected swabs for high-risk HPV DNA testing in female-to-male trans masculine patients. *PLoS One* 13(3):e0190172.

94. Asscheman, H., Giltay, E.J., Megens, J.A., de Ronde, W.P., van Trosenburg, M.A. and Gooren, L.J. (2011). A long-term follow-up study of mortality in transsexuals receiving treatment with cross-sex hormones. *European Journal of Endocrinology* 164:635–642.

95. Asscheman, H., T'Sjoen, G., Lemaire, A., Mas, M., Meriggiola, M.C., Mueller, A., et al. (2014). Venous thrombo-embolism as a complication of cross-sex hormone treatment of male-to-female transsexual subjects: A review. *Andrologia* 46:791–795.

96. Pomp, E.R., Rosendaal, F.R. and Doggen, C.J. (2008). Smoking increases the risk of venous thrombosis and acts synergistically with oral contraceptive use. *American Journal of Hematology* 83:97–102. Suchon, P., Al Frouh, F., Henneuse, A., Ibrahim, M., Brunet, D., Barthet, M.C., et al. (2016). Risk factors for venous thromboembolism in women under combined oral contraceptive. The PILI Genetic Risk Monitoring (PILGRIM) Study. *Thrombosis and Haemostasis* 115:135–142.

97. Asscheman, H., Gooren, L.J. and Eklund, P.L. (1989). Mortality and morbidity in transsexual patients with cross-gender hormone treatment. *Metabolism* 38:869–873.

98. Stadel, B.V. (1981). Oral contraceptives and cardiovascular disease. *New England Journal of Medicine* 305:612–618 and 305:672–677.

99. van Kesteren, P.J., Asscheman, H., Megens, J.A. and Gooren, L.J. (1997). Mortality and morbidity in transsexual subjects treated with cross-sex hormones. *Clinical Endocrinology (Oxford)* 47:337–342.

100. Seal, L.J., Franklin, S., Richards, C., Shishkareva, A., Sinclaire, C. and Barrett, J. (2012). Predictive markers for mammoplasty and a comparison of side effect profiles in transwomen taking various hormonal regimens. *Journal of Clinical Endocrinology and Metabolism* 97:4422–4428.

101. Baglin, T., Gray, E., Greaves, M., Hunt, B.J., Keeling, D., Machin, S., et al. and the British Committee for Standards in Haematology. (2010). Clinical guidelines for testing for heritable thrombophilia. *British Journal of Haematology* 149:209–220.

102. Olié, V., Canonico, M. and Pierre-Yves, S. (2010). Risk of venous thrombosis with oral versus transdermal estrogen therapy among postmenopausal women. *Current Opinion in Hematology* 17:457–463.

103. Renoux, C., Dell'aniello, S., Garbe, E. and Suissa, S. (2010). Transdermal and oral hormone replacement therapy and the risk of stroke: A nested case-control study. *BMJ* 3:c2519.

104. Elbers, J.M., Asscheman, H., Seidell, J.C. and Gooren, L.J. (1999). Effects of sex steroid hormones on regional fat depots as assessed by magnetic resonance imaging in transsexuals. *American Journal of Physiology* 276:E317–E325.

105. Gooren, L.J., Wierckx, K. and Giltay, E.J. (2014). Cardiovascular disease in transsexual persons treated with cross-sex hormones: Reversal of the transitional sex difference in cardiovascular disease pattern. *European Journal of Endocrinology* 170:809–819.

106. Lapauw, B., Taes, Y., Simoens, S., van Caenegem, E., Weyers, S., Goemaere, S., et al. (2008). Body composition, volumetric and areal bone parameters in male-to-female transsexual persons. *Bone* 43:1016–1021.

107. Elamin, M.B., Garcia, M.Z., Murad, M.H., Erwin, P.J. and Montori, V.M. (2010). Effect of sex steroid use on cardiovascular risk in transsexual individuals: A systematic review and meta-analyses. *Clinical Endocrinology (Oxford)* 72:1–10.

108. Maraka, S., Sing Ospina, N., Rodriguez-Gutierrez, R., Davidge-Pitts, C.J., Nippoldt, T.B., Prokop, L.J., et al. (2017). Sex steroids and cardiovascular outcomes in transgender individuals: A systematic review and meta-analysis. *Journal of Clinical Endocrinology and Metabolism* 102:3914–3923.

109. Giltay, E.J., Lambert, J., Gooren, L.J., Elbers, J.M., Steyn, M. and Stehouwer, C.D. (1999). Sex steroids, insulin, and arterial stiffness in women and men. *Hypertension* 34:590–597.

110. Elamin, M.B., Garcia, M.Z., Murad, M.H., Erwin, P.J. and Montori, V.M. (2010). Effect of sex steroid use on cardiovascular risk in transsexual individuals: A systematic review and meta-analyses. *Clinical Endocrinology (Oxford)* 72:1–10.

111. Lips, P., Asscheman, H., Uitewaal, P., Netelenbos, J.C. and Gooren, L. (1989). The effect of cross-gender hormonal treatment on bone metabolism in male-to-female transsexuals. *Journal of Bone and Mineral Research* 4:657–662.

112. Mueller, A., Zollver, H., Kronawitter, D., Oppelt, P.G., Claassen, T., Hofmann, I., et al. (2011). Body composition and bone mineral density in male-to-female transsexuals during cross-sex hormone therapy using gonadotrophin-releasing hormone agonist. *Experimental and Clinical Endocrinology & Diabetes* 119:95–100.

113. van Kesteren, P., Lips, P., Gooren, L.J., Asscheman, H. and Megens, J. (1998). Long-term follow-up of bone mineral density and bone metabolism in transsexuals treated with cross-sex hormones. *Clinical Endocrinology (Oxford)* 48:347–354.

114. Singh-Ospina, N., Maraka, S., Rodriguez-Gutierrez, R., Davidge-Pitts, C., Nippoldt, T.B., Prokop, L.J., et al. (2017). Effect of sex steroids on the bone health of transgender individuals: A systematic review and meta-analysis. *Journal of Clinical Endocrinology and Metabolism* 102:3904–3913.

115. van Caenegem, E., Taes, Y., Wierckx, K., Vanderwalle, S., Toye, K., Kaufman, J.M., et al. (2013). Low bone mass is prevalent in male-to-female transsexual persons before the start of cross-sex hormonal therapy and gonadectomy. *Bone* 54:92–97.

116. Seal, L.J., Franklin, S., Richards, C., Shishkareva, A., Sinclaire, C. and Barrett, J. (2012). Predictive markers for mammoplasty and a comparison of side effect profiles in transwomen taking various hormonal regimens. *Journal of Clinical Endocrinology and Metabolism* 97:4422–4428.

117. Asscheman, H., Gooren, L.J., Assies, J., Smits, J.P. and de Slegte, R. (1988). Prolactin levels and pituitary enlargement in hormone-treated male-to-female transsexuals. *Clinical Endocrinology (Oxford)* 28:583–588.

118. Gooren, L.J., Assies, J., Asscheman, H., de Slegte, R. and van Kessel, H. (1988). Estrogen-induced prolactinoma in a man. *Journal of Clinical Endocrinology and Metabolism* 66:444–446. Kovacs, K., Stefaneanu, L., Ezzat, S. and Smyth, H.S. (1994). Prolactin-producing pituitary adenoma in a male-to-female transsexual patient with protracted estrogen administration: A morphologic study. *Archives of Pathology & Laboratory Medicine* 118:562–565. Serri, O., Noiseux, D., Robert, F. and Hardy, J. (1996). Lactotroph hyperplasia in an estrogen treated male-to-female transsexual patient. *Journal of Clinical Endocrinology and Metabolism* 81:3177–3179. Bunck, M.C., Debono, M., Giltay, E. J., Verheijen, A.T., Diamant, M. and Gooren, L. J. (2009). Autonomous prolactin secretion in two male-to-female transgender patients using conventional oestrogen dosages. *BMJ Case Reports* bcr02.2009. Garcia-Malpartida, K., Martin-Gorgojo, A., Rocha, M., Gómez-Balaguer, M. and Herández-Mijares, A. (2010). Prolactinoma induced by estrogen and cyproterone acetate in a male-to-female transsexual. *Fertility and Sterility* 94:1097. Cunha, F. S., Domenice, S., Câmara, V.L., Sircili, M.H., Gooren, L.J., Mendonça. B.B., et al. (2015). Diagnosis of prolactinoma in two male-to-female transsexual subjects following high-dose cross-sex hormone therapy. *Andrologia* 47:680–684.

119. Rogers, A., Karavitaki, N. and Wass, J.A. (2014). Diagnosis and management of prolactinomas and non-functioning pituitary adenomas. *BMJ* 10:g5390.

120. Mueller, A. and Gooren, L. (2008). Hormone-related tumors in transsexuals receiving treatment with cross-sex hormones. *European Journal of Endocrinology* 159:197–202.

121. Gethins, M. (2012). Breast cancer in men. *Journal of the National Cancer Institute* 104:436–438.

122. Gooren, L.J., van Trotsenburg, M.A., Giltay, E.J. and van Diest, P.J. (2013). Breast cancer development in transsexual subjects receiving cross-sex hormone treatment. *Journal of Sexual Medicine* 10:3129–3134.

123. Brown, G.R. and Jones, K.T. (2015). Incidence of breast cancer in a cohort of 5,135 transgender veterans. *Breast Cancer Research and Treatment* 149:191–198.

124. Tai, Y.C., Domchek, S., Parmigiani, G. and Chen, S. (2007). Breast cancer risk among male BRCA1 and BRCA2 mutation carriers. *Journal of the National Cancer Institute* 99:1811–1814.

125. van Kesteren, P., Meinhardt, W., van der Valk, P., Geldof, A., Megens, J., et al. (1996). Effects of estrogens only on the prostates of aging men. *Journal of Urology* 156:1349–1353.

126. Deebel, N.A., Morin, J.P., Autorino, R., Vince, R., Grob, B. and Hampton, L J. (2017). Prostate cancer in transgender women: Incidence, etiopathogenesis, and management challenges. *Urology* 110:166–171.

127. Gooren, L. and Morgentaler, A. (2014). Prostate cancer incidence in orchidectomised male-to-female transsexual persons treated with oestrogens. *Andrologia* 46:1156–1160.

128. Silverberg, M.J., Nash, R., Becerra-Culqui, T.A., Cromwell, L., Getahun, D., Hunkeler, E., et al. (2017). Cohort study of cancer risk among insured transgender people. *Annals of Epidemiology* 27:499–501.

129. Richards, C., Bouman, W.P., Seal L., Barker, M.J., Nieder, T.O. and T'Sjoen, G. (2016). Non-binary or genderqueer genders. *International Review of Psychiatry* 29:95–102.

130. Bouman, W.P., Richards, C., Addinall, R.M., Arango de Montis, I., Arcelus, J., Duisin, I., et al. (2014). Yes and yes again: Are standards of care which require two referrals for genital reconstructive surgery ethical? *Sexual and Relationship Therapy* 29:377–389.

131. Sineath, R.C., Woodyatt, C., Sanchez, T., Giammattei, S., Gillespie, T., Hunkeler, E., et al. (2016). Determinants of and barriers to hormonal and surgical treatment receipt among transgender people. *Transgender Health* 1:129–136.

132. Wiepjes, C.M., Nota, N.M., de Blok, C.J.M., Klaver, M., de Vries, A.L.C., Wensing-Kruger, S.A., et al. (2018). The Amsterdam Cohort of Gender Dysphoria Study (1972–2015): Trends in prevalence, treatment, and regrets. *The Journal of Sexual Medicine* 15:582–590.

133. Peitzmeier, S., Gardner, I., Weinand, J., Corbet, A. and Acevedo, K. (2017). Health impact of chest binding among transgender adults: A community-engaged, cross-sectional study. *Culture, Health & Sexuality* 19:64–75.

134. Monstrey, S., Selvaggi, G., Ceulemans, P., Van Landuyt, K., Bowman, C., Blondeel, P., et al. (2008). Chest-wall contouring surgery in female-to-male transsexuals: A new algorithm. *Plastic and Reconstructive Surgery* 121:849–859.

135. Bluebond-Lagner, R., Berli, J.U., Sabino, J., Chopra, K., Singh, D. and Fischer, B. (2017). Top surgery in transgender men: How far can you push the envelope? *Plastic and Reconstructive Surgery* 139:873e–882e.

136. Kanhai, R.C., Hage, J.J. and Mulder, J.W. (2000). Long-term outcome of augmentation mammoplasty in male-to-female transsexuals: A questionnaire survey of 107 patients. *British Journal of Plastic Surgery* 53:209–211.

137. Kanhai, R.C., Hage, J.J. and Karim, R.B. (2001). Augmentation mammoplasty in male-to-female transsexuals: Facts and figures from Amsterdam. *Scandinavian Journal of Plastic and Reconstructive Surgical Hand Surgery* 35:203–206.

138. Hage, J.J., Kanhai, R.C., Oen, A.L., van Diest, P.J. and Karim, R.B. (2001). The devastating outcome of massive subcutaneous injection of highly viscous fluids in male-to-female transsexuals. *Plastic and Reconstructive Surgery* 107:734–741.

139. Rachlin, K. (1999). Factors which influence individuals' decisions when considering female-to-male genital reconstructive surgery. *International Journal of Transgenderism* 3. Downloaded from https://cdn.atria.nl/ezines/web/IJT/97-03/numbers/symposion/ijt990302.htm on November 15, 2018.

140. Wierckx, K., Van Caenegem, E., Elaut, E., Dedecker, D., Van de Peer, F., Toye, K., et al. (2011). Quality of life and sexual health after sex reassignment surgery in transsexual men. *Journal of Sexual Medicine* 8:3379–3388.

141. van der Sluis, W.B., Smit, J.M., Pigot, G.L.S., Buncamper, M.E., Winters, H.A.H., Mullender, M.G., et al. (2017). Double flap phalloplasty in transgender men: Surgical technique and outcome of pedicled anterolateral thigh flap phalloplasty combined with radial forearm free flap urethral reconstruction. *Microsurgery* 37:917–923.

142. Frey, J.D., Poudrier, G., Chiodo, M.V. and Hazen, A. (2016). A systematic review of metoidoplasty and radial forearm flap phalloplasty in female-to-male transgender genital reconstruction: Is the "ideal" neophallus an achievable goal? *Plastic and Reconstructive Surgery Global Open* 4:e1131.

143. Perovic, S.V., Stanojevic, D.S. and Djordjevic, M.L. (2000). Vaginoplasty in male transsexuals using penile skin and a urethral flap. *British Journal of Urology International* 86:843–850.

144. De Cuypere, G., T'Sjoen, G., Beerten, R., Selvaggi, G., De Sutter, P., Hoebeke, P., et al. (2005). Sexual and physical health after sex reassignment surgery. *Archives of Sexual Behavior* 34:679–690.

145. Horbach, S.E., Bouman, M.B., Smit, J.M., Özer, M., Buncamper, M.E. and Mullender, M.G. (2015). Outcome of vaginoplasty in male-to-female transgenders: A systematic review of surgical techniques. *Journal of Sexual Medicine* 12:1499–1512.

146. Jiang, D., Witten, J., Berli, J. and Dugi, D., 3rd (2018). Does depth matter? Factors affecting choice of vulvuloplasty over vaginoplasty as gender-affirming genital surgery for transgender women. *Journal of Sexual Medicine* 15:902–906.

147. Robinson, G.E., Burren, T., Mackie, I.J., Bounds, W., Walshe, K., Faint, R., et al. (1991). Changes in haemostasis after stopping the combined contraceptive pill: Implications for major surgery. *British Medical Journal* 302:269–271.

148. Douketis, J. (2005). Hormone replacement therapy and risk for venous thromboembolism: What's new and how do these findings influence clinical practice? *Current Opinion in Hematology* 12:395–400.

CHAPTER 8

1. De Sutter, P., Verschoor, A., Hotimsky, A. and Kira, K. (2002). The desire to have children and the preservation of fertility in transsexual women: A survey. *International Journal of Transgenderism* 6. Downloaded from https://cdn.atria.nl/ezines/web/IJT/97-03/numbers/symposion/ijtvo06no03_02.htm on November 12, 2018.

2. Wierckx, K., van Caenegem, E., Pennings, G., Elaut, E., Dedecker, D., van de Peer, F., et al. (2012). Reproductive wish in transsexual men. *Human Reproduction* 27:483–487.

3. Dietckx, M., Motmans, J., Mortelmans, D. and T'Sjoen, G. (2015). Families in transition: A literature review. *International Review of Psychiatry* 28:36–43.

4. Knudson, G. and De Sutter, P. (2017). Fertility options in transgender and gender diverse adolescents. *Acta Obstetricia et Gynecologica Scandinavica* 96:1269–1272.

5. Coleman, E., Bockting, W., Botzer, M., Cohen-Kettinis, P., DeCuypere, G., Feldman, J., et al. (2011). Standards of Care for the health of transsexual, transgender, and gender-nonconforming people, Version 7. *International Journal of Transgenderism* 13:165–232. Hembree, W.C., Cohen-Kettenis, P.T., Gooren, L., Hannema, S.E., Meyer, W.J., Murad, M.H., et al. (2017). Endocrine treatment of gender-dysphoric/gender-incongruent persons: An Endocrine Society Clinical Practice Guideline. *Journal of Clinical Endocrinology and Metabolism* 102:3869–3903.

6. Hoffkling, A., Obedin-Maliver, J. and Sevelius, J. (2017). From erasure to opportunity: A qualitative study of the experiences of transgender men around pregnancy and recommendations for providers. *BMC Pregnancy and Childbirth* 17:332.

7. Hamada, A., Kingsberg, S., Wierckx, K., T'Sjoen, G., De Sutter, P., Knudson, G., et al. (2015). Semen characteristics of transwomen referred for sperm banking before sex transition: A case series. *Andrologia* 47:832–838. Lübbert, H., Leo-Rossberg, I. and Hammerstein, J. (1992). Effects of ethinyl estradiol on semen quality and various hormonal parameters in a eugonadal male. *Fertility and Sterility* 58:603–608.

8. De Sutter, P. (2001). Gender reassignment and assisted reproduction: Present and future reproductive options for transsexual people. *Human Reproduction* 16:612–614. Schulze, C. (1988). Response of the human testis to long-term estrogen treatment: Morphology of Sertoli cells, Leydig cells and spermatogonial stem cells. *Cell Tissue Research* 251:31.

9. Ahmad, S. and Leinung, M. (2017). The response of the menstrual cycle to initiation of hormonal therapy in transgender men. *Transgender Health* 2:176–179.

10. van den Broecke, R., van der Elst, J. and Dhont, M. (2001). The female-to-male transsexual patient: A source of human ovarian cortical tissue for experimental use. *Human Reproduction* 16:145–147.

11. Light, A.D., Obedin-Maliver, J., Sevelius, J.M. and Kerns, J.L. (2014). Transgender men who experienced pregnancy after female-to-male gender transitioning. *Obstetrics & Gynecology* 124:1120–1127. Veale, J., Watson, R.J., Adjei, J. and Saewyc, E. (2016). Prevalence of pregnancy involvement among Canadian transgender youth and its relation to mental health, sexual health, and gender identity. *International Journal of Transgenderism* 17:107–113.

12. Martinez, F., on behalf of the International Society for Fertility Preservation-ESHRE-ASRM Expert Working Group (2017). Update on fertility preservation from the Barcelona International Society for Fertility Preservation-ESHRE-ASRM 2015 expert meeting: Indications, results and future perspectives. *Fertility and Sterility* 108:407–415.

13. Jay, N., Mansfield, M.J., Blizzard, R.M., Crowley, W.F., Jr, Schoenfeld, D., Rhubin, L., et al. (1992). Ovulation and menstrual function of adolescent girls with central precocious puberty after therapy with gonadotropin-releasing hormone agonists. *Journal of Clinical Endocrinology and Metabolism* 75:890–894.

14. Finlayson, C., Johnson, E.K., Chen, D., Dabrowski, E., Gosiengfiao, Y., Campo-Engelstein, L., et al. (2016). Proceedings of the Working Group Session on Fertility Preservation for Individuals with Gender and Sex Diversity. *Transgender Health* 1:99–107.

15. Leibowitz, S. and de Vries, A.L.C. (2016). Gender dysphoria in adolescence. *International Review of Psychiatry* 28:21–35.

16. Chen, D., Simons, L., Johnson, E.K., Lockart, B.A. and Finlayson, C. (2017). Fertility preservation for transgender adolescents. *Journal of Adolescent Health* 61:120–123.

17. Nahata, L., Tishelman, A.C., Caltabellotta, N.M. and Quinn, G.P. (2017). Low fertility preservation utilization among transgender youth. *Journal of Adolescent Health* 61:40–44.

18. Strang, J.F., Jarin, J., Call, D., Clark, B., Wallace, G.L., Anthony, L.G., et al. (2018). Transgender Youth Fertility Attitudes Questionnaire: Measure development in nonautistic and autistic transgender youth and their parents. *Journal of Adolescent Health* 62:128–135.

19. Mahfouda, S., Moore, J.K., Siafarikas, A., Zepf, F.D. and Lin, A. (2017). Puberty suppression in transgender children and adolescents. *The Lancet Diabetes and Endocrinology* 5:816–826.

20. Bertelloni, S., Baroncelli, G.I., Ferdeghini, M., Menchini-Fabris, F. and Saggese, G. (2000). Final height, gonadal function and bone mineral density of adolescent males with central precocious puberty after therapy with gonadotropin-releasing hormone analogues. *European Journal of Pediatrics* 159:369–374.

21. Wallace, S.A., Blough, K.L. and Kondapalli, L.A. (2014). Fertility preservation in the transgender patient: Expanding oncofertility care beyond cancer. *Gynecological Endocrinology* 30:868–871.

22. Martinez, F., on behalf of the International Society for Fertility Preservation-ESHRE-ASRM Expert Working Group (2017). Update on fertility preservation from the Barcelona International Society for Fertility Preservation-ESHRE-ASRM 2015 expert meeting: Indications, results and future perspectives. *Fertility and Sterility* 108:407–415.

23. Maxwell, S., Noyes, N., Keefe, D., Berkeley, A.S. and Goldman, K.N. (2017). Pregnancy outcomes after fertility preservation in transgender men. *Obstetrics & Gynecology* 129:1031–1034.

24. Demeestere, I., Simon, P., Dedeken, L., Moffa, F., Tsépélidis, S., Brachet, C., et al. (2015). Live birth after autograft of ovarian tissue cryopreserved during childhood. *Human Reproduction* 30:2107–2109.

25. Donnez, J. and Dolmans, M.M. (2015). Ovarian cortex transplantation: 60 reported live births bring the success and worldwide expansion of the technique towards routine clinical practice. *Journal of Assisted Reproduction and Genetics* 32:1167–1170.

26. Xiao, S., Zhang, J., Romero, M.M., Smith, K.N., Shea, L.D. and Woodruff, T.K. (2015). *In vitro* follicle growth supports human oocyte meiotic maturation. *Scientific Reports* 5:17323.

27. Martinez, F., on behalf of the International Society for Fertility Preservation-ESHRE-ASRM Expert Working Group (2017). Update on fertility preservation from the Barcelona International Society for Fertility Preservation-ESHRE-ASRM 2015 expert meeting: Indications, results and future perspectives. *Fertility and Sterility* 108:407–415.

28. Szell, A.Z., Bierbaum, R.C., Hazelrigg, W.B. and Chetkowski, R.J. (2013). Live births from frozen human semen stored for 40 years. *Journal of Assisted Reproduction and Genetics* 30:743–744.

29. Wierckx, K., Stuyver, I., Weyers, S., Hamada, A., Agarwal, A., De Sutter, P., et al. (2012). Sperm freezing in transsexual women. *Archives of Sexual Behavior* 41:1069–1071.

30. Martinez, F., on behalf of the International Society for Fertility Preservation-ESHRE-ASRM Expert Working Group (2017). Update on fertility preservation from the Barcelona International Society for Fertility Preservation-ESHRE-ASRM 2015 expert meeting: Indications, results and future perspectives. *Fertility and Sterility* 108:407–415.

31. Ibid.

32. Ethics Committee of the American Society for Reproductive Medicine (2015). Access to fertility services by transgender persons: An Ethics Committee opinion. *Fertility and Sterility* 104:1111–1115.

33. Committee on Health Care for Underserved Women (2011). Committee Opinion no. 512: Health care for transgender individuals. *Obstetrics & Gynecology* 118:1454–1458.

34. De Roo, C., Tilleman, K., T'Sjoen, G. and De Sutter, P. (2016). Fertility options in transgender people. *International Review of Psychiatry* 28:112–119.

35. Trebay, G. He's pregnant. You're speechless. *NY Times,* June 22, 2008. Beatie, T. (2009). *Labor of love: The story of one man's extraordinary pregnancy.* Berkeley, CA: Seal Press.

36. Light, A.D., Obedin-Maliver, J., Sevelius, J.M. and Kerns, J.L. (2014). Transgender men who experienced pregnancy after female-to-male gender transitioning. *Obstetrics & Gynecology* 124:1120–1127.

37. Obedin-Maliver, J. and Makadon, H. J. (2016). Transgender men and pregnancy. *Obstetric Medicine* 9:4–8.

38. Light, A.D., Obedin-Maliver, J., Sevelius, J.M. and Kerns, J.L. (2014). Transgender men who experienced pregnancy after female-to-male gender transitioning. *Obstetrics & Gynecology* 124:1120–1127.

39. Ellis, S. A., Wojnar, D.M. and Pettinato, M. (2015). Conception, pregnancy, and birth experiences of male and gender variant gestational parents: It's how we could have a family. *Journal of Midwifery & Women's Health* 60:62–69.

40. Brännstroöm, M., Johannesson, L., Bokström, H., Kvarnström, N., Mölne, J., Dahm-Kähler, P., et al. (2015). Live birth after uterus transplantation. *Lancet* 385:607–616.

41. Jones, B. P., Williams, N. J., Saso, S., Thum, M. Y., Quiroga, I., Yazbek, J., et al. (2018). Uterine transplantation in transgender women. *BJOG* https://doi.org/10.1111/1471-0528.15438.

42. Light, A.D., Obedin-Maliver, J., Sevelius, J.M. and Kerns, J.L. (2014). Transgender men who experienced pregnancy after female-to-male gender transitioning. *Obstetrics & Gynecology* 124:1120–1127.

43. MacDonald, T., Noel-Weiss, J., West, D., Walks, M., Biener, M., Kibbe, A., et al. (2016). Transmasculine individuals' experiences with lactation, chestfeeding, and gender identity: A qualitative study. *BMC Pregnancy and Childbirth* 16:106.

44. Obedin-Maliver, J. and Makadon, H. J. (2016). Transgender men and pregnancy. *Obstetric Medicine* 9:4–8.

45. Glaser, R.L., Newman, M., Parsons, M., Zava, D. and Glaser-Garbrick, D. (2009). Safety of maternal testosterone therapy during breast feeding. *International Journal of Pharmaceutical Compounding* 13:314–317.

46. Reisman, T. and Goldstein, Z. (2018). Case Report: Induced lactation in a transgender woman. *Transgender Health* 3:24–26.

47. Phelps, D. L. and Karim, A. (1977). Spironolactone: Relationship between concentrations of dethioacetylated metabolite in human serum and milk. *Journal of Pharmaceutical Sciences* 66:1203.

CHAPTER 9

1. Oates, J.M. and Dacakis, G. (1983). Speech pathology considerations in the management of transsexualism—A review. *British Journal of Disorders of Communication* 18:139–151.

2. King, J.B., Lindstedt, D.E., Jensen, M. and Law, M. (1999). Transgendered voice: Considerations in case history management. *Logopedics Phoniatrics Vocology* 24:14–18.

3. Oates, J. and Dacakis, G. (1997). Voice change in transsexuals. *Venereology* 10:178–187.

4. Günzberger, D. (1995). Acoustic and perceptual implications of the transsexual voice. *Archives of Sexual Behavior* 24:339–348.

5. Dacakis, G. (2002). The role of voice therapy in male-to-female transsexuals. *Current Opinion in Otolaryngology & Head and Neck Surgery* 10:173–177.

6. Brown, M., Perry, A., Cheesman, A.D. and Pring, T. (2000). Pitch change in male-to-female transsexuals: Has phonosurgery a role to play? *International Journal of Language & Communication Disorders* 35:129–136.

7. White, C.T. (1998). On the pragmatics of an androgynous style of speaking (from a transsexual's perspective). *World Englishes* 17:215–223.

8. Kulick, D. (1999). Transgender and language: A review of the literature and suggestions for the future. *Gay & Lesbian Quarterly* 5:605–622.

9. Byrne, L.A., Dacakis, G. and Douglas, J.M. (2003). Self-perceptions of pragmatic communication abilities in male-to-female transsexuals. *Advances in Speech-Language Pathology* 5:15–25.

10. de Bruin, M.D., Coerts, M.J. and Greven, A.J. (2000). Speech therapy in the management of male-to-female transsexuals. *Folia Phoniatrica et Logopaedica* 52:220–227.

11. Dacakis, G. (2000). Long-term maintenance of fundamental frequency increases in male-to-female transsexuals. *Journal of Voice* 14:549–556.

12. King, R.S., Brown, G.R. and McCrea, C.R. (2012). Voice parameters that result in identification or misidentification of biological gender in male-to-female transgender veterans. *International Journal of Transgenderism* 13:117–130.

13. Leung, J., Oates, J. and Chan, S.P. (2018). Voice, articulation, and prosody contribute to listener perceptions of speaker gender: A systematic review and meta-analysis. *Journal of Speech, Language, and Hearing Research* 61:266–297.

14. van Borsel, J., De Cuypere, G., Rubens, R. and Bestaerke, B. (2000). Voice problems in female-to-male transsexuals. *International Journal of Language and Communication Disorders* 35:427–442.

15. Owen, K. and Hancock, A.B. (2010). The role of self- and listener perceptions of femininity in voice therapy. *International Journal of Transgenderism* 12:272–284.

16. Carew, L., Dacakis, G. and Oates, J. (2007). The effectiveness of oral resonance therapy on the perception of femininity of voice in male-to-female transsexuals. *Journal of Voice* 21:591–603.

17. Neumann, K., Welzel, C. and Gonnermann, U. (2002). Satisfaction of MtF transsexuals with operative voice therapy—A questionnaire-based preliminary study. *International Journal of Transgenderism* 6. Downloaded from https://cdn.atria.nl/ezines/web/IJT/97-03/numbers/symposion/ijtvo06no04_02.htm on August 24, 2018.

18. Kanagalingam, J., Georgalas, C., Wood, G.R., Suki, A., Guri, S. and Cheesman, A.D. (2005). Cricothyroid approximation and subluxation in 21 male-to-female transsexuals. *Laryngoscope* 115:611–618.

19. Pickuth, D., Brandt, S., Neumann, K., Berghaus, A., Spielmann, R.P. and Heywang-Köbrunner, S.H. (2000). Value of spiral CT with cricothyroid approximation. *British Journal of Radiology* 73:840–842.

20. Matai, V., Chessman, A.D. and Clarke, P.M. (2003). Cricothyroid approximation and thyroid chondroplasty: A patient survey. *Otolaryngology—Head and Neck Surgery* 128:841–847.

21. Wagner, I., Fugain, C., Monneron-Girard, L., Cordier, B. and Chabolle, F. (2003). Pitch-raising surgery in fourteen male-to-female transsexuals. *Laryngoscope* 113:1157–1165.

22. Yang, C.Y., Palmer, A.D., Murray, K.D., Meltzer, T.R. and Coen, J.I. (2002). Cricothyroid approximation to elevate vocal pitch in male-to-female transsexuals: Results of surgery. *Annals of Otolaryngology, Rhinology and Laryngology* 111:477–485.

23. Van Borsel, J., van Eynde, E., de Cuypere, G. and Bonte, K. (2008). Feminine after cricothyroid approximation? *Journal of Voice* 22:379–384.

24. Kim, H.-T. (2014). The new technique of voice feminization surgery: Vocal fold shortening and recreation of anterior commissure. Paper presented at the WPATH Conference, Bangkok, Thailand.

25. Shenenberger, D.W. and Utecht, L.M. (2002). Removal of unwanted facial hair. *American Family Physician* 66:1907–1911.

26. Azziz, R., Carmina, E. and Sawaya, M.E. (2000). Idiopathic hirsutism. *Endocrine Reviews* 21:347–362.

27. Paquet, P., Fumal, I., Piérard-Franchimont, C. and Piérard, G.E. (2002). Long-pulsed ruby laser-assisted hair removal in male-to-female transsexuals. *Journal of Cosmetic Dermatology* 1:8–12.

28. Schroeter, C.A., Groenewegen, J.S., Reineke, T. and Neumann, H.A.M. (2003). Ninety percent permanent hair reduction in transsexual patients. *Annals of Plastic Surgery* 51:243–248.

29. Capitán, L., Simon, D., Berli, J.U., Bailón, C., Bellinga, R.J., Santamaria, J.G., et al. (2017). Facial gender confirmation surgery: A new nomenclature. *Plastic and Reconstructive Surgery* 140:766e–767e.

30. Hage, J.J., Becking, A.G., de Graaf, F.H. and Tuinzing, D.B. (1997). Gender-confirming facial surgery: Considerations on the masculinity and femininity of faces. *Plastic and Reconstructive Surgery* 99:1799–1807.

31. Barone, M., Cogliandro, A. and Persichetti, P. (2017). Role of rhinoplasty in transsexual patients. *Plastic and Reconstructive Surgery* 140:624e–625e.

32. Bellinga, R.J., Capitán, L., Simon, D. and Tenóro, T. (2017). Technical and clinical considerations for facial feminization surgery with rhinoplasty and related procedures. *JAMA Facial Plastic Surgery* 19:175–181.

CHAPTER 10

1. Hughto, J.M.W, Reisner, S.L. and Pachankis, J.E. (2015). Transgender stigma and health: A critical review of stigma determinants, mechanisms, and interventions. *Social Science & Medicine* 147:222–231.

2. A sample response reported on page 7 of Van Doussa, H., Power, J. and Riggs, D.W. (2017). Family matters: Transgender and gender diverse people's experience with family when they transition. *Journal of Family Studies*. https://doi.org/10.1080/13229400.2017.1375965

3. Lesser, J.G. (1999). When your son becomes your daughter: A mother's adjustment to a transgender child. *Families in Society* 80:182–189.

4. The following conversations, including the interviewer's questions and the young person's replies, both in quotations, are adapted from interviews reported in Green, R. (1998). Transsexuals' children. *International Journal of Transgenderism* 2. Downloaded from https://cdn.atria.nl/ezines/web/IJT/97-03/numbers/symposion/ijtc0601.htm on August 25, 2018.

5. Freedman, D., Tasker, F. and Di Ceglie, D. (2002). Children and adolescents with transsexual parents referred to a specialist gender identity development service: A brief report of key developmental features. *Clinical Child Psychology and Psychiatry* 7:423–432.

6. White, T. and Ettner, R. (2007). Adaptation and adjustment in children of transsexual parents. *European Journal of Child and Adolescent Psychiatry* 16: 215–221.

7. Riggs, D.W., Power, J. and von Doussa, H. (2016). Parenting and Australian trans and gender-diverse people: An exploratory survey. *International Journal of Transgenderism*. https://doi.org/10.1080/15532739.2016.1149539

8. White, T. and Ettner, R. (2004). Disclosure, risks and protective factors for children whose parents are undergoing a gender transition. In Leli, U. and Drescher. J. (eds.), *Transgender subjectivities: A clinician's guide*. The Haworth Medical Press, pp. 129–145.

9. Wren, B. (2002). "I can accept my child is transsexual but if I ever see him in a dress I'll hit him": Dilemmas in parenting a transgendered adolescent. *Clinical Child Psychology and Psychiatry* 7:377–397.

10. Levine, S.B. and Davis, L. (2002). What I did for love: Temporary returns to the male gender role. *International Journal of Transgenderism* 6. Downloaded from https://cdn.

atria.nl/ezines/web/IJT/97-03/numbers/symposion/ijtvo06no04_04.htm on August 25, 2018.

11. Gagné, P., Tewksbury, R. and McGaughey, D. (1997). Coming out and crossing over: Identity formation and proclamation in a transgender community. *Gender & Society* 11:478–508. Gagné, P. and Tewksbury, R. (1998). Conformity pressures and gender resistance among transgendered individuals. *Social Problems* 45:81–101.

12. Nuttbrock, L., Rosenblum, A. and Blumenstein, R. (2002). Transgender identity affirmation and mental health. *International Journal of Transgenderism* 6. Downloaded from https://www.researchgate.net/publication/289048859_Transgender_identity_affirmation _and_mental_health on August 25, 2018.

13. Van Beusekom, G., Bos, H.M.W., Overbeek, G. and Sandfort, T.G.M. (2015). Same-sex attraction, gender nonconformity, and mental health: The protective role of parental acceptance. *Psychology of Sexual Orientation and Gender Diversity* 2:307–312.

14. Katz-Wise, S.L., Ehrensaft, D., Vetters, R., Forcier, M. and Austin, B. (2018). Family functioning and mental health of transgender and gender-nonconforming youth in the Trans Teen and Family Narratives Project. *Journal of Sex Research* 55:582–590.

15. Ullman, J. (2017). Teacher positivity towards gender diversity: Exploring relationships and school outcomes for transgender and gender-diverse students. *Sex Education* 17:276–289.

16. Pflum, S.R., Testa, R.J., Balsam, K.F., Goldblum, P.B. and Bongar, B. (2015). Social support, trans community connectedness, and mental health symptoms among transgender and gender nonconforming adults. *Psychology of Sexual Orientation and Gender Diversity* 2:281–286.

17. Nuttbrock, L., Bockting, W., Rosenblum, A., Hwahng, S., Mason, M., Macri, M., et al. (2015). Transgender community involvement and the psychological impact of abuse among transgender women: Transgender community involvement and the psychological impact of abuse among transgender woman. *Psychology of Sexual Orientation and Gender Diversity* 2:386–390.

18. Marciano, A. (2014). Living the VirtuReal: Negotiating transgender identity in cyberspace. *Journal of Computer-Mediated Communication* 19:824–838.

19. Lewins, F. (2002). Explaining stable partnerships among FTMs and MTFs: A significant difference? *Journal of Sociology* 38:76–88.

20. Aramburu, C. and Ballard-Reisch, D. (2013). Gender expression as a reflection of identity reformation in couple partners following disclosure of male-to-female transsexualism. *International Journal of Transgenderism* 14:49–65.

21. Lindroth, M., Zeluf, G., Mannheimer, L.N. and Deogan, C. (2017). Sexual health among transgender people in Sweden. *International Journal of Transgenderism* 18:318–327.

22. This quotation comes from page 467 of Galupo, M.P., Henise, S.B. and Davis, K.S. (2014). Transgender microaggressions in the context of friendship patterns of experience. *Psychology of Sexual Orientation and Gender Diversity* 1:461–470.

23. Stryker, S. (1998). The transgender issue: An introduction. *Gay & Lesbian Quarterly* 4:145–158.

24. Kirksey, K.M., Williams, B. and Garza, D.J. (1995). Thoughts on caring for transsexual patients. *Journal of Emergency Nursing* 21:519–520.

25. Lombardi, E.L. and van Servellen, G. (2000). Building culturally sensitive substance use prevention and treatment programs for transgendered populations. *Journal of Substance Abuse Treatment* 19:291–296.

26. Witten, T.M. and Whittle, S. (2004). Transpanthers: The greying of transgender and the law. *Deakin Law Review* 9:503–522.

27. Roen, K. (2001). "Either/or" and "both/neither": Discursive tensions in transgender politics. *Signs: Journal of Women in Culture and Society* 27:501–522.

28. Bornstein, K. (1994). *Gender outlaw.* New York: Routledge.

29. Roen, K. (2001). "Either/or" and "both/neither": Discursive tensions in transgender politics. *Signs: Journal of Women in Culture and Society* 27:517.

30. The phrase *true selves* forms part of the title of the excellent book: Brown, M.L. and Rounsley, C.A. (2003). *True selves: Understanding transsexualism—For families, friends, coworkers, and helping professionals.* New York: Jossey-Bass.

31. Gagné, P., Tewksbury, R. and McGaughey, D. (1997). Coming out and crossing over: Identity formation and proclamation in a transgender community. *Gender & Society* 11:501.

32. Ibid., p. 502.

33. Benjamin, H. (1966). *The transsexual phenomenon.* New York: The Julian Press. Downloaded from http://www.mut23.de/texte/Harry%20Benjamin%20-%20The%20 Transsexual%20Phenomenon.pdf on August 25, 2018.

34. Wojdowski, P. and Tebor, I.B. (1976). Social and emotional tensions during trans-sexual passing. *Journal of Sex Research* 12:193–205.

35. Meier, S.C., Sharp, C., Michonski, J., Babcock, J.C. and Fitzgerald, K. (2013). Romantic relationships of female-to-male trans men: A descriptive study. *International Journal of Transgenderism* 14:75–85.

36. Boza, C. and Perry, K.N. (2014). Gender-related victimization, perceived social support, and predictors of depression among transgender Australians. *International Journal of Transgenderism* 15:35–52.

37. Mizock, L., Woodrum, T.D., Riley, J., Sotilleo, E.A., Yuen, N. and Ormerod, A.J. (2017). Coping with transphobia in employment: Strategies used by transgender and gender-diverse people in the United States. *International Journal of Transgenderism* 18:282–294.

38. Ruggs, E.N., Martinez, L.R., Hebl, M.R. and Law, C.L. (2015). Workplace "trans"-actions: How organizations, coworkers, and individual openness influence perceived gender identity discrimination. *Psychology and Sexual Orientation and Gender Diversity* 4:404–412.

39. Reed, O.M., Franks, A.S. and Scherr, K.C. (2015). Are perceptions of transgender individuals affected by mental illness stigma? A moderated mediation analysis of anti-transgender prejudice in hiring recommendations. *Psychology of Sexual Orientation and Gender Diversity* 2:463–469.

40. Mizock, L. and Mueser, K.T. (2014). Employment, mental health, internalized stigma, and coping with transphobia among transgender individuals. *Psychology of Sexual Orientation and Gender Diversity* 1:146–158.

41. Kolakowski, V.S. (1997). Toward a Christian ethical response to transsexual persons. *Theology & Sexuality* 6:10–31.

42. O'Donovan, O. (1983). Transsexualism and Christian marriage. *Journal of Religious Ethics* 11:135–162.

43. Ibid., p. 150.

44. UNDP, MSDHS (May 2018). *Legal gender recognition in Thailand: A legal and policy review.*

45. Finlay, H. (2003). Corbett to Kevin: Legal recognition of transsexualism in England and Australia. *13th Commonwealth Law Conference*, Melbourne, Australia, p. 13.

46. Ibid., p. 24.

47. Monro, S. (2002). Transgender trouble: Legislation beyond binaries? *Res Publica* 8:275–283.

48. Family Court of Australia (2001). Re Kevin (validity of marriage of transsexual) FamCA 1074. The following paragraph references in the text apply to this legal document. Paragraph 329.

49. Ibid. Paragraph 208.

50. Clough, A.S. (2001). The illusion of protection: Transsexual employment discrimination. *Georgetown Journal of Gender and the Law* 1:849–886.

51. Kirkland, A. (2003). Victorious transsexuals in the courtroom: A challenge for feminist legal theory. *Law and Social Inquiry* 28:21.

52. Kirkland, A. (2003). Victorious transsexuals in the courtroom: A challenge for feminist legal theory. *Law and Social Inquiry* 28:1–37.

53. Ungar, M. (2000). State violence and lesbian, gay, bisexual and transgender (LGBT) rights. *New Political Science* 22:61–75.

54. Dworkin, S.H. and Yi, H. (2003). LGBT identity, violence, and social justice: The psychological is political. *International Journal for the Advancement of Counselling* 25:269–279.

55. Witten, T.M. and Eyler, A.E. (1999). Hate crimes and violence against the transgendered. *Peace Review* 11:461–468.

56. Davy, Z., Sorlie, A. and Schwend, A.S. (2018). Democratising diagnoses? The role of the depathologisation perspective in constructing corporeal trans citizenship. *Critical Social Policy* 38:13–34.

57. Kara, S. (2017). *Gender is not an illness. How pathologizing trans people violates international human rights law.* GATE.

58. Witten, T.M. (2009). Graceful exits: Intersection of aging, transgender identities, and the family/community. *Journal of GLBT Family Studies* 5:36–62.

59. Witten, T.M. (2016). The intersectional challenges of aging and of being a gender non-conforming adult. *Generations* 40:63–70.

60. Guillamon, A., Junque, C. and Gómez-Gil, E. (2016). A review of the status of brain structure research in transsexualism. *Archives of Sexual Behavior* 45:1615–1648.

61. Hunter, C. and Bishop, J.-A. (2016). The complexity of trans*/gender identities: Implications for dementia care. In Westwood, S. and Price, E. (Eds.), *Lesbian, gay, bisexual and trans* individuals living with dementia: Concepts, practice and rights* (pp. 124–137). London: Routledge.

62. Fredriksen-Goldsen, K.I., Cook-Daniels, L., Kim, H.-J., Erosheva, E.A., Emlet, C.A., Hoy-Ellis, C.P., et al. (2013). Physical and mental health of transgender older adults: An at-risk and underserved population. *The Gerontologist* 54:488–500.

63. Witten, T.M. (2014). It's not all darkness: Robustness, resilience, and successful transgender aging. *LGBT Health* 1:24–33.

64. Witten, T.M. (2014). End of life, chronic illness, and trans-identities. *Journal of Social Work in End-of-Life & Palliative Care* 10:1–26.

65. Porter, K.E., Ronneberg, C.R. and Witten, T.M. (2013). Religious affiliation and successful aging among transgender older adults: Findings from the Trans Metlife Survey. *Journal of Religion, Spirituality & Aging* 25:112–138.

CHAPTER 11

1. Heath, R.A. (2006). *The Praeger handbook of transsexuality: Changing gender to match mindset.* Westport, CT: Praeger.

2. These articles about transgender health were published in the June 17, 2016 issue of *The Lancet* magazine.

3. Information about the Trans Youth Project at the University of Washington is available via http://depts.washington.edu/scdlab/research/transyouth-project-gender-development/

4. Newhook, J.T., Winters, K., Pyne, J., Jamieson, A., Holmes, C., Feder, S., et al. (2018). Teach your patients and providers well: Call for refocus on the health of trans and gender-diverse children. *Canadian Family Physician* 64:332–335.

5. Pimenoff, V. and Pfäfflin, F. (2011). Transsexualism: Treatment outcome of compliant and noncompliant patients. *International Journal of Transgenderism* 13:37–44.

6. Norton, J. (1997). "Brain says you're a girl, but I think you're a sissy boy": Cultural origins of transphobia. *Journal of Gay, Lesbian, and Bisexual Identity* 2:152.

7. Osborne, M. (2003). Beyond gatekeeping: Truth and trust in therapy with transsexuals. *IFGE Conference, Philadelphia, PA.* Downloaded from http://library.transgenderzone. com/?page_id=2106 on August 24, 2018.

8. Carroll, L., Gilroy, P.J. and Ryan, J. (2002). Counseling transgendered, transsexual, and gender-variant clients. *Journal of Counseling and Development* 80:131–139.

9. Lombardi, E. (2010). Transgender health: A review and guidance for future research: Proceedings from the Summer Institute at the Center for Research on Health and Sexual Orientation, University of Pittsburgh. *International Journal of Transgenderism* 12:211–229.

10. dickey, l.m., Hendricks, M.L. and Bockting, W.O. (2016). Innovations in research with transgender and gender nonconforming people and their communities. *Psychology of Sexual Orientation and Gender Diversity* 3:187–194. Adams, N., Pearce, R., Veale, J., Radix, A., Castro, D., Sarkar, A., et al. (2017). Guidance and ethical considerations for undertaking transgender health research and institutional review boards adjudicating this research. *Transgender Health* 2:165–175.

11. Heath, R.A. and Murray, G. (2016). Multifractal dynamics of activity data in Bipolar Disorder: Towards automated early warning of manic relapse. *Fractal Geometry and Nonlinear Analysis in Medicine and Biology* 2:140–149. Zulueta, J., Piscitello, A., Rasic, M., Easter, R., Pallavi, B., Langenecker, S.A., et al. (2018). Predicting mood disturbance severity with mobile phone keystroke metadata: A BiAffect digital phenotyping study. *Journal of Medical Internet Research* 20:e241.

12. Hirst, J. (2015). *The gender fairy*. Balaclava, Victoria: Oban Road Publishing.

13. Booth, C.R., Brown, H.L., Eason, E.G., Wallot, S. and Kelty-Stephen, D.G. (2018). Expectations on hierarchical scales of discourse: Multifractality predicts both short- and long-range effects of violating gender expectations in text-reading. *Discourse Processes* 55:12–30.

INDEX

About the Authors

RACHEL ANN HEATH, BSc (Hons), PhD, is conjoint associate professor of psychology, University of Newcastle, Australia. Rachel has over 40 years' experience in psychological research, having earned an Honor's degree and University Medal in Psychology from the University of Newcastle, Australia, and a PhD in Psychology from McMaster University in Canada. Author of *The Praeger Handbook of Transsexuality* (Praeger, 2006), for the last 15 years Rachel has been evaluating the scientific and lifestyle aspects of transsexuality. She has given numerous talks and courses to the general public, students, and professionals on various aspects of gender diversity and was cofounder of a gender center in the Newcastle/Hunter region in Australia. Rachel was formerly professor of psychology at the University of Sunderland and Kingston University, London, and honorary professor of psychology at the University of Newcastle in Australia. Her work has been publicized in the New York media as well as in *New Scientist* magazine and on the BBC Radio 4 science show *The Material World*. Rachel is developing technology for detecting the early signs of relapse in depression and other mood disorders using wearable and mobile devices. These developments may be useful for minimizing the impact of these health problems on gender-diverse people of all ages.

KATIE WYNNE, MA (Hons Cantab), MBBS, MRCP, PhD, FRACP, is a senior staff specialist in endocrinology and diabetes at John Hunter Hospital and the Hunter Medical Research Institute and holds a conjoint position at the University of Newcastle, Australia. She qualified in medicine from King's College London, having completed a degree in experimental psychology from Cambridge University. Her PhD was awarded in physiology from Imperial College London in 2005. Since moving to Australia in 2012, she has developed a HealthPathway for delivering transgender health in primary care and has provided education to a wide range of health professionals in New South Wales, Australia. She is the current chair of the community advocacy group the Hunter Gender Alliance, is on the ACON Trans and Gender Diverse Health Advisory Committee, and is a member of ANZPATH and WPATH. Dr. Wynne is one of the authors of the 2019 Australian "Position Statement on the Hormonal Management of Adult Transgender and Gender Diverse Individuals" endorsed by the Australian and New Zealand Professional Association for Transgender Health, the Royal Australasian College of Physicians, the Australasian Chapter of Sexual Health Medicine, and the Endocrine Society of Australia. Her research over the last 15 years has focused on hormonal disorders and metabolic health.

About the Sex, Love, and Psychology Series Editor

JUDY KURIANSKY, PhD, is a licensed clinical psychologist and adjunct faculty in the Department of Clinical Psychology at Columbia University Teachers College and the Department of Psychiatry at Columbia University College of Physicians and Surgeons, as well as a visiting professor at Peking University Health Sciences Center and honorary professor in the Department of Psychiatry of the University of Hong Kong. A diplomate of the American Board of Sexology and fellow of the American Academy of Clinical Sexology, she was awarded the AACS Medal of Sexology for Lifetime Achievement.

Kuriansky is a pioneer of sex diagnosis, dating back to being on the DSM-III committee; sex therapy evaluation, including early Masters and Johnson therapy; and call-in advice about sex on the radio and TV. A cofounder of the Society for Sex Therapy and Research and past board member of the American Association of Sex Educators, Counselors and Therapists (AASECT), she has authored hundreds of articles in professional journals, including the *Journal of Marital and Sex Therapy* and SIECUS reports, and mass market articles including those for *Cosmopolitan* and *Family Circle* magazines. She has written sex advice columns worldwide, including for the *South China Morning Post*, *Singapore Straits Times*, *Sankei Shinbun* newspaper, and the *New York Daily News*. She has developed and led hundreds of workshops about sexuality around the world from China and Japan to India, Israel, Iran, Austria, and Argentina, including on an integration of Eastern and Western techniques for safe sex and for relationship enhancement.